Palliative Care for People With Cancer

Third Edition

Edited by

Jenny Penson MA(Ed), SRN, HV Cert, Cert Ed, RNT, Cert Counselling
Education Manager, North Devon Hospice, Devon, UK

and

Ronald Fisher MA, FRCA
Lecturer in Palliative Care, and formerly Consultant Physician in
Continuing Care at the first Macmillan Unit, Christchurch Hospital,
Dorset, UK

A member of the Hodder Headline Group
LONDON · NEW YORK · NEW DELHI

First edition published in Great Britain in 1991
Second edition published in Great Britain in 1995
Third edition published in 2002 by Arnold,
a member of the Hodder Headline Group,
338 Euston Road, London NW1 3BH

http://www.arnoldpublishers.com

Distributed in the United States of America by
Oxford University Press Inc.,
198 Madison Avenue, New York, NY 10016

Whilst the advice and information in this book are believed to be true and accurate
at the date of going to press, neither the authors nor the publisher can accept any
legal responsibility or liability for any errors or omissions that may be made. In
particular (but without limiting the generality of the preceding disclaimer) every
effort has been made to check drug dosages; however, it is still possible that errors
have been missed. Furthermore, dosage schedules are constantly being revised and
new side-effects recognized. For these reasons the reader is strongly urged to
consult the drug companies' printed instructions before administering any of the
drugs recommended in this book.

British Library Cataloguing in Publication Data
A catalogue record for this book is available from the British Library

Library of Congress Cataloguing-in-Publication Data
A catalogue record for this book is available from the Library of Congress

ISBN 0340 76396 5

1   2   3   4   5   6   7   8   9   10

Commissioning Editor: Georgina Bentliff
Development Editor: Heather Smith
Production Editor: Anke Ueberberg
Production Controller: Bryan Eccleshall
Cover Design: Terry Griffiths

Typeset in 10/13 pts Sabon by Integra Software Services Pvt. Ltd., Pondicherry, India
www.integra-india.com
Printed and bound in Malta by Gutenberg Press

What do you think about this book? Or any other Arnold title?
Please send your comments to feedback.arnold@hodder.co.uk

CONTENTS

PART 1   SYMPTOM MANAGEMENT: THE CORNERSTONE OF CARE

PART 2   MEETING NEEDS: ART AND SCIENCE

FOREWORD

A recent circular from the UK Department of Health (HCS 1998/115) recommends that:

> the principles and practice of palliative care for all those facing life-threatening illnesses need to be integrated into the whole of National Health Service (NHS) practice. Health authorities and NHS Trusts are asked to... consider how palliative care can be made an integral component of all their services'

This reflects a remarkable evolution of palliative care in the short time since the foundation of St Christopher's Hospice, where it all started in the late 1960s, to this acceptance and integration into the mainstream of health care. There is often a gap between NHS circulars and what actually happens 'on the ground', but this at least reflects an official view of the potential contribution of palliative care to the modern NHS. So how has this come about?

Palliative care embodies a change in approach to the management of patients with incurable and advanced disease, allowing a positive but realistic strategy to be devised. Patient- and family-centred care and a concern for psychological, social and spiritual as well as physical problems underpin the philosophy of palliative care. Rehabilitation is a priority, but within an achievable framework whose objective is to improve the quality of life for the individual and his or her family, however limited their time may be.

This philosophy of care reflects the complex needs of patients nearing the end of life, but also developed in part as a reaction to the burgeoning technology of modern health care. It in some ways represents a return to more basic principles of 'caring for the sick' and recognizes that drugs, procedures or complex treatment can never be enough when used in isolation. There is an essential corollary to the development of 'whole-person' care: that it should be based on the best possible scientific evidence. Palliative care should thus integrate 'science and compassion'.

Over the past 30 years, there has been enormous development of specialist palliative care services, not just in the UK, but also in many other parts of the world. At the same time, there has been a recognition of the need for the more widespread application of 'non-specialist' palliative care, or the so-called palliative care approach. All professionals who may be involved in end-of-life care should be familiar with the basic principles of care, have a knowledge of the control of common symptoms and possess an understanding of psychosocial needs and how they may be managed. This should be part of all good clinical practice.

Palliative care is increasingly being included in undergraduate curricula for doctors and pre-registration courses for nurses. As far as doctors are concerned, we are now at the point at which every clinical medical school in the UK includes aspects of palliative care in its undergraduate curriculum. We are also, however, still at a stage at which many health-care professionals may miss out on the formal teaching and learning of palliative care.

This book is aimed at those who may have missed out or those who are just embarking on a course in palliative care. It provides a concise and readable introduction to the subject, with practical and pithy information for those working at the coalface, as well as some thoughtful and thought-provoking discussions of difficult dilemmas that are faced in palliative care. The book contains much distilled wisdom and experience founded on a sound knowledge base. It will certainly serve the non-specialist, but will also act as a springboard for those wanting to delve more deeply.

The editors, Jenny Penson and Ronald Fisher, are to be congratulated on having nurtured their baby to a third edition. This is testimony to the usefulness and success of the previous editions, and I am sure that this will not be the last.

Geoffrey Hanks
University of Bristol
February 2002

PREFACE TO THE THIRD EDITION

> The Nurse is the main communicator between the patient, the relatives and the doctors and has the function of not only giving care but of co-ordinating the care of others.[1]
>
> Hockey (1989)

Palliative care requires a multi-disciplinary approach, this once again being reflected in the new edition of this book. The text is aimed primarily at nurses, but, in view of the multi-disciplinary approach, doctors, social workers, physio-therapists, medical students, occupational therapists, teachers, administrators, volunteers and others will find much to interest them.

It has, quite rightly, been pointed out that palliative care also encompasses other progressive diseases that are not specifically covered in the book. Covering these would demand a not inconsiderable enlargement of the book and a con-sequent increase in cost, and we feel that we must abide by our original policy. This dilemma is, however, by no means unique. Around 1000 years ago, Aelfric, schoolmaster of Cerne Abbas (*c.* AD 995–1020) responded: 'we dare not lengthen this book much more, lest it be out of moderation and should stir up man's anti-pathy because of its size.'

The National Health Service has embarked on a 10-year plan of moderniza-tion, and performance must be improved. We do not disagree with this, providing that performing well means improving quality rather than merely productivity.

When we delve into the past, it not infrequently seems to be like the present or even a projection of the future. We were recently reminded of this when read-ing a passage from *Aphorisms of his Bedside Teachings and Writings*, by Sir William Osler:

> By far the most dangerous foe we have to fight is apathy – indifference from whatever cause, not from lack of knowledge, but from carelessness, from absorption in other pursuits, from a contempt bred of self-satisfaction.

These words were written nearly a hundred years ago, when there were obviously misgivings in the air and a concern for the future. Today there is also unease, not helped by headlines in the media that breed distrust. There is certainly no place for indifference in palliative care; it is quite foreign to our philosophy and is the essence of inhumanity.

---

[1] Hockey, L. 1989: Medical education. In: *The Edinburgh Symposium – pain control.* Edinburgh: Royal Society of Medicine.

Sadly, our colleague and friend, Ann Newbury, died of cancer in September 1999. Her admirable chapter in previous editions 'The care of the patient near the end of life' is an example not only of her sensitivity, but also of her expertise. We remember well her fitting opening quotation:

I shall live a year, barely longer. During that year let as much as possible be done.

Joan of Arc

Jenny Penson and Ronald Fisher
2002

ACKNOWLEDGEMENTS

We are greatly indebted to our contributors. They have 'scorned delights and lived laborious days', not only to meet their deadlines, but also to share with us their knowledge and expertise. We are most grateful. Our thanks also go to those 20 anonymous reviewers who not only encouraged us to update this book, but also made helpful suggestions.

LIST OF CONTRIBUTORS

THE EDITORS

Jenny Penson MA(Ed), SRN, HV Cert, Cert Ed, RNT, Cert Counselling

Jenny Penson began her involvement with palliative care in 1975 when she became a Macmillan nurse, attached to the first Macmillan unit, at Christchurch in Dorset. She has written extensively on many aspects of palliative care and has been involved in research on the care of relatives and on bereavement issues. Her other main interests lie in complementary approaches to care and in the use of helping skills. She has contributed to conferences and courses all over the UK and abroad, working with many different professional and volunteer groups.

She has recently returned to the palliative care field, as Education Manager at North Devon Hospice, after several years of working in multi-disciplinary education in general and nurse education in particular.

Ronald A. Fisher MA, FRCA

Lecturer in Palliative Care, and formerly Consultant Physician in Continuing Care at the first Macmillan unit, Christchurch Hospital, Dorset.

Ronald Fisher introduced hospice medicine into the National Health Service at Christchurch Hospital in January 1975. This included the first NHS home-care service for cancer patients, the forerunner of the present Macmillan Nursing Service, and a support and advisory team for the district general hospitals. In 1977, a day-care service was started.

From 1977 to 1980 he was Chairman of a Select Committee of Experts at Strasbourg at the invitation of the Council of Europe to study 'Problems related to death'. He has been long associated with Cancer Relief, was its Honorary Consultant and is now a vice President of that charity.

THE CONTRIBUTORS

Sam Ahmedzai FRCP
Professor of Palliative Medicine and Head of Academic Palliative Medicine Unit, University of Sheffield, Royal Hallamshire Hospital and Director of Trent Palliative Care Centre, Sheffield, South Yorkshire, UK

Jane Brewer MA (Ed), SRN, RCNT, RNT, DN, Cert Ed, DPH, CPH, Reflexology Cert
Senior Lecturer, Institute of Health Studies, University of Plymouth, Taunton, Somerset, UK

Sheila Cassidy MB ChB, MA (Oxon), DSc (Hons), D Lit (Hon), CNA, UKCP
Psycho-oncologist and Psychotherapist, Plymouth Oncology Centre, Plymouth,
Devon, UK

Maggie Fisher RCN, MA, MSc, Adv Dip in Transpersonal Psychotherapy, PG Dip in
Counselling, PCI Dip in Systemic Mgs, Dip Life Sci Nurs, Dip Anat Physiol Body
Massage, Cert Ed, Cert Onc Nurs
Nurse, Counsellor, Psychotherapist, Consultant and Trainer; Formerly Nursing and
Counselling Director, St Catherine's Specialist Palliative Care Centre, Crawley,
West Sussex, UK

Charlette Gallagher-Allred PhD, RD, LD
Volunteer Nutritionist, Kobacker House Hospice, Riverside, Columbus, Ohio, USA and
Manager, Geriatrics and Long Term Care, Ross Products Division, Columbus, USA

Elizabeth Grigg MA, Post Grad Dip (Ed), BA, SRN, RNT, Cert FPA, Cert Midwif,
Cert Intens Care Nurs
Principal Lecturer, Institute of Health Studies, Somerset Centre, University
of Plymouth

Susanna R. Hill MB ChB, DCH, MRCGP, Dip Pall Med
Caen Medical Centre, Braunton, Devon, UK

Denise Hodson SRN, RSCN
Clinical Nurse Specialist, Regional Paediatric Oncology and Haematology Unit,
St James's University Hospital Trust, Leeds, UK

Ann Hopper PhD, MEd, MTD, RGN, RM
Honorary Research Fellow, University of Exeter, Exeter, Devon, UK

Tim Hunt MD, DSc, MRCP
Consultant Physician in Palliative Medicine, Arthur Rank Home, Macmillan Continuing
Care Unit, Cambridge, Cambridgeshire, UK

Karen Jenns MSc, RGN, Onc Cert, Dip HS
Clinical Nurse Specialist, Oxford Lymphoedema Service, Churchill Hospital, Oxford,
Oxfordshire, UK

Suzanne Mace BA (Hons), Dip Man Stud, RGN
Patient Services Manager, North Devon Hospice, Barnstaple, Devon, UK

Kerry Macnish BSc (Hons) Pall Nurs, RGN
Community Palliative Nurse Specialist, Hospiscare, Exeter, Devon, UK

Kathryn Mannix MB BS, MRCP
Consultant in Palliative Medicine, Marie Curie Centre, Newcastle upon Tyne,
Northumberland, UK

Mark Napier MB BS, MRCP
Consultant Medical Oncologist, Exeter Oncology Centre, Royal Devon and Exeter
Hospital, Exeter, Devon, UK

Anne Pelham MB ChB, MRCGP, Dip Cog Ther
Specialist Registrar in Palliative Medicine, St Oswald's Hospice, Newcastle upon Tyne, Northumberland, UK

Rajaguru Srinivasan MB, MRCP
Specialist Registrar in Oncology, Exeter Oncology Centre, Royal Devon and Exeter Hospital, Exeter, Devon, UK

The Reverend David Stoter
Senior Chaplain, Queen's Medical Centre, and Manager, Bereavement Centre, Queen's Medical Centre Nottingham, University Hospital, NHS Trust, Nottinghamshire, UK

John Sweeney MA (Hons), RMN, RGN, RNT, MNSPH
Palliative Homecare Nurse, Prince and Princess of Wales Hospice, Glasgow, UK

Vandana Vora MRCP
Specialist Registrar in Palliative Medicine, Sheffield Teaching Hospitals Trust, Sheffield, South Yorkshire, UK

Alan Winchester MA, RGN
Clinical Nurse Specialist, Taunton and Somerset NHS Trust/St Margaret's Somerset Hospice Palliative Care Team, Taunton, Somerset, UK

PALLIATIVE CARE FROM THE FIRST MILLENNIUM – TURNING DARKNESS INTO LIGHT

Ronald A. Fisher

This introduction is a mixture of old and new, a bridge between the past and the future. It will, I hope, have some historical interest for new readers and show how palliative care has evolved.

But, first, what was life like at the turn of the first millennium? Robert Lacey and Danny Danziger, in their book *The Year 1000*, describe life as it was 1000 years ago. It was, it seems, an era of fervent religious faith, the people embracing the Church and believing in the powers of the Saints. There was a rebirth of monasteries that resulted in an increase in the number of establishments being built. Instead of a Millennium Dome, there was a monastic boom.

Adjacent to each monastery, there would have been an infirmary, the medical institution of the time, so there would be a refuge for all, a place of rest for travellers and pilgrims, for the sick and dying. Anyone in need was welcomed; no one was turned away. This spirit was embodied in the words of Saint Benedict, the father of Western monasticism (*c.* AD 480–547): 'Let all guests who come to the monastery be entertained like Christ himself. He will say "I was a stranger and you took me in".' Such was the spirit of the times.

In the monasteries, monks worked, prayed and studied. As Sheila Cassidy reminds us in her chapter, monks who had left the mainstream of society were perhaps able 'to see things more clearly, to reflect and then to comment on what is seen.' The poem *Pangur Bán*, written by an Irish monk in St Gallen, Switzerland, towards the end of the first millennium, is certainly indicative of the search for enlightenment.

PANGUR BÁN
I and Pangur Bán my cat
'Tis a like task we are at:
Hunting mice is his delight
Hunting words I sit all night.

Better far than praise of men
'Tis to sit with book and pen;
Pangur bears me no ill will
He too plies his simple skill.

Oftentimes a mouse will stray
In the hero Pangur's way;
Oftentimes my keen thought set
Takes a meaning to its net.

'Gainst the wall he sets his eye
Full and fierce and sharp and sly;
'Gainst the wall of knowledge I
All my little wisdom try.

Practice every day has made
Pangur perfect in his trade;
I get wisdom day and night
Turning darkness into light.

And turning darkness into light is, after all, the purpose of this book.

So, did palliative care begin 1000 years ago? Nothing begins at the time one imagines, and palliative care certainly did not exist then as we know it today. There are, however, some clues. We know, for example, that the word 'hospice' derives from the Latin word *hospes*, meaning a host or guest and was used by Cicero (*c.* 106 BC–AD 43) (Manning, 1984). We know also that the word 'palliate' is a derivative of the medieval Latin word *palliatio*, to cloak or disguise. So there were two words waiting to be blended some time in the future into a label or title for a philosophy that had yet to develop and would take a few hundred years to evolve.

Over the past 30 years or so, the terminology has varied between 'terminal care', 'hospice care', 'continuing care' and 'palliative care'. The words 'terminal care' are the most insensitive ones in our medical jargon. They obscure rather than clarify, they mislead, and they are inadequate. So why add to the distress of patients and families by using such ill-chosen words? The expression 'palliative care' is far more acceptable and carries with it a hint of hope. Yet doctors and nurses, as well others associated with cancer care, add to the confusion by using both phrases as if they are synonymous.

It can be argued that, since incurable cancer is a terminal disease, the care given must also be terminal, but to carry this argument to its logical and perhaps ridiculous conclusion, all care is terminal since life is made up of partial deaths and we begin to die from the moment we are born. Terminal care is only a part of the palliative care programme and comes at the end of life, that is, in the last hours or days. 'Ultimate care' would perhaps be a better expression.

We can now go on to define palliative medicine as being that which relieves suffering when cure is impossible, suffering that can be physical, psychological, social and spiritual, and which involves both the patient and the family.

It is appropriate to enrich this definition with the words of Barbara McNulty, who was once the nurse in charge of the home-care service at St Christopher's

Hospice in London. In the early 1970s, I was privileged to accompany her on her round in the community, during which she taught me so much.

> In caring for the dying patient one cannot separate his needs from those of his family – they are a unit whose individual members interact; what affects one will react upon another. One cannot treat a dying patient's physical symptoms and ignore his emotional needs. The home with all its problems, the patient with all his fears and pain, are the objects of our concern.

I have already pointed out that palliative care may well start at the moment at which the patient is informed of the diagnosis of cancer. Peter Maguire has written that the emotional upheaval that occurs at this time often goes unrecognized (Maguire and Faulkner, 1988); consequently, there is no psychological intervention and psychiatric morbidity goes untreated. It should not be forgotten either:

> that death from cancer is never instantaneous. It occurs in stages, it is a process, and there are variations in the rate at which the final point approaches. Total final death is merely the last in a series of functional organic partial deaths, since although the organs live together they die separately.
>
> Fisher (1980)

What I am suggesting here is that dying from cancer can be a prolonged affair, which means that the period of palliative care is highly variable in length. Nor should it be forgotten that medicine is not an exact science: we are not always sure what will happen next.

As drug therapy improves, we can be cautiously optimistic that, although cure may not be achieved, the progress of the disease will be slowed and life prolonged. So we should always give hope as long as it is reasonable to do so, hope, not for the cure of the cancer, but to enable the patient to achieve goals and live a life full of meaning in whatever environment the patient may inhabit. Without hope, there is no endeavour.

Medical historians will report in due course that it was not until well into the second half of the twentieth century that the fortunes of the chronic cancer patient began to improve. Until then, many patients with advancing malignant disease had suffered unnecessarily. Millions had, for example, suffered unalleviated cancer pain, and tragically many died in pain. This is now generally accepted with regret, but then history is full of regrets.

So why has this been such a neglected area of medicine? It has been said the fault lies with the education that nurses and doctors have or have not received, an education that has been orientated towards cure, so that when we failed to cure, we did not know how to cope with our failures and therefore tended to retreat from the situation. What I call the 'Eeyore syndrome' takes over:

> *Said Eeyore*: 'I make it seventeen days come Friday since anyone spoke to me.'
> *Said Rabbit*: 'I was here myself a week ago.'

'Not conversing', *said Eeyore.* 'Not first one and then the other. You said "Hallo" and *flashed past!*'

Milne (1928)

Life-sustaining treatments ranging from antibiotics to organ transplants have, it is argued, caused us to concentrate on the disease rather than the patient. The philosopher Ivan Illich calls this 'the medicalization of life', the opening sentence of his book *Limits of Medicine: Medical Nemesis* rather startlingly stating that 'the Medical Establishment has become a threat of life' (Illich, 1974). By this he means that health-care professionals have taken over so completely that the patient loses his or her independence. Professor Karl Ziegler of Switzerland, also commenting on the omnipotence of doctors, has coined the words 'thanatocrats' to describe those who have the power to prolong life or terminate it.

Another interesting thought is that doctors and nurses have inherited this attitude of neglect over the centuries, that it is a 'hangover' from the past. Is this theory so wild? We have after all inherited and accepted much that is in the *Corpus Hippocratum*, the (Hippocratic collection). Hippocrates (*c.* 460–377 BC) is universally known as the 'father of medicine', many of the clinical observations in use today being there, clearly stated, in his ancient manuscripts. As W.H.S. Jones (1945) writes:

> There is within the corpus the work of a medical genius, perhaps the greatest genius among all the physicians whose writings have come down to us. He *inherited* much from his predecessors but either personally or through his pupils he bequeathed far more to his successors. Whether or not his name was Hippocrates the inheritance is still ours.

Over the centuries, contributions by Galen, William Harvey, John Hunter, Edward Jenner, Joseph Lister, Alexander Fleming, Frederick Banting and Charles Best, Richard Bright, Thomas Addison, William Osler, Florence Nightingale and Cicely Saunders, to name but a very, very few, have added to that inheritance to create medicine as it is today.

Let us now look at a part of that inheritance, at one of its bequests.

> First I will define what I conceive Medicine to be. In general terms it is to do away with the sufferings of the sick, to lessen the violence of their disease, *and to refuse to treat those who are overmastered by their disease, realising that in such cases such medicine is powerless.*

Corpus Hippocraticum

We have totally accepted the first half of that definition, but did we not also accept the second half, and was it not only recently that we began to reject it?

Fascinating though these theories are, the fact remains that we were ignorant of what could be done: 'Wisdom is prevented by ignorance and delusion is the result' (*Bhagaradgta, 5 tr P. Lal*). And delusion certainly was the result because generations of nurses and doctors deluded themselves into believing that nothing could be done for the patient with an incurable cancer, with the result that we took refuge in those all too familiar statements 'We have done all we can' or 'There is nothing more to be done.'

In retrospect, I suppose we should be grateful for such delusions because if there had been no doubts, there would have been no questioning and no enlightenment. We therefore had a neglected area of medicine. Health services worldwide were failing to improve the care of these unfortunate patients, failing to satisfy their physical, emotional, social and spiritual needs. It was not until we were alerted by Dame Cicely Saunders to this famine of care that hospices and continuing care units began to appear in the UK. We, the editors, were privileged to introduce hospice care into the National Health Service in January 1975 at Christchurch Hospital in Dorset. At the same time, we started a home-care service that was the prototype of today's Macmillan nursing service and a peripatetic 'support team' for the hospitals in the district. Two years later we introduced day care. From these specialist units, with their growing expertise and scientific approach, was born palliative medicine, now recognized by the Royal College of Physicians as a speciality. The emergence of palliative medicine is one of the best things that has happened to medicine in the twentieth century.

When lecturing in the early 1970s, I used to remind audiences that since dying is part of living, *care of the dying is also care of the living*. This is a vital statement that follows the aphoristic style adopted by the early Greek philosophers, an aphorism being encapsulated wisdom, a device used 'to arrest attention and assist the memory'. '*Care of the dying is care of the living*' is totally acceptable today, but in those earlier days, there was much more talk of helping people to die well, to die with dignity, to have a good death. This thanatological terminology was, however, deceptive, full of promise but signifying very little. Better surely to speak of a 'tranquil death'.

Nursing care of the dying patient is care for the patient who is still living; it is helping that patient to live his or her life to the fullest, whether at home or in hospital. It is care that is not just centred on the individual but includes members of the family. The nurse in a palliative care team, whether in the community or hospital, is in the unique position of being able to spend most time with the patient and the family and, by virtue of this intimacy, acquire a wide knowledge of the patient. This knowledge can be shared with other members of the caring team, the patient and the family thus receiving total harmonious care. As Lisbeth Hockey (1989) says: 'the nurse is the main communicator between the patient, the relatives and the doctors and has the function of not only giving care but of co-ordinating the care of others'.

What then is the role of the specialist unit and the specialist nurse? Both are of vital importance. They are there to advise on difficult problems, to take over the care of the patient if necessary, to research and evaluate, and to teach. Given the right tools, community and hospital nurses will be able to play their natural roles. It is important that, as far as 'family nurses' are concerned, this role should not be stolen from them. After all, nurses have worked in the community for some considerable time, in fact from 1859 when that socially conscious philanthropist William Rathbone started the District Nursing Service in Liverpool (Hardy, 1981). There is a wealth of know-how inherent in this service.

It should also be remembered that palliative care does not necessarily end with the death of the patient. Until life begins to glow again, some surviving relatives may need support during the bereavement period. Similarly, for those patients whose disease has been controlled as a result of treatment, there may be a transition period during which the family nurse and the family doctor will need to 'map the middle ground of survivorship and provide psycho-social support' (Loescher et al., 1989). As Mullen (1985) reflects, 'there is no moment of cure but rather an evolution from the phase of extended survival into a period when the activity of the disease or the likelihood of its return is sufficiently small that the cancer can now be considered permanently arrested'. It is only then that palliative care can end.

REFERENCES

Fisher, R. 1980: *Problems related to death: care of the dying*. Report of the European Public Health Committee. Strasbourg: Council of Europe.

Hardy, G. 1981: *William Rathbone and the early history of district nursing*. Ormskirk: G.W. & A. Hesketh.

Hockey, L. 1989: Medical education. In: *The Edinburgh symposium – pain control*. Royal Society of Medicine.

Illich, I. 1974: *Limits of medicine: medical nemesis*. Harmondsworth: Penguin.

Jones, W.H.S. 1945: Hippocrates and the *Corpus Hippocraticum*. In: *Proceedings of the British Academy*, Vol. XXXI. London: Geoffrey Cumberledge.

Lacey, R. and Danziger, D. 1999: *The year 1000*. London: Little, Brown.

Loeschler, L.J., Welch-McCaffrey, D., Leigh, S.A. et al. 1989: Surviving adult cancers. Pts 1 and 2. *Annals of Internal Medicine* 111, 411–32, 517–24.

Maguire, P. and Faulkner, A. 1988: How to communicate with cancer patients. Pt 2: Handling uncertainty: collusion and denial. *British Medical Journal* 297, 972–4.

Manning, M. 1984: *The hospice alternative – living with dying*. London: Souvenir Press.

Milne, A.A. 1928: *The house at Pooh corner*. London: Methuen.

Mullen, F. 1985: Seasons of survival: reflections of a physician with cancer. *New England Journal of Medicine* 313, 270–3.

Part 1

SYMPTOM MANAGEMENT: THE CORNERSTONE OF CARE

chapter 1

THE MANAGEMENT OF PAIN

Tim Hunt

All pain is subtle, variable and shifting. We are all unskilled in describing our pain. Few patients talk with their doctors, rather doctors and patients talk at each other. Of all health professionals, the nurse is unique in having close, trusted, prolonged contact. This position is one of enormous responsibility and opportunity. At a minimum, the nurse is in the position of translator. ...At a maximum, the nurse is in a position of a research worker....To liberate this crucial subject, nurses must first educate themselves and then the rest of us.

Wall (1987)

It is pain and the unknown that people most fear in advanced cancer, pain often being inextricably bound up with the word 'cancer'. There is a concept that pain increases with the duration of illness, although one out of four patients do not experience significant pain. In developed countries, it is estimated that between 60 per cent and 90 per cent of patients with advanced cancer experience debilitating pain. The World Health Organization (WHO) estimated in 1990 that, globally, at least 4 millon people had suffered from cancer pain. This makes it mandatory for all carers, even without specialist knowledge, to recognize the problem of pain. The American Pain Society recently proposed that pain should be the fifth vital sign, to be considered alongside pulse, respiration, blood pressure and temperature in forming the basis of monitoring the quality of patient care.

To help patients, it is first necessary accurately to assess their pain and to recognize the many factors that may cause and influence the perception of pain. We as carers also need to enhance our understanding of the wide range of treatments available and to select what is appropriate treatment with the fewest adverse effects.

THE AETIOLOGY OF PAIN

The cause of pain may be physical or emotional, often both, so it is necessary to know the relative importance of each and tailor the treatment accordingly. Both components are present in nearly every case of pain. The most valuable diagnostic tool is listening, and listening again, to the patient: open and unbiased listening will provide clues to the cause of the pain.

PHYSICAL CAUSES OF PAIN

The primary site of a malignancy is only one factor that may determine pain, of greater importance being the further dissemination of the disease, that is, where other organs or tissues may be involved (Table 1.1). Nearly three out of five patients had two or three different sites of pain, while just under one-third described four or more different sites of pain. This adds to the problems and importance of the correct assessment of pain.

EMOTIONAL, PSYCHOLOGICAL AND SOCIAL CAUSES OF PAIN

Patients and relatives suffer considerable anxiety and stress following a diagnosis of cancer and are therefore particularly vunerable at this time. The hallmark of good palliative care is a holistic approach, that is, one dealing with the whole person and considering the many influences on that person. In practice, this means that cancer pain should be considered as being influenced by many factors rather than only by the patient's physical state. These factors commonly include anxiety, fear of the unknown, fear of death, a sense of profound hopelessness and reactive depression. We know that these influences can lower the threshold for pain, so pain that would normally be tolerable now becomes unbearable. Anxiety itself may intensify pain. A holistic approach provides the opportunity to explore what may alter the pain threshold and may in turn allow intervention to relieve pain in ways that would not always be possible if we considered only the physical pathology of the disease.

Table 1.1 Causes of pain in 284 patients with known malignant tumours*

	Percentage of cases
Tumour, the tumour itself e.g. extending into soft tissue, nerve compression, intracranial pressure	38.4
Bone involvement e.g. bone metastases, fractures	21.1
Intraperitoneal involvement e.g. intestinal obstruction, ascites	12.4
Related to treatment e.g. dysphagia, constipation, infection	11.9
Related to illness, particularly debility e.g. pressure sores	4.6
Concurrent pathology not directly related to the tumour e.g. osteoarthroses, migraine	11.7
Cause of pain(s) uncertain	2.9

*A patient may have more than one cause of pain.

Pyschological distress and its influence on pain is variable and depends on the personality and coping ability of the patient, the family structure and often the social fabric. There is no doubt that anxiety and depression intensify pain, depression in a patient often being a better predictor of pain than the site or nature of the malignancy. Just over half of all patients appear to adjust normally to the stress of cancer, but of the other half, nearly 70 per cent may have severe reactive anxiety and depression, and about 13 per cent major depression. Further more, certain types of chemotherapy and medication may cause confusion or distressed states that are often difficult to recognize. Psychological distress may start because of the unsatisfactory control of pain, and a normal personality may become mentally distressed when severe pain continues to be present.

The range of possible psychosocial problems is immense; it may include financial worries, the concerns of a young mother over who will look after her children when she becomes more ill and after her death, the guilt arising from previous personal relationships, being the parent of illegitimate children when no one else knows, and the guilt and fear associated with religious attitude and conflict.

There are some patients for whom medicines to relieve pain persistently fail, and the patient, relatives and carers look to further changes in medication to provide solutions. The response of the patient to the pain and the medication may suggest an underlying psychological factor influencing the intensity and frequency of the pain. The pain may involve several body systems, it may be dramatic at times, or there may be an abnormal preoccupation with minor symptoms or an exaggerated dependence on medication or on the clock determining the reporting of pain. It is important for carers to recognize these often overlooked signs of psychological overlay and to help the patient and relatives to consider a new attitude and way of coping, as well as to adjust to the progression of the illness.

ASSESSMENT

The word 'pain' has numerous implications, from the discomfort arising from a single mouth ulcer to the extreme severity of acute pain in renal colic. We must first understand what a patient may mean by using the word 'pain' as this word means different things to different people. What is 'pain' to one person may be 'a grumble' to another. Unless we understand what a patient means by 'pain', it is not possible to evaluate whether the treatment is reducing his or her pain.

THE DETAILED HISTORY

The taking of a detailed history requires considerable time, an hour or more not infrequently being required for the first consultation. In addition, the longer the patient has experienced pain, the more time is required to unravel the true cause of that pain. The key to taking a detailed history is unhurried time, empathy and suspicion.

- Write down in the patient's own words the details of the pain. Is it just one pain or more than one?
- Mark on a diagram of the body the site of the various pains and where these pains may radiate or move to. It may help to show this diagram to the patient.
- What is the frequency and duration of the pain? Once a day? When? How long does it last? Does the intensity change, as in colicky pain, or is it constant?
- Describe the pain? Stabbing, burning, tearing, aching?
- How severe is the pain? Does it prevent some activity or prevent sleep?
- Is it difficult to talk about pain? Some patients may conceal their pain or not fully indicate its extent because their admission may suggest weakness or bring about a confrontation with their illness. Declaring pain may lead to medication, with the fear of possible addiction or clouding of the mind.
- What does the patient think may bring about the pain? Eating? Lying down? Movement?
- What does the patient do at the onset of the pain?
- Is there anything that relieves or removes the pain?
- What medicines does the patient take for the pain? Do the medicines help? How long do the medicines take to work, and for how long do they help? Do they help instantly? Examine the actual medicine containers, the dates, the instructions. Is the patient taking his or her medicines?
- What does the patient's partner or family think about the pain?
- Consider speaking to close relatives or other carers to obtain supportive or further information. Does the pain become less serious or less intense when the patient is with others?

MEASUREMENT OF PAIN

There is no overall acceptable way of measuring pain. There are extreme cases such as young children, of whom the mother is the best barometer, and aged or psychiatric patients, with whom communication may be impossible. Methods of measuring pain were first introduced as a research tool, many systems now being available. Measuring pain from one day to the next is a way of establishing whether treatment is effective. It is important to select a simple system, one that can be understood and carried out by the patient wherever possible.

With a visual analogue scale, the patient is asked to place a mark, or indicate to someone where a mark should be made, on a scale similar to the scale on a ruler. This line is often based on a 10 cm line with equally spaced vertical lines between the two ends, one end being marked 'No pain' and the other 'Extreme pain'.

If a numerical rating (numerical analogue) scale is used, the patient is asked to grade the pain from, for example, 1 to 5, or more commonly from 1 to 10, the higher number representing the more severe pain.

A verbal expression (verbal analogue) scale can be used when it is more appropriate to ask a patient to indicate in some way the degree of pain and to record this. Patients may show this in the distance between their hands or fingers: the larger the distance, the greater the pain.

Diagrams of facial expressions can be used, severe pain being indicated by a face with a downturned mouth and closed eyes, contrasting with a smiling face to reflect no pain. This is sometimes used for children. Colours and drawings can also be employed to express and record pain, red colours suggesting severe pain, blues and greens being used for little pain.

Carers must be particularly careful not to bias the reporting or recording of pain by patients. Bias may be easily and unintentionally introduced by a nurse calling out, 'How is your pain? You look better. Is it about 2 or 3? Yesterday, it was 5.' More meaningful information may be provided if the patient or carer recording the pain is unaware of the previous pain score, for example from the day before, as such an awareness may introduce bias.

The elderly present particular problems in the use of such recording techniques as there are frequent problems in understanding questions and in reading and making appropriate marks on forms. Much patience may be required if these records are to be of any real use.

REASONS FOR A FAILURE TO RELIEVE PAIN

There are many causes of inadequate pain relief, these being best overcome by the increased education of those in the caring professions.

Lack of knowledge

Many carers are unaware of the importance of pain in the overall well-being of the patient and have a poor factual knowledge of the correct use of appropriate analgesics.

Problems of addiction

Some patients are aware that morphine and other opioids are associated with drug addiction and may not want to take morphine, whereas some professional carers are ignorant and feel that tolerance to opioids precludes their early use. There are also unfounded fears concerning respiratory depression.

Inaccurate assessment and infrequent reassessment

A common error lies in the initial assessment, which then leads to prescribing inappropriate treatment. There must be frequent reassessment to prevent a return of unacceptable pain and to identify any new pain.

Inadequate emotional and psychological support

These are real problems and are not remediable by using drugs. They may be more influential than any physical causes of pain, and a failure to recognize them may make the correct assessment of the pain very difficult. A failure to recognize the psychological element, particularly in terms of fear and panic attacks, is not uncommon in hospitals.

It may not lie within the capabilities of most nurses and doctors to address these problems so they may need to rely on a competent social worker, a clinical psychologist, a minister of religion or a person who is not directly involved with the everyday care of the patient. An experienced volunteer can be of great value in such circumstances.

Poor relationship between patient and carer

Good communication is an absolute necessity as, without this, the professional adviser is disadvantaged when assessing pain. If there is a poor rapport between both parties, there is nearly always a poor control of the pain. Similarly, poor communication between carers can lead to important information not being passed on within the professional team, thus preventing the correct recognition and treatment of pain. Such problems are more likely to occur the larger teams become.

Focus on prolonging life and cure

If prolonging life and cure are the aims of professional carers, attention to the quality of life, and in turn the alleviation of pain, is often lost.

Inappropriate treatment and prescribing

Not all pain responds to drug therapy so the wider aspects of treatment need to be considered. These may extend from providing emotional and family support, and occupational and diversion therapy, to palliative radiotherapy and surgery. Even within the choice of drugs available, inappropriate prescribing is not uncommon; an antispasmodic may, for example, be more suitable than an opioid for pain arising from excessive colonic wind.

TYPES OF PAIN

Understanding the main types of pain helps to determine treatment, but there is also the danger that schemes to represent pain may be too simplistic and overlook the fact that there is an overlap of causes and that many factors may influence the perception of pain. Much interest is currently invested in whether the pain is nociceptive or neuropathic (see below).

Somatic and visceral pain

Somatic and visceral pain are examples of nociceptive pain and result from a stimulus, which may be chemical, thermal or pressure, that triggers normal nerve endings. This is the most common type of pain. Injury to the skin and deeper tissues is called somatic pain, whereas malignancy involving the deep abdominal and thoracic structures produces visceral pain, which may sometimes cause referred pain, the pain being perceived as lying away from the site of the actual pathology. An example of this is pain from the gall bladder or pancreas being perceived between the shoulder blades.

Most nociceptive pain responds to analgesics ranging from paracetamol to opioids depending on the severity of the pain.

Neuropathic pain

Neuropathic pain is often the result of partial damage to a nerve, such pain frequently being not particularly sensitive to opioids. Neuropathic pain is often characterized by abnormal sensations such as allodynia, which is pain resulting from a stimulus that does not normally cause pain, for example putting on a shirt, when the underlying skin feels a burning sensation. Other examples are hyperalgesia, when something that causes minimal pain now causes considerable pain. In many cases of neuropathic pain, the patient will describe the sensation as 'burning', 'pins and needles' or 'a red-hot poker' pain.

This is a difficult pain to relieve and responds best to a number of drugs that were formerly not regarded as being analgesics, including tricyclic antidepressants (e.g. amitryptline), steroids (e.g. prednisolone), anticonvulsants (e.g. carba-mazepine) and antiarrhythmic preparations (e.g. flecainide).

Bone pain

Bone pain is often associated with bone metastases and may respond to one of the many drugs derived from aspirin, the non-steroidal anti-inflammatory drugs (NSAIDs), radiotherapy and those drugs which influence bone metabolism, such as calcitonin and the bisphosphonates. This pain was previously considered to be not particularly responsive to the opioids, but oxycodone, a recently reintro-duced opioid, may provide considerable pain relief in bone pain. Bone, and in particular joint, pain are common irrespective of cancer.

Breakthrough pain

Breakthrough pain, sometimes called incident pain, has recently received much interest. A number of terms have been used to describe this pain, including 'transient' pain, 'flare-up', 'episodic' or 'movement' pain. Such pain may be triggered on weight-bearing or movement, another example being pain on swallowing or coughing. Although there is no clear definition of this type of pain, it generally refers to an intermittent exacerbation of pain that can occur spontaneously or in relation to a specific activity. For this type of pain, it is best to use an analgesic that is both quick acting and of short duration so that any adverse effects of giving additional analgesia, such as drowsiness, are kept to a minimum.

A few years ago, the term 'breakthrough' pain was used with another mean-ing, as was seen when a patient, taking modified-release morphine or another analgesic, suffered pain before taking the next dose of analgesic. This was often the result of a decline in the plasma level of the analgesic. Today, many carers still use the term 'breakthrough pain' with this meaning so it is necessary to be careful in the use of the terms.

SPECIAL PROBLEMS RELATING TO PAIN

Particular problems may arise when a patient experiences severe, unexpected pain; this could be an emergency situation. The key considerations must be empathy, good communication, calmness and companionship, the latter being achieved by someone staying with the patient all the time until the problem has been resolved. A mental checklist is useful here.

First, has the patient been taking the prescribed analgesia? If the patient is receiving a subcutaneous infusion from a syringe driver, check that the device is working, that the line is patent and the cannula site is not indurated or inflamed.

Next, review the situation calmly, making certain that the patient is in a comfortable position. If relatives and friends are present, reassure them that the situation is being reviewed, and dissuade a large number of relatives from remaining at the bedside.

Third, is this a panic attack? Does the patient seem frightened or extremely anxious? Do not give opioids, but consider giving a suitable anxiolytic such as midazolam 2–5 mg intravenously or 5 mg subcutaneously or intramuscularly. Make certain that a carer remains with the patient all the time; an independent carer may provide more reassurance than a close relative.

Is the pain increased with movement? Is there a bone fracture or spinal cord compression? Is the patient known to have bone secondaries? Has there been a recent fall? If the patient is in severe pain, or is to be moved, consider giving a bolus dose of opioid via an intramuscular or slow intravenous route, which may have to be at least 50 per cent above the regular 4-hourly dose or equivalent. The subcutaneous route is often the slowest to show a response. Explain the findings to the patient and relatives. Consider giving a small dose of an anxiolytic by mouth, with some warm water, until the matter has been further investigated. Before any emergency transport journey, review whether an antiemetic is necessary.

If the pain is caused by respiratory distress, consider oxygen and give an opioid by injection. Provide a carer to stay with the patient.

If there is abdominal pain, consider intestinal obstruction and/or perforation, particularly if there is a history of intestinal cancer. With the pain of subacute obstruction and colic, consider hyoscine butylbromide 20 mg given by injection, via the intravenous, intramuscular or subcutaneous route.

With chest pain, consider a cardiac problem. If this is accompanied by cardiac difficulty in breathing, pallor and sometimes an indescribable feeling of being very unwell, pulmonary embolus should be included in the differential diagnosis.

The patient may be unable to express his or her pain, or may indicate that the pain is present 'all over'. Although there may be no overt signs of agitation or panic, some but not all of these situations reflect fear, anxiety and even anger. Careful thought must be given to the patient's psychological state. The use of an anxiolytic rather than an analgesic may give the patient some mental respite.

When the pain persists and every effort has been made to determine its cause, a complete review is required. This review should look at psychological and social problems, including fear, anxiety and loneliness, which are often much more difficult to identify than physical causes of pain and are hidden by continual reference to the pain.

Chronic pain can become a problem with cancer patients. It may result from the repeated stimulation of the receptors by an unpleasant stimulus that persists to such a degree that the sensation of pain becomes permanent. These cases require reassessment using a multi-disciplinary approach. In some cases, there may be no means of alleviating the pain.

PAIN IN THE ELDERLY

Understanding and ameliorating pain in the elderly may be difficult. Illness and pathology are often multiple, and it may be difficult to differentiate a chronic from a new pain. There is also the little-known but frequent pain that occurs after a stroke. Any relevant medical history from many decades ago may not be recalled or recorded. The patient may also find it difficult to decribe or localize the pain. Many elderly people are hard of hearing. They are often set in their ways, and the expressions and language used by many professionals may be alien to them and often not understood. Then there is the real pain of loneliness, apprehension, lack of security and real or imaginary worries. All these difficulties may frustrate and make the busy professional intolerant. This is where time, empathy and skill supersede textbook knowledge.

Many elderly people have existing problems of dehydration, reduced renal function, a low albumin level and cerebrovascular problems that may be manifest as slight confusion or forgetfulness. These often amplify the adverse effects of drugs, the most commonly encountered being increased drowsiness and confusion. A patient in this state is less inclined to drink, which leads to further dehydration and renal problems. The individual response to analgesia is more unpredictable than for the younger patient.

Because of the complexities of understanding pain in the elderly, professionals are often forced to give unconsidered opinions, which are often recorded, conveyed to other professionals and accepted as being the reason behind the pain. Because of this, the effects of any treatment cannot be properly assessed. Many elderly patients are unable to articulate or challenge the views of professionals. In every case, there should be scrutiny and re-examination of earlier conclusions and decisions.

Certain guidelines should be followed:

- Patience is an absolute requirement in trying to understand pain problems in the elderly, but some professionals are unsuited to this task.
- Multiple pathology and existing conditions require particular caution when prescribing.
- In general, all drug doses should be reduced, it being prudent to use a lower dose when introducing any drug.
- If there is a change in the condition of the patient, first be suspicious of the medication and consider all its possible adverse effects.
- As difficult as it may be, encourage an increased fluid intake.
- If an elderly patient does not want to take a particular medicine, there may be a very good reason for this. He or she may, for example, have previously experienced a side-effect of which you are unaware.
- Review each case and the drugs being used frequently, more often than for a younger patient.
- Major pathology in the elderly may not always cause pain, as is recognized for intestinal perforation or fractures of the head of femur. This results from central

autonomic dysfunction, which may lead to a loss of the appreciation of pain. An absence of pain does not, however, mean an absence of pathology.

PHARMACOLOGICAL AND RELATED APPROACHES TO THE MANAGEMENT OF PAIN

MAIN GROUPS OF DRUGS AND INTERVENTIONS

There are seven main groups of drug and related interventional approaches for the relief of pain, each group having many subgroups. More than one treatment is often used simultaneously because the pain seen in patients with cancer may arise from more than one cause. Morphine remains the standard by which all other analgesics are assessed.

Opioid

Opioids are the naturally occuring substances derived from the opium poppy that provide morphine. With further processing, morphine is converted into diamorphine (heroin). Many substances, including codeine, have been derived from morphine, and in recent years many synthetic or laboratory-designed opioids have become available.

Anti-inflammatory agents

There are two groups of drug that have the general properties of relieving inflammation and pain:

1 NSAIDs, many of which are derived from asprin;
2 corticosteroids (or steroids, such as prednisolone and dexamethasone), which are the most potent anti-inflammatory drugs.

Adjuvant drugs

Adjuvant drugs encompass a wide range of agents whose primary use is not analgesia; these include antidepressants, anticonvulsants and antiarrhythmic drugs. They ameliorate pain by interfering with normal nerve transmission and are widely used for neuropathic pain. These drugs were originally used as a second-line choice, alongside the opioids, to relieve pain, but they are now often used as a first-line approach. Our knowledge on this group of drugs and their side-effects is, however, very limited.

Neurolytic agents

Neurolytic agents are used to block nerves. The relief from their use may only be temporary, but it is very worthwhile. A well-known example is using a local anaesthetic to block the subcostal nerve for pain experienced from a rib fracture. A long-acting anaesthestic, such as bupivacaine, is commonly injected, with or without steroids, into or near a nerve. Examples are coeliac plexus and related blocks that are most useful to block pain from abdominal malignancies, such as carcinoma of the pancreas, whereas spinal blocks are useful for suppressing the pain of a pelvic tumour. Other chemicals, such as alcohol or phenol, may sometimes cause semi-permanent or even permanent nerve blockade. Cryotherapy, the use of very low temperatures to ablate nerves, is less used nowadays.

Radiotherapy

Radiotherapy is employed for severe bone pain arising from bony metastases. It is often very effective, but there is a limit to the amount of radiotherapy that may be given to the same area of bone. It may be of value in shrinking a tumour mass, or malignant lymph nodes, which will lessen the pain. Similarly, it may lower the intracranial pressure associated with brain tumours, thereby relieving pressure pain.

Electrical stimulation

An electrical current is used to stimulate the nerve, and with some appliances, patients may control the degree of stimulation themselves. In cancer patients, electrical stimulation is used for neuropathic pain. Trans-electrical nerve stimulation (TENS), also known as transcutaneous nerve stimulation, in which the electrodes are placed on the skin, is the more common form of this technique. Major procedures include dorsal and spinal cord stimulation. Although our knowledge of how such stimulation works is incomplete, it is thought to work within the model of the gate theory of pain. This model suggests that the stimulation of certain small nerve fibres tends to open the 'gate' and promote pain, whereas stimulation of the larger nerve fibres tends to close the 'gate' and inhibit pain. Electrical stimulation is thought to work by stimulating the larger nerve fibres.

Surgery

Surgical ablation or the sectioning of a nerve is sometimes used for intractable pain but is often associated with serious side-effects such as paralysis. Chordotomy is an example of this procedure.

THE 'ANALGESIC LADDER'

In the mid-1980s, the WHO introduced the concept of a ladder to promote the adequate use of analgesics in cancer. The first step of the ladder was asprin or paracetamol; if pain continued, a move was made to the second step, essentially giving mild opioids as codeine. If necessary, the third step, the use of strong opioids, was invoked. The original concept was a three-step ladder, but in recent years, with the increasing use of interventional therapy such as nerve blocks, it may be reasonable to introduce an additional, fourth step. Other ladders or steps have more recently been proposed, one idea being that the second step involves NSAIDs, the third step corticosteroids, and the fourth opioids.

The ladder concept is a simplistic and stylised approach to encourage the progression from one group of drugs to another until there is a respite from the pain. The analgesic ladder will continue to evolve and be redesigned as our understanding of pain increases. It should, however, always be used in parallel with the knowledge that certain sources of pain respond best to certain medications.

ANALGESICS

PARACETAMOL AND ASPIRIN

Paracetamol (available as tablets, dissolvable tablets, suspension and suppositories) remains the first choice for mild-to-moderate pain and has minimal side-effects, except on the liver if taken in large doses for a long time. Because it is relatively short acting, it needs to be taken every 4–6 hours to achieve a continuous therapeutic effect. Although it is often prescribed as a 1 g dose (two 500 mg tablets), there is a therapeutic value from taking 500 mg alone.

Paracetamol combined with a 'weak' opioid is available in several preparations. Such combinations include adding dihydrocodeine (=co-dydramol), codeine phosphate (=co-codamol) and dextropropoxyphene (=co-proxamol). It is debatable whether these combinations are more effective than paracetamol alone as the side-effects of the 'weak' opioid can sometimes be greater than those which arise from taking paracetamol alone. For example, detropropoxyphene, although possessing analgesic properties, may cause serious constipation in the elderly.

Aspirin (acetylsalicylic acid) was for many years the most frequently used analgesia, often being combined with morphine to provide an effective analgesic. Aspirin is still invaluable in tackling pain caused by inflammatory conditions, for example of the joints, but side-effects including bronchospasm, thereby excerbating asthma, and gastrointestinal ulceration have made it less popular as a first-step or long-term analgesic in cancer patients.

OPIOIDS

There are currently nearly two dozen opioid preparations available on the UK market, some being available in several formulations. Morphine remains the standard by which all other analgesics are compared. There is an indistinct arbitary division of the opioids into weak and strong opioids, weak ones including codeine and dihydrocodeine. One characteristic of the weak opioids is that they are considered to have a 'ceiling effect'. In practice, this means that if a high dose is used to provide analgesia, the side- or adverse effect of the drug will exceed its possible value as an analgesic. This in turn means that, for severe or strong pain, the weak opioid is stopped and the patient started on a stronger opioid.

Morphine

Morphine as tablets, capsules, solution, intermediate release, modified-release suspension and injection remains the first choice for oral medication. It is well absorbed from the small bowel, after which it is converted mainly in the liver into an active metabolite that provides potent analgesia. When taken orally, it generally provides analgesia for about 4 hours. It is available in either immediate-release or sustained-release, now generally referred to as modified release or MR, formulations, the latter being taken either every 12 hours (e.g. MST) or every 24 hours (e.g. MXL). Morphine rectal suppositories have more recently been reintroduced, the strength of which should be the same as the oral dose. Suppositories are useful if the patient cannot take medication by mouth, although rectal absorption is more variable than absorption via the oral route. Morphine may be given by injection (intramuscular, intravenous or subcutaneous), but because it has a relatively poor solubility, diamorphine is the first choice, if injection is required (see below).

Starting morphine For the elderly and opioid-naive patient, a suitable starting dose is 2.5 mg every 4 hours, but for most patients it is possible to start at 5 mg every 4 hours. The patient should be reassessed as often as possible and the dose increased if the pain persists.

Reassessment should also include reviewing the possible adverse effects of the drug. About one-third of patients experience drowsiness and/or nausea in the first few days; in the latter case, a regular antiemetic should be prescribed to be taken with the morphine. About one-half of patients suffer from constipation so a suitable laxative at an effective dose should be prescribed, at the same time that morphine is started, the laxative dose being rapidly increased and titrated to minimize the constipation.

Modified-Release Formulations Prescribers are increasingly commencing morphine-naive patients immediately on MR formulations of morphine, but with the very ill and elderly, it may be prudent first to use immediate-acting morphine on a 4-hourly basis until the pain has been controlled and any side-effects ameliorated, conversion to an MR formulation then taking place.

Titrating the Dose of Morphine The dose of morphine should be increased until adequate analgesia has been obtained. An approximate rule is to increase the dose by about one-third to one-half. For example, if the previous dose is 10 mg 4-hourly and the pain persists, increase the dose to 15 mg 4-hourly. Most pain, if opioid sensitive, can be controlled on about 20–30 mg 4-hourly.

'Rescue' Medication The patient should be given clear instructions, if possible in legible writing, on what to do if the pain is troublesome before the next dose of morphine, whether this is 4- or 12-hourly. For this, the patient is provided with immediate-acting morphine, as tablets or a solution. The general rule is that patients should take the same dose as they are taking every 4 hours if the pain becomes apparent.

They should make a written note of how often such 'rescue' medication is taken so that the daily dose can be adjusted upwards at the next review. It should be stressed that they should continue taking their regular 4-hourly dose of morphine, irrespective of when they took their rescue medication. When the 4-hourly dose is next increased, the rescue medication should also be increased to the new 4-hourly dose. A modification of this should be worked out for those taking MR morphine each 12 or 24 hours.

Even when patients have been stabilized on an MR preparation, they should still be provided with an immediate-acting morphine to use when necessary.

Conversion from Immediate-Release to Modified-Release Preparations Immediate release preparations are usually prescribed to be taken 4-hourly, but in practice patients tend to take such morphine four or five, rather than six, times a day because they sleep for 6–8 hours. Therefore a 10 mg 4-hourly dose should be multiplied by four or five to establish the approximate 24 hour equivalent; the 12 hour MR preparation will thus be between 20 mg and 25 mg, and the 24 hour MR preparation 40–50 mg.

Diamorphine

Diamorphine is available in tablet form, but the most common use of diamorphine is as an injection (subcutaneous or intramuscular) because of its better solubility than morphine, from which it is derived. It can either be given by injection, every 4 hours, or more appropriately by continuous subcutaneous infusion (see below).

It is a common misconception that diamorphine is a 'stronger' analgesic than morphine. Diamorphine is converted to morphine within the body, but when adminstered, it is, dose for dose, more potent than morphine. Therefore, 3 mg oral morphine is approximately equivalent to 1 mg diamorphine given by (subcutaneous or intramuscular) injection. The oral dose of morphine is divided by three to give the approximate equal strength of the diamorphine injection.

Buprenorphine

Buprenorphine (as SL tablets) has a longer duration of action than morphine, the slow-release sublingual tablet of 200 µg being held and dissolved in the mouth and absorbed through the buccal mucosa. It occupies a place mid-way in the analgesic ladder and at higher doses may antagonize morphine, this supporting the recommendation that it may be unwise to use two different opioids simultenously.

Buprenorphine was widely used about 20 years ago, but it has three possible disadvantages. First, some patients find that it is uncomfortable to retain the tablet in a very dry mouth while it is absorbed, and if it is swallowed, this inactivates most of the opioid. Second, when buprenorphine is given by this route, it is often associated with nausea and vomiting, although this claim has not been throughly substantiated. Third, there is a probable 'ceiling effect', which suggests that increasing the dose above 12 or more tablets per day does not provide greater analgesia.

Codeine phosphate

Codeine phosphate (as tablets, syrup or intramuscular injection) is used for mild-to-moderate pain. Its main use is to slow gut peristalsis and help to relieve diarrhoea; because of this, it causes severe constipation at higher doses. It is also used as an anti-tussive.

Dihydrocodeine

Dihydrocodeine (as tablets, a solution or a subcutaneous injection) is probably a better analgesic than its close relation codeine phosphate, from which it is derived. It is likely to possess about the same potency as codeine phosphate when given by mouth and is used for moderate-to-severe pain, but it is constipating. In an injectable form, it is twice as potent as codeine phosphate.

Dextromoramide

Dextromoramide (as tablets or suppositories) is effective for severe pain, is quick acting, often within 15–20 minutes, and provides pain relief for 3–6 hours. Because of these characteristics, it is given for anticipated breakthrough or incident pain, for example before re-dressing a painful wound.

Dipipanone with Cyclizine

This combination (as tablets) is used for severe pain and has a duration of action of about 6 hours. It suits patients who are prone to nausea because it is combined with cyclizine, which is a potent antiemetic. This combined preparation of an opioid and an antiemetic may, however, oversedate many patients. It is available in only one strength.

Fentanyl Citrate

Fentanyl citrate (available as a transmucosal lozenge) was recently developed in this formulation especially for the relief of breakthrough pain in patients receiving maintenance opioid therapy for chronic pain. It is known as transmucosal fentanyl citrate (TMFC).

The drug is held in a sugary matrix, with a slight fruity flavour, the lozenge being on a small stick. The stick of the lozenge is held by the patient and gently rubbed and rotated against the buccal mucosa of the mouth, inside the cheek. There is a quick absorption through the buccal mucosa, which leads to a first plasma peak in about 20 minutes, although the analgesic effect may occur within 10–15 minutes. About three-quarters of the fentanyl citrate contained in the lozenge is swallowed in the saliva and absorbed in the gut, this giving rise to a further plasma peak. The analgesic effect may last from 2 to 6 hours.

It is available in six strengths, 200 µg, 400 µg, 600 µg, 800 µg, 1200 µg and 1600 µg (Actiq). The approximate equivalent of 200 µg of TMFC is 2 mg intravenous morphine or 6 mg oral morphine, but as the bioavailability of TMFC is 50 per cent, the actual clinical equivalent of a 200 µg lozenge is nearer 3 mg oral morphine.

There is no clear relationship between the oral dose of opioid that is being taken and the strength of the fentanyl citrate lozenge required to relieve breakthrough pain, so the optimum strength of TMFC has to be titrated for each patient. One suggestion is to start giving the patient a 200 µg strength lozenge. If there is no pain relief in 15–20 minutes, remove the first lozenge and give a second 200 µg lozenge. If pain relief is shall not obtained, check that the instructions to the patient are clear and that the patient is rolling or plating the lozenge across his or her buccal surface. The next time TMFC is used, give a 400 µg or 600 µg lozenge depending on the results of the previous use.

This is a novel drug delivery system, and there are a number of suggested guidelines that should be followed in its use. First, patients should ideally already be receiving opioids before being introduced to TMFC. Second, patients must be properly instructed in its use. Third, it is important that there should be a reasonable amount of saliva in the mouth to make the lozenge soluble to allow absorption. If the mouth is dry, it should be well moistened with either water or artificial saliva before using the lozenge.

There are several adverse effects of using TMFC, the most frequent being facial flushing and pruritus. Other side-effects associated with higher doses include headache, nausea, occasional vomiting, a slowing of heart rate and constipation. The practical significance of these reports will, however, only be assessed from further experience in its use. Finally, in common with all opioids, the side-effects are generally increased in those who are dehydrated or have impaired renal function. The potential role of TMFC in breakthrough pain is being further evaluated.

Fentanyl

Fentanyl (available as a transdermal patch or injection) has been used for many years in an injectable form to augment anaesthesia and is suitable for severe pain. There is a current vogue for drug formulations to be available in patch form, using a transdermal delivery system (FTDP), as for hormonal replacement therapy and nicotine substitutes.

The fentanyl is contained in a reservoir that is part of a 'patch' that adheres to the skin. The adhesive itself is saturated with fentanyl, and this additional fentanyl gives a boost in absorption when the patch is first applied. Fentanyl is released from the reservoir to permeate and diffuse through the skin, where it is absorbed into the blood circulation. The larger the surface area of the patch, the greater the strength of the patch; Therefore the higher strength applications are the larger patches.

Fentanyl works on the same receptor sites as morphine, but it is not a more potent analgesic than morphine. If morphine does not relieve a pain, it is most unlikely that it will be relieved by fentanyl. FTDP is not designed for acute pain or for when a quick response is required by frequent titration of the drug.

It may take up to 2 days for the plasma level of fentanyl to reach a steady state, and between a few and 24 hours to provide analgesia. Because of this, it is recommended that the patient is first started on morphine or another opioid, being transferred to after pain relief has been obtained. The patch requires changing each 72 hours, the new patch being placed on a new site.

When transferring the patient from another opioid to FTDP, there should be a period of overlap with the previous analgesic for about 12 hours as it takes about this time for the fentanyl level to build up in the body. During this time, there will be changes in the plasma levels of both drugs, and about one-half of patients may experience some pain during the first day or two of initiating FTDP. Patients should be warned about this and be provided with an immediate-release opioid to take at such times. For the same reasons, some patients may experience depressive symptoms during this transitional period.

Because this is a relatively new method of drug delivery, our knowledge of its characteristics is considerably less than for oral morphine. We do not, for example, know why a few patients require a new patch every day, or some every second day, when the majority find renewal each third day satisfactory. Further more, it is unclear why some patients consistently experience transient bizzare thoughts and depression on the third day. These unusual features are probably related to the complex diffusion of fentanyl through the skin and how it is then attracted to, and then released from, the fat reservoirs of the body.

Patients using FTDP should be advised to refrain from taking very hot baths and avoid exposure to local heat such as would result from placing a heat pad near the patch. Where the patient has fever, or there is a chronic skin disorder, it may not be appropriate to use FTDP. Patches can cause local pruritis, particularly in those with sensitive skin. This may be reduced by placing the patch on skin sites that are thicker and less sensitive, but it is uncertain how this may affect absorption of the fentanyl.

The strength of a patch is expressed as the amount of fentanyl delivered each hour. Patches are available in four strengths, which, together with the approximate equivalent oral morphine, and suggested 'breakthrough' doses of immediate-acting morphine, are listed in Table 1.2. To achieve a higher level of fentanyl, two or more patches may be applied, but they should all be changed at the same time each third day. The patch should not be cut or folded over with the idea of reducing the dose of fentanyl.

Special consideration needs to be given before starting FTDP in elderly patients or those with poor renal function because the lowest strength of FTDP (25 µg per hour) is equal to oral morphine 135 mg per 24 hours or about 23 mg oral morphine each 4 hours. FTDP may in general not be suitable for patients taking low doses of oral morphine because the lowest dose of FTDP may be too high and lead to drowsiness and related side-effects.

In the terminal stages of illness, it is sometimes preferable to use an immediate-acting opioid for pain, this often being achieved by setting up a syringe driver and using subcutaneous diamorphine. A general guideline for establishing the dose of diamorphine required for continuous subcutaneous delivery is to divide the strength of the patch by two. This provides the diamorphine dose required for the first 24 hours. The patch is then removed. For the second 24 hours

Table 1.2 Fentanyl and morphine dosages

FTDP strength µg/hour	Oral morphine over 24 hours (mg)	Approximate 'breakthrough' dose of oral morphine (mg)
25	135	15
50	225	30
75	315	45
100	404	60

and subsequently, after review, the diamorphine strength can be increased by two. This strategy is used because fentanyl is still present in the body for some time after removal of the patch. Therefore if a dose of FTDP of 50 µg per hour is being used, remove the FTDP and start subcutaneous diamorphine 25 mg per 24 hours for the first day. For the second and each subsequent day, the dose of subcutaneous diamorphine will be 50 mg per 24 hours.

Fentanyl patches are considerably more expensive than most other formulations of opioid, because of which some palliative care departments have brought out guidelines on the most appropriate use of the patch. These include the patient who cannot take medicine by mouth, and when there is dysphagia or pain on swallowing, poor compliance with taking oral medication or intractable vomiting.

It has been suggested that the adverse effects associated with FTDP are considerably fewer than those seen with morphine and other opioids, especially as far as constipation is concerned. Delirium and confusion have been noted, probably as frequently as with morphine, but there have been no definitive studies to assess possible significant differences.

The present formulation of the FTDP is the first generation of this type of drug delivery system. Current developments are moving towards more sophisticated patches to provide more predictable and variable absorption, using matrix reservoirs, iontophoresis and other electrical systems. Some approaches are considering using other analgesics in this delivery system.

Hydromorphone
Hydromorphone (as capsules and intermediate-release and MR preparations) is a strong opioid that is closely related to morphine, although it is 5–10 times more potent than morphine. Of particular interest is that it may have fewer side-effects than morphine and other opioids, and it can be used more safely than other opioids in cases of poor renal function. Hydromorphone has been the first choice when the side-effects of morphine encourage a change to a different opioid. With a rapid onset of action and a short half-life, the MR form is most suitable for cancer pain. It is probably more effective than many other opioids for providing relief for breathlessness.

Methadone
Methadone (as a solution, tablets or an injection) is a strong but complex opioid in terms of pharmokinetics, working on both the mu and delta receptors, morphine working only on the mu receptors. Its main characteristic is a long half-life of 24 hours, but this can vary considerably in some patients, predisposing to complications of possible drug accumulation. Therefore, methadone is not recommended for use in the elderly. Renal or hepatic impairment is not a contraindication to its use. Methadone has been employed for some time as a substitute opioid for registered drug addicts.

Several years ago, methadone was used for neuropathic pain and for patients in whom there was an inadequate response to morphine or the side-effects of high doses of morphine were unacceptable. This property of helping neuropathic pain may result from a weak NMDA antagonistic activity. There is a considerable variability in the dose required between patients. Many drugs, including all the antiepileptics and anticonvulsants, interact with methadone and result in greater side-effects and respiratory depression.

Oxycodone

This strong semi-synthetic opioid analgesia (available as suppositories, intermediate-release and MR preparations, and tablets) was used in the UK for many years in suppository form (oxycodone pectinate). Although similar to morphine in many respects, it probably has a wider therapeutic use than morphine because it acts on both the mu and kappa opioid receptors. The oral form is about 1.5–2-fold more potent than oral morphine, and it is suggested that the possible side-effects, including hallucinations, are fewer than with morphine. Its plasma half-life is considerably increased in renal failure, and it may be prudent to reduce the dose of oxycodone in such cases by approximately one-quarter.

Oxycodone has been used in North America for a wide range of non-cancer pains, particularly those arising from musculoskeletal disorders such as rheumatoid conditions and arthroses, and overlaps in some clinical usage with NSAIDs without having their adverse effects of gastric erosion and haemorrhage. Oxycodone is also of use in some of the neuropathic pain situations, such as post-herpetic neuralgia, not only managing the allondynia, but also reducing the number of episodes of breakthrough pain associated with herpetic pain.

Laboratory studies have more recently suggested that the co-adminstration of oxycodone and morphine may provide very effective pain relief with fewer central effects. If this is substantiated in clinical experience, it will introduce new interest in the synergistic activity of opioids.

Phenazocine

This mu agonist (available in tablet form) has been used as a useful alternative to strong opioids when the central nervous system side-effects of morphine, such as hallucinations and nausea, have been intolerable. It is about five times more potent than morphine, with a longer action of duration, providing pain relief for 6–8 hours. Phenazocine can be absorbed through the buccal mucosa if it is held for long enough in the mouth, although absorption is slow and the taste is acceptable but not outstanding. It is potentially a most useful opioid, but its clinical value is limited because it is now available in only one strength 5 mg tablet, each being equivalent to approximately 25 mg oral morphine.

Tramadol

For many years, tramadol (as an injection, capsules or tablets) has been one of the most commonly used opioids in mainland Europe. It is a weak opioid, and has found a place in clinical practice between dihydrocodeine and the stronger opioids. It has opioid and non-opioid properties as it inhibits both norepinephrine and 5-hydroxytryptamine uptake. This contributes to the not uncommon side-effect of orthostatic hypertension and causes it to interact with tricyclic and selective serotonin reuptake inhibitor antidepressants. Some of the side-effects, such as constipation, are probably slightly milder than those seen with morphine. Unlike the opioids in general, the effects of tramadol are only partly reversed by naloxone. It is believed to have a 'ceiling effect'.

NON-STEROIDAL ANTI-INFLAMMATORY DRUGS (NSAIDs)

About 25 different drugs are currently classed as NSAIDs. These are generally more potent than paracetamol and aspirin. Paracetamol often remains the first choice for mild pain because its adverse effects are considerably fewer than those of most NSAIDs. Like aspirin, most NSAIDs are analgesic, anti-inflammatory and antipyretic, but NSAIDs differ in their relative properties. The NSAIDs are the most commonly prescribed non-opioid analgesics, and because of their wide use, they are associated with many adverse effects and are the most important cause of iatrogenic gastrointestinal haemorrhage. This has brought about an interest in those preparations with fewer adverse effects.

Choice of non-steroidal anti-inflammatory drug

If gastrointestinal problems are present, either paracetamol or one of the older NSAIDs, for example ibuprofen, should be chosen. Increase the dose of NSAID to that recommended in the current edition of the *British National Formulary*. When there is regular supervision to monitor any possible adverse effects, consider one of the more potent NSAIDs, such as as diclofenac, flurbiprofen or naproxen, or even a high dosage of dispersible aspirin. Ketorolac should be used only with specialist advice. If there is recent or active gastrointestinal pathology, consider rofecoxib, one of the newer cyclo-oxygenase-2 (COX-2) preparations.

When inflammation is present and may be contributing to the pain, higher doses of NSAIDs are required. If there is no response to a higher dose, consider changing to another NSAID because there are distinct differences in their properties. Like aspirin, some NSAIDs may cause bronchoconstriction in asthmatic patients, and some NSAIDs may affect the blood coagulation time.

If there is any suspicion of gastrointestinal adverse effects and NSAID treatment needs to be continued, consider the concurrent prescription of one of the protective drugs, such as protein pump inhibitors (omeprazole or lansoprazole) and prostaglandin analogues (misoprostol). Omeprazole is probably the protective agent of choice once adverse gastrointestinal symptoms arise. The H_2-receptor antagonists (cimetidine and ranitidine) do not provide very effective protection.

Ibuprofen

Ibuprofen (as tablets, intermediate-release and MR preparations, syrup or gel) is one of the earliest and most 'tried and tested' NSAIDs. It is particularly useful for pain associated with inflammatory conditions and has one of the lowest incidences of adverse effects. It is about three times more potent than aspirin, analgesia being provided within 30 minutes and lasting for up to 6 hours. The average daily dose for pain relief ranges from 1200 mg to twice that dose, divided into three or four equal doses throughout the day. A disadvantage for some patients is the large size of the tablets, but it is available in both syrup and effervescent granule formulations. In gel form, it is applied to the skin over small joints and may provide some pain relief in these situations.

Diclofenac

Diclofenac (as tablets, MR preparations, suppository and injection) is a relatively widely prescribed NSAID. Probably fewer than 10 per cent of patients report adverse effects, the most common of which is nausea. The incidence of these adverse effects, as with other NSAIDs, increases with renal impairment.

Diclofenac is available in immediate-release (50 mg) tablets, which are associated with a slightly lower incidence of adverse effects than the MR capsules (75 mg and 100 mg). The dispersible tablets (50 mg) are thought to provide significant pain relief within 20 minutes and may be suitable for certain incident pain. Most of the preparations provide analgesia for up to 8 hours. Some patients are prescribed a total of 200 mg daily for pain, but it is prudent to lower this if it is the intention is to use the NSAID for some time.

The injection, as the suppository, is useful for those unable to take oral medication; it can be administered via a subcutaneous continuous infusion (75–150 mg daily), but it is not compatible in the same syringe with most other drugs and should be administered via a separate syringe. The suppository is sometimes incorrectly used in the belief that there will be fewer adverse effects than with oral diclofenac. It is however, just as likely to cause adverse effects in those with such a predisposition.

Diclofenac is also available in tablet form combined with the prostaglandin analogue misoprostol to provide gastrointestinal protection.

Ketorolac

Ketorolac (as tablets or injection) is a relatively new and highly potent NSAID, being about 350 times more potent than aspirin. This potency, however, increases the risk of serious adverse effects, and the drug must be used with caution. It is not a first-line NSAID and should not be used concurrently with other NSAIDs or anticoagulants, being avoided if there is hepatic impairment.

Ketorolac is best administered by continuous subcutaneous infusion using a syringe driver, starting with 50 mg per 24 hours and increasing each day by 10 mg per 24 hours up to about 100 mg per 24 hours. It is compatible in the same syringe with diamorphine but not with many other drugs, including cyclizine, haloperidol, midazolam and morphine.

Misoprostol, lansoprazole or omeprazole should be prescribed and taken by mouth concurrently to provide some gastrointestinal protection. A useful function is to help to relieve severe bone pain for the patient awaiting radiotherapy.

Cyclo-oxygenase-2 (COX-2) inhibitors

NSAIDs inhibit the COX enzymes, which in turn inhibits the production of prostaglandins; these protect much of the body, including the gastric mucosa. Because this protection is diminished when taking NSAIDs, there may be erosion of the gut mucosa and bleeding.

There are two forms of COX in the body. COX-1 is present in all normal tissues of the body, particularly the gastrointestinal tract. COX-2 becomes important when there is gross inflammation within the body. Present drug developments are to produce selective COX inhibitors because these have fewer adverse effects on the gastrointestinal system, the two present preparations being rofecoxib and celecoxib. These new NSAIDs are more expensive than the older preparations but are important for the patient with a proven predisposition towards gastric pathology.

CORTICOSTEROIDS

Corticosteroids relieve pain in several ways. As potent anti-inflammatory drugs, they reduce the amount of inflammatory substances that excite nerve endings. In the case of the headache associated with a cerebral tumour and metastases, they reduce oedema and in turn pressure, which may be causing pain. They may reduce the pressure exerted by tumours on nerves, particularly large pelvic tumours that cause pressure on the main nerves supplying the legs. Similarly, a large dose of corticosteroids (for example, dexamethasone 12–16 mg daily) is the first-line treatment for reducing the pain and symptoms of the lower vertebrae that may suggest developing spinal cord compression. Here the pain is increased on coughing, and the sensory system of the legs loses the ability to discriminate between hot and cold, later also losing the ability to sense when to empty the bladder or bowel. Corticosteroids are also useful in dampening the pain arising from bone metastases until radiotherapy or other treatment can be arranged.

Several corticosteroid preparations are now available in tablet and injectable forms. Their equivalence in terms of anti-inflammatory effect is outlined in the current edition of the *British National Formulary*. Of these corticosteroids, prednisolone and dexamethasone remain the first choice when considering pain. Prednisolone is in general used when relatively low doses of corticosteroids are required, and dexamethazone for higher doses. The dose of corticosteroids depends on the urgency and magnitude of the symptoms, high doses being used for the pain associated with potentially emergency situations, such as cord compression, and lower doses for bone and liver capsule pain.

There are some general guidelines for the use of corticosteroids:

- After the initial dose of corticosteroids has been given, and once the major symptom has been controlled, reduce the dose as soon as possible.
- If corticosteroids are being used for more than a few weeks, it is advisable to keep the daily dose to 7.5 mg or less of prednisolone in order to minimize the adverse effects.
- There are many adverse effects, and many drug interactions, of corticosteroids. These adverse effects cover every system of the body and in 1–2 per cent of patients cause steroid agitation or psychoses, which become apparent within a day or two of starting the drug. In long-term use, they do not help to prevent pressure sores.

ADJUVANT ANALGESICS

These are mainly, but not entirely, the antidepressants and antiepileptics (anti-convulsants). Their principal use is not for pain, although they are used for neuropathic pain. Some neuropathic pain responds well to certain types of drug but not others. Oxycodone, for example, which is a strong opioid, provides good relief for post-herpetic pain, whereas tramadol, a weak opioid, is useful for the pain of diabetic neuropathy.

A general guideline for neuropathic pain is as follows:

- *First line*:   if an opioid does not relieve the pain, add an NSAID.
- *Second line*:   if there is no improvement in 2 weeks, consider using one of the new opioids, such as oxycodone, either on its own or added to the existing opioid, although both should be in a low dose as there will be a synergistic affect

    or

    commence a tricyclic antidepressant or antiepileptic. Decrease the opioid dose, and monitor for adverse effects. Slowly increase the dose of the adjuvant drug.
- *Third line*:   if no improvement is seen in 3 weeks, stop the therapy and use one of the newer antiepileptics, for example gabapentin. Monitor for adverse effects, and check for drug interaction.

Antidepressants or antiepiletics?

The choice between antidepressants and antiepileptics depends on experience and local custom. Amitryptyline has long been the first choice, the starting dose and dose increment depending on the presence of adverse effects. If the adverse effects outweigh any potential advantage, consider another antidepressant. If there is no response within 3 weeks, replace the antidepressant with an antiepileptic or add the antiepileptic to the antidepressant, carefully monitoring for adverse effects.

Antidepressants

Tricyclic antidepressants have long been used for chronic pain but have not been found useful for acute pain; in the past few years, they have also been used for neuropathic pain. It was first thought that antidepressants worked by elevating mood, but it is now thought that they have their own analgesic properties. A much lower therapeutic dose is required for pain relief than for the treatment of depression. Two main groups of antidepressant are used for pain – the tricyclic agents and the newer SSRIs. Both may potentiate opioids.

Amitryptyline Amitryptyline is the main representative of the tricyclic anti-depressant family, and more is known about its properties in relation to pain than for any other antidepressant. Most patients can be started at a dose of 10–25 mg, usually given as a single dose at night, this being increased by 25 mg per 24 hours every 3–5 days. In some cases, a dosage as high as 160 mg daily is used.

The dose required to relieve neuropathic pain must be titrated for each patient, the increments and maximum dose being highly dependent on the adverse effects, which are the main disadvantage of all antidepressants. They are seen especially in the elderly, with mental dulling, ataxia and serious falls. Dry mouth and constipation may be particularly troublesome. These effects may be insidious and require frequent and thoughtful monitoring.

If the adverse effects become intolerable or dangerous, consider using an antidepressant with fewer side-effects, such as imipramine or lofepramine, the latter being especially good when postural hypotension or ataxia is a problem. Lofepramine and imipramine are the first choice before amitryptyline in some centres. Only one antidepressant should be used at a time, and known drug interactions should be checked in the current edition of the *British National Formulary* before starting antidepressants. There is a suggestion that antidepressants may reduce the effect of antiepileptics.

All the tricyclic antidepressants may be of value in reducing neuropathic pain, those with the most adverse effects, such as amitryptyline, probably providing the best pain relief. Similarly, each antidepressant may have its own advantages and disadvantages, which vary between patients, so the antidepressant should be carefully selected for each individual.

Citalopram, fluxatine and paroxetine These drugs are among the newer SSRIs and are also being tried in neuropathic pain, but it is not yet known how effective these new antidepressants will be in this situation. There is no absolute advice that can be given on doses as our present knowledge is limited, but pain relief will probably be achieved at the lower end of the range of therapeutic doses recommended for depression. The adverse effects of these drugs, albeit fewer than with the older tricyclics, should not be overlooked.

Mitazapiz Mitazapiz is a member of another class of antidepressants, the norepinephrine and selective serotonin antidepressants. It may have considerably fewer side-effects than amitryptline and help equally with neuropathic pain. It is however, about 15 times more expensive than amitryptline and more evidence is needed to assess its role in neuropathic cancer pain.

If antidepressants do not help neuropathic pain within 3–4 weeks, some centres advocate that an antiepileptic such as sodium valproate or carbamazepine should be added. This approach is, however, contentious because it is suggested that antidepressants may lower the effect of antiepileptics. Alternatively, the antidepressant can be stopped and substituted with an antiepileptic. If antidepressants are used for more than about 8 weeks, suddenly stopping them may cause withdrawal symptoms so there is a general recommendation that they should be reduced slowly over a few weeks.

Antiepileptics
Antiepileptics are sometimes the first choice for neuropathic pain, for example when there is sudden cutting, lancinating or sharp, stabbing pain. They may act on the damaged neurones and prevent them from overactivity, slowing down or inhibiting certain nervous transmission.

All antiepileptics have complex interactions with other drugs, and any addition to the patient's medication should always be checked for known interaction in the current edition of the *British National Formulary*. There are further complex interactions between the antiepileptics themselves so a general rule is to use only one class of this drug at a time.

Sodium valproate Sodium valproate (as tablets, MR tablets, syrup, liquid and intravenous injection) is probably the first choice of antiepileptic for neuropathic pain. As one of the common side-effects when starting antiepileptics is sedation, it should be used as a single dose at night, starting with 200 mg and increasing this each week by about 200 mg. A reduction in pain should be noted when the daily dose is between 500 mg and 800 mg, although a response may be noted at a much lower dosage.

Sodium valproate may affect urinary testing in diabetics, giving false-positive results, and may potentiate the effects of many antipsychotics, including haloperidol, levomepromazine (methotrimeprazine) and prochlorperazine, which are all commonly used in palliative medicine. The effect of sodium valproate may be decreased if the patient is taking aspirin, and it is ideally avoided if there is hepatic dysfunction; the dose should be lowered when there is renal insufficiency. Sedation may be a problem in some patients, but many patients conversely feel more alert taking sodium valproate and may become slightly hyperactive with an increased appetite.

Carbamazepine This drug (as tablets, MR tablets, liquid or suppositories) is effective for neuropathic pain, although the individual dose requirement varies considerably. It should be built up from about 100 mg taken as a single dose at night, a further 100 mg taken in the morning being added after a week. The daily dose can be increased every 2 weeks by 100–200 mg, and some response should be obtained before the daily dose is 100 mg. For many patients, a dose of about 200 mg two or three times a day helps their neuropathic pain. If carbamazepine suppositories are used, the total dose should be about 25 per cent above the oral dose.

This drug should be used with extreme caution if there is bone marrow depression or cardiac conduction abnormalities, and all patients should be monitored for anaemia and the clinical signs of leucopenia and resulting infection. Liver function tests, particularly the gamma glutanyl transpeptidase level, can appear abnormal when taking carbamazepine, but the drug does not need to be stopped.

Many drugs can potentiate the effect of carbamazepine, including co-proxamol and erythromycin, and it decreases the clinical effects of drugs such as haloperidol, tramadol, tricyclic antidepressants and corticosteroids.

Gabapentin Gabapentin (as capsules) is of recent introduction and was first used as an 'add-on' drug to another antiepileptic when certain epileptic seizures could not be controlled. Relatively little is known about the optimum level or dose increment when used for neuropathic pain, and there is much discrepancy in the proposed level. Some studies suggest that doses as high as 3600 mg a day may be required, starting at 600 mg and increasing by about 400 mg each day in divided doses twice or three times daily. It should, however, be stressed that these levels are above the recommended levels for its use as an antiepileptic, and that some patients have experienced severe adverse effects, including disorientation, when given only 100 mg gabapentin. A more cautious approach is to start with 100 mg twice daily, increasing this every 5–6 days by the same amount until relief is obtained.

Gabapentin may have a strong synergistic action with opioids such as oxycodone but not with morphine. Caution is required in patients with poor renal function. Withdrawl symptoms have been noted with an abrupt decrease or cessation of the drug. The common side-effects include headaches, drowsiness, dizziness and weight gain. Gabapentin is not a first-choice antiepileptic for pain as it is a relatively expensive drug, being approximately 10 times dearer than sodium valproate, which, together with carbamazepine, is the first choice.

Biphosphonates

Bisphosphonates are calcium-regulating hormones and, like calcitonin, which has been used for pain relief, inhibit bone resorption. They are used to treat hypercalcaemia and bone pain caused by osteolytic bone metastases.

Disodium pamidronate, 60–90 mg, is given by intravenous infusion in 500 ml saline over 1–2 hours, although some centres choose a slower infusion rate. It is essential that the patient is well hydrated at the time of infusion; if there is any doubt, the patient must first be hydrated with intravenous fluids. The pamidronate infusion may be repeated every 2–3 weeks according to the bone pain symptoms, and there is often a reported reduction in pain within a week of the infusion.

Some centres use a maintainence dose of an oral bisphosphonate, such as sodium clodronate. This is usually 1.6 g daily, but it may sometimes be increased to 3 g in tablet form to reduce bone pain and prevent hypercalcaemia. Food should be avoided for 1 hour both before and after taking these tablets.

Nitrous oxide and oxygen

The combination of nitrous oxide and oxygen, often referred to as Entonox or Equanox, involves a mixture of equal volumes of the two gases and has long been used in emergency ambulances and obstetric practice to provide quick analgesia. The gas is inhaled through a demand valve, but many very ill and frail patients find this difficult to use. Entonox is useful for short painful procedures, such stitching skin lacerations. It works within a few minutes but is not intended to provide analgesia for more than several minutes.

Ketamine

Ketamine is principally used as an intravenous anaesthetic and, over the past decade, has occasionally been used for neuropathic pain and pain unresponsive to opioids. It blocks the NMDA receptor sites, which are part of an important pain channel.

Ketamine is also used where there is extreme pain such as may result from intestinal perforation or arterial embolus. The dose used for such situations is between 20 mg and 100 mg, depending on body weight, and is given by either intravenous or intramuscular injection. It should not be used when there is the possibility of increased intercranial pressure or fits, and it should be used with caution in cardiac illness and hypertension. Because ketamine may cause restlesness and agitation, it is sometimes given with a small dose of midazolam or other benzodiazepine to counteract this tendency. It can also be given by continuous subcutaneous infusion at a dose of between 100 mg and 500 mg per 24 hours, but because it is an irritant, it should be diluted with the largest practical volume of sodium chloride 0.9 per cent to fit a syringe driver.

Ketamine is not a first-line analgesic. Relatively little is known about the drug and its adverse effects, which include cardiological and severe behavioural changes, some of the latter include disturbing nightmares and hallucinations.

The Ketamine injection formulation has more recently been used to provide a solution for oral adminstration. As the drug is not licenced for this use, it is available on a named patient basis only. To obtain supplies of ketamine in the community for oral adminstration, the patient's general practitioner needs to contact the community pharmacist and the manufacturer to initiate the necessary paperwork. The injection of ketamine is diluted in a ratio of 50 mg ketamine to 5 ml purified water. The starting dose is about 25 mg three times a day, being increased every few days by 10 mg with each dose. The maximum reported dose is about 800 mg in 24 hours, but most patients gain pain relief at a level of about 300–500 mg daily. Because the solution has an unpleasant taste, it needs to be masked with a suitable flavour, such as a fruit juice.

Cannabinoids

Cannabinoids are extracted from the cannabis plant. They were used many years ago by the French army to relieve pain from surgery in battle, being known in recent times more as potent antiemetics, and being used for dyspnoea and some of the problems associated with neurological illnesses. Most of the claims relating to cannabis have been anecdotal as its general use has been illicit. One study on the use of certain cannaboid extracts given orally suggests that it had an analgesic effect similar to about 60 mg codeine but that higher doses caused severe adverse effects. The complex chemical structure of cannabis provides a substance with many effects, including hallucinatory, which makes it difficult to identify its real analgesic properties.

OPIOID SUBSTITUTION AND ROTATION

If an opioid causes unacceptable adverse effects, especially when this results from increasing the dose to counteract increasing pain, or if the opioid has been used for some time and there is no apparent benefit from increasing the dose, it is often appropriate to change or substitute that opioid for another. This substitution may be repeated if the second opioid gives rise to similar problems. The continuation of this sequence is often refered to as opioid rotation. Hydromorphone was introduced with this idea in mind as a substitute for morphine sulphate.

SUBCUTANEOUS INFUSION AND SYRINGE DRIVERS

The subcutaneous route for the administration of medication using syringe drivers has become widely used over the past decade. Continuous infusion removes the need for frequent injections and provides a way of maintaining a stable blood level of a drug.

ADVANTAGES

The indications for using the continuous subcutaneous infusion route include the following:

- a patient who is too ill or frail to take medication by mouth;
- intractable vomiting;
- dysphagia and swallowing difficulties;
- gastrointestinal obstruction or other pathology preventing the absorption of oral medication;
- a psychological reluctance to take oral medication.

This method provides a resonable assurance that the drug is being absorbed and that a stable plasma level is maintained.

DISADVANTAGES

This method is frequently used in the comatose and dying patient, and many view its use as being a precursor to a terminal phase. Furthermore, there has been adverse comment in the press suggesting that this method may be a means of accelerating death. If it is necessary to use a syringe driver, the matter should be discussed with and explained to both the patient and the relatives.

One practical difficulty of subcutaneous infusion is that it is necessary to determine the patient's drug requirements for the next 24 hours. There must also be a good understanding of the drugs that can be administered using this method.

SYRINGE DRIVERS

The medication is delivered by the syringe driver, which is a small, battery-powered pump. This holds the syringe, the mechanism moving the plunger of the syringe at a set rate in order to deliver the medication via a fine-gauge infusion line and cannula that is sited in the subcutaneous tissue. There are different makes of syringe driver, and professionals should be particularly aware of the make and model they are using for a particular patient: serious errors have been made when professionals have confused models. The two models most commonly encountered are:

1 The Graseby M16A, recognized by its blue front panel and being calibrated for drug delivery in millimeters per hour;
2 The Graseby MS26, which has a green front panel and is calibrated for drug delivery in millimeters per 24 hours. This is the model that is most widely used in palliative care.

The delivery rate of each model is adjustable; the length of the syringe barrel is measured in millimeters and divided by the total time in hours over which drug delivery is required. Each driver is supplied with detailed instructions, and the manufacturers provide tuition and educational material. Professionals should receive proper instruction before using syringe drivers.

In the first preparation of the syringe driver, an allowance should be made for the solution to fill the dead space of the infusion connecting line and cannulae.

SUITABILITY OF DRUGS FOR THE SYRINGE DRIVER

There are a number of general recommendations relating to the drugs that may be infused by this method.

- Drugs with an acidic pH should generally be avoided as these may cause pain and irritation at the site of the cannula.
- It is preferable to keep the number of drugs in a single syringe to two as the more drugs that are used together in a syringe, the more likely adverse reactions are to occur.
- Temperature may affect the stability of drugs so the syringe driver should not be kept in a warm place, for example under the pillow.
- The syringe driver should be protected from excessive light as this may affect drug stability.
- The contents of the syringe driver should, where possible, be replaced each 24 hours, especially if antiemetics are contained in the solution.

The most suitable analgesics for delivery in this way are diamorphine and hydromorphone because of their good solubility. The maximum recommended dose of diamorphine is probably in the region of 250 mg/ml, although higher concentrations are frequently used; these may, however, cause increased skin induration and require more frequent changes of site of the cannula.

The compatibility of drugs within the same syringe is important as it may affect the stability of the drugs and cause skin irritation. Compatibility depends on a number of complex factors, including the pH and concentration of each drug, the length of time and the temperature at which the drugs are together in the syringe, and the diluent. It is unfortunately not possible to provide absolute guidelines regarding compatibility because of the many variables. Furthermore, a number of drugs may be used by this route but are not licensed for such use. To confirm the compatability of drugs, the local palliative care unit or hospital pharmacy should be contacted.

The following drugs, in injection form, are usually compatible with diamorphine and hydromorphone: fentanyl, glycopyrrolate, haloperidol, hyoscine butylbromide, hyoscine hydrobromide, ketamine, levomepromazine (methotrimeprazine), and midazolam.

Caution is advocated in using the following with other drugs: metoclopramide and cyclizine (at high doses), ketrolac, and octreotide (at high doses).

Diclofenac and dexamethasone should not be mixed with other drugs and should be delivered via a separate syringe.

As a general rule, water for injection is the standard diluent, but saline for injection 0.9 per cent is recommended for ketamine, ketorolac, octreotide and diclofenac.

Once a solution has been prepared, it should be examined in a good light to determine whether there is any cloudiness, precipation, change in colour or crystallization. This will give a crude idea of incompatability, and such a syringe and contents should be discarded.

The syringe driver is provided with a boost button, which the patient may wish to use for breakthrough pain, although to encourage the patient to use this may promote problems. Each boost will cause a shortening of the 24 hour infusion time by about 7–10 minutes, and indiscriminate use may result in confusion regarding the timing of renewal of the syringe. Furthermore, this may confuse the actual situation regarding breakthrough pain unless records are kept.

PROBLEMS WITH SUBCUTANEOUS INFUSION

Some patients may suffer repeated irritation or induration at the site of the cannula. In such cases, consider the following:

- Insert the cannula more deeply towards an intermuscular level instead of at the normal subcutaneous level.
- Use the flexor, or inner, aspect of the arm to site the cannula as this allows an easier flow of any drug; the cannula is usually sited on the extensor or outer surface of the arm.
- Dilute the drug with a large volume of diluent, which will require using a 20 ml instead of the usual 10 ml syringe.
- Consider, where appropriate, a trial of saline for injection 0.9 per cent instead of water as the diluent.
- Use a teflon (plastic) cannula instead of the metal cannula that is found with butterfly-type cannulae.
- Consider adding either hyaluronidase (1500 units) or a corticosteroid (e.g.hydrocortisone 100 mg) to each syringe of the infusion. This should delay or reduce an inflammatory response at the site of the cannula.
- Review the drugs that are in the infusion mixture to ensure that there are no known allergic or other adverse reactions.

ROUTES OF DRUG ADMINSTRATION

Taking a drug by mouth remains the first choice route. Probably more is known about the characteristics of a drug taken orally than via any other route, and

Table 1.3 Drug delivery with difficulty of swallowing

	Delivery system
Normal swallowing	Tablets, capsules
Mild swallowing difficulties or other problems	Liquids, solutions, suspensions, 'sprinkling'
Serious swallowing difficulties	Suppositories and pessaries – rectal or vaginal, Buccal absorption, transdermal delivery systems, injections – subcutaneous, intravenous, intramuscular, continuous infusion

this route is simple and acceptable to most patients. In addition, the cost is significantly lower than the more in-vogue routes.

There are certain situations in which an alternative to the oral route becomes necessary. Examples are where there are swallowing problems, pain or obstruction caused by tumour, muscle incoordination on swallowing, as seen with certain neurological states, or intractable vomiting. The choice of routes and delivery systems in relation to swallowing difficulties is shown in Table 1.3.

It is often necessary to devise methods of administration that are unlicensed or 'unofficial', for example taking out the matrix containing the drug and mixing this with, or sprinkling it on, jam, yoghurt or a similar acceptable food. Such methods have also been used to wash down a drug into a nasogastric, polyethylene glycor or other feeding tube. Soft coated tablets have been used per rectum, or per vaginum, although the absorption via these routes is sometimes erratic. The use of suppositories has not been popular in the UK, but these should be considered if this route is acceptable to the patient. Morphine and other analgesics are now available again in this form. The use of the continuous subcutaneous route and syringe driver is considered below.

NERVE BLOCKS

Nerve blocks are an important adjunct to pain control, particularly when the usual pharmacological means do not relieve pain. They range from the relatively simple infiltration of intercostal nerves when the pain is caused by a rib fracture to complex regional blocks in cases of pancreatic carcinoma.

A trial of a local anaesthetic injected into or around the nerve is usually first carried out in order to assess the response, and if this provides some relief, a semi-permanent block is effected by using a long-acting anaesthetic agent such as bupivacaine together with a steroid. More permanent ablation may be carried out using a chemical agent such as phenol, cryotherapy or surgical section.

The most frequent nerve blocks used in palliative medicine include:

- coeliac plexus blockade, which often provides excellent relief from pancreatic and hepatic pain;
- brachial plexus blockade for axillary involvement, often the result of carcinoma of the breast;
- dorsal root ganglion blockade for back pain, which may result from mechanical changes as a result of bone metastases;
- lumbar sympathectomy for pain associated with pelvic tumours.

SPINAL ANALGESIA

When opioids, adjuvant drugs, radiotherapy and other interventions have been tried and there is no relief from the pain, especially when the pain involves the lower half of the body, spinal analgesia may be appropriate, this being provided via the epidural or intrathecal route. The choice of route will depend largely on the opinion of an anaesthetist with a special interest in pain.

The intrathecal route requires approximately one-tenth the dose of opioid that would be required using the epidural route, which in turn requires one-tenth of the dose injected via the subcutaneous route. This means that lower doses of drugs are required with the spinal route, resulting in fewer adverse effects. The analgesic drug is best provided using a continuous infusion with a boost facility, the pumps used being more precise than those used for subcutaneous infusions. If opioids are being given via other routes, their doses should be reduced in steps as the spinal route analgesia starts to be effective. There must be a monitoring of the motor and sensory systems of the lower legs in case an excess amount of drug is being given, in which case the strength or rate of drug delivery should be reduced.

Spinal anaesthesia is not without problems, including hypotension, pruritis and sensory loss. Morphine or diamorphine, together with bupivacaine, is the drug most frequently used for spinal anaesthesia. There are maintenance problems with spinal anaesthesia, one of the most common being catheter displacement, but the incidence of this can be reduced using various methods of securing the catheter. Less common is infection, and there are also occasional leaks of cerebrospinal fluid from the portal used for entry of the catheter.

Spinal blocks are overall, very useful for drug delivery, especially when large doses of opioids given via other routes cause intolerable adverse effects. This is sometimes the only way of providing satisfactory pain relief. Skilled staff are however, required to carry out these procedures and to supervise their maintenance, and the technique is costly in economic terms.

NON-PHARMACOLOGICAL APPROACHES TO THE MANAGEMENT OF PAIN

Many non-drug treatments are available for pain, some of which are used for cancer pain (see Ch. 10). These extend from simple and traditional treatments to the magnets and complex electrical devices advertised in the daily newspapers, but there are no definitive studies to evaluate many of these approaches. Some may work by distraction therapy, others as counter-irritants or by providing a placebo response, as is found with some drugs. Their mechanism of action is not understood, but some may work within the model of the gate theory of pain (see below). Many, but not all, patients do obtain pain relief from these interventions, but it is usually not possible to identify who will obtain help.

The demand for non-pharmacological alternatives for pain relief is increasing. There are many possible reasons for this, but a consistent finding is that the practitioners of complementary medicine are often able to give more time to patients, which encourages both empathy and communication.

ACUPUNCTURE

Needles are inserted through the skin at specific body sites in line with traditional treatment methods. These needles are twirled rapidly, or a low-strength electrical current is applied through them to provide a stimulus. This stimulus is thought to stimulate endorphins, which are the natural opioids produced within the brain, which in turn provides analgesia. The mechanics of how this may work are not understood, but it does provide some, but not all, patients with pain relief, especially from nerve, bone and soft tissue pain. When it helps the pain associated with malignant conditions, the effects are usually much shorter acting than those seen in non-malignant pain.

MASSAGE AND AROMATHERAPY

Massage has long been used to sooth inflammation and local pain. It may relax contracted or tense soft tissue such as muscle by generating mild heat and encouraging an increased local lymphatic flow. Aromatherapy, which involves the use of essential oils extracted from plants, has recently come into a renewed vogue. Many patients benefit from the soporific feeling induced by massage, which may in turn cause a feeling of total relaxation and well-being. In many patients, this reduces the overall dimensions of pain.

HEAT AND COLD

There is no strict rule on whether heat or cold should be applied to an area of local pain. In general terms, cold is often used for an acute, sudden-onset pain, as seen with a muscle cramp, and heat for more chronic pain. Cold is applied by ice packs or refrigerant spray, which cools by evaporation and works fairly quickly. Heat increases the local blood flow and often relaxes soft tissue such as muscle. It may be applied either superficially from infrared heat lamps, or deeply by the use of heat packs that may be warmed in microwave ovens, and by the simple but effective hot-water bottle or its modern equivalent. Warmth also relieves the pain associated with acute colic.

TRANSCUTANEOUS ELECTRICAL NERVE STIMULATION

This concept uses an electrical device that provides a low-strength current at low-frequency oscillations, this being transmitted through two electrodes applied to the skin. There is a complex relationship between the stimulation produced by the TENS machine and certain nerve fibres, TENS probably working within the gate theory of pain (see above).

TENS causes a tingling sensation and may allieviate pain, especially that arising from musculoskeletal problems and even bone secondaries. It is often necessary to try different sites for the electrodes and different settings of the TENS machine to fully exploit its potential. The technique probably helps three-quarters of chronic pain sufferers when first used, but with continual use, the number obtaining any relief is considerably reduced. It should not be used on patients with a pacemaker or serious cardiac condition.

COUNTER-IRRITANTS

Rubefacients, which are chemical substances that irritate and in turn warm the skin by increasing its blood flow, for example capsium-containing creams, have been used for centuries to relieve local pain. They have a place in controlling pain in those cancer patients experiencing muscle, tendon and joint pain, and if neuropathic pain involves the skin.

PSYCHOLOGICAL CONSIDERATIONS

The cause of most pain in cases of advanced cancer can be understood, but there are cases in which the causes and associations of the pain may be difficult or even impossible to understand. One must be scrupulous before labelling a pain as being psychological in origin because to do this may preclude a reasoned and careful assessment and prevent effective treatment. There are particular problems in patients who have two or more pains, one clearly being related to a physical cause but the other having no apparent cause on repeated assessment. Whatever the conclusion, such patients may actually be experiencing pain even though the cause may remain uncertain. Anaglesics can be used to treat psychophysiological pain but are ineffective if used alone.

In many cases in which a psychological or emotional element, as distinct from a physical or sensory element, is the main contributor to the pain, cognitive techniques of pain control should be introduced. The more basic of these include relaxation, distraction therapy and hypnosis. Examples of relaxation include organized fantasies to evoke calm, for example thinking one is lying on a beach with pleasant sounds around. Distraction could take the form of painting, jigsaws or occupational therapy. Hypnosis works to reduce pain in some but not all patients, but it usually requires repetition at frequent intervals. A small group of patients can be helped by self-hypnosis, but this requires tuition.

THE IMPORTANCE OF THE CARER

Well-meaning carers may express an overconcern about pain, conversation that is intended to be supportive unintentionally reinforcing the importance and perception of the pain. Carers should not make overfrequent enquiry into or exaggerated reference to pain, or centre all the well-being of the patient on the pain. If patients discover that they only receive time and empathy from nurses or doctors when they complain about pain, it is no surprise that pain becomes the fulcrum of patient–carer relationships. It is easier to ask about pain than to ask a patient how she feels about her family not wanting her home. A carer can shift the pain threshold by providing encouragment and empathic strength to the patient so that pain assumes a different importance in the patient's life. Both professional and volunteer carers have an important role in this area, and their aim should be to help the patient rather than make the patient dependent on, or magnify, any symptom.

CONCLUSION

It was not until the 20th century was well advanced that the welfare of the chronic cancer patient began to improve. A mere 30 years ago, millions of patients throughout the world suffered unalleviated cancer pain, many tragically dying in pain. Now, however, research and education have largely removed the myths surrounding morphine treatment as well as the belief that cancer pain is inevitable and uncontrollable. Experience has replaced ignorance, and a choice of treatments is now available. This chapter covers the wide range of pharmacological and non-pharmacological approaches available for the relief of pain; no patient should now have to suffer needlessly.

FURTHER READING

Davis, B.D. 2000: *Caring for people in pain*. London: Routledge.
Doyle, D., Hanks, G.W.C. and MacDonald, N. (eds) 1998: *Oxford textbook of palliative medicine*. Oxford: Oxford Medical Publications.
Regnard, C. and Tempest, S. 1998: *A guide to symptom relief in abdominal disease*, 4th edn. Manchester: Haigh & Hochland.
Twycross, R. 1997: *Symptom management in advanced cancer*, 2nd edn. Oxford: Radcliffe Medical Press.
Wall, P. 1999: *Pain: the science of suffering*. London: Orion.

chapter 2

OTHER SIGNIFICANT SYMPTOMS

Susanna R. Hill

You cannot prevent the birds of sorrow flying overhead;
but you can prevent them building nests in your hair!

Chinese proverb

Pivotal in the development of palliative medicine as a speciality has been the emphasis on holistic care for both patients facing a terminal illness and their families. Central to this concept is the control of the various physical symptoms presented by these patients. If palliative medicine is to be carried out effectively, the health-care team involved in patient care must have a clear understanding of the symptoms the patient displays. This includes a knowledge of their possible causes and treatments, looking at the physical, social, psychological and spiritual dimensions, as well as the ability to recognize when more specialized help is needed. There should be a personalized management plan that maximizes the patient-determined quality of life, and family-orientated care that extends through the time of bereavement (Billings, 2000).

Despite the variety of primary diagnoses, many of the symptoms encountered (Table 2.1) are common to these patients and can be managed in a similar way. This chapter discusses the symptoms most commonly presented by patients with progressive incurable illness (excluding pain, breathlessness, terminal restlessness and oedema, which are covered in other chapters), considering the causes, diagnosis and treatment options.

Certain common principles apply to the management of all symptoms, and it is helpful to look at these before examining specific examples.

COMMON PRINCIPLES OF SYMPTOM CONTROL

An attention to detail, especially during history-taking, is vital if one is trying to establish why a patient is having a particular problem (Table 2.2). It is helpful to list, with patients, their current symptoms, asking them to prioritize the severity of these. Many doctors might, for example, consider pain to be the

Table 2.1 Prevalence of common symptoms in patients with advanced cancer (Donnelly and Walsh, 1995)

	Percentage of patients
Pain	82
Nausea and vomiting	59
Dyspnoea	51
Constipation	51
Weakness	64
Anorexia	64
Depression	40
Confusion	20

worst problem for a patient, but if asked, the patient may be more concerned about constipation.

Once a priority list has been established, a careful history of each symptom should be taken – when did it start, what precipitates it, what helps to relieve it, is it present all the time or only intermittently? The patient should then be carefully examined.

Using all this information, it should in most cases be possible to form a hypothesis about the cause of the symptom. It is helpful to consider symptoms in terms of

Table 2.2 Outline of symptom management

- List the symptoms

- Establish priorities with the patient

- Take a careful history

- Examine the patient

- Postulate the diagnosis – caused by illness, past or present treatment, or concurrent illness

- Investigate if appropriate – balance benefit versus patient cost

- Diagnosis

- Align with the patients – what do they understand about the symptoms, what are their fears, etc.? Speak 'on the same level' without using medical jargon

- Discuss the treatment options, individualizing care

- Continually evaluate the situation

whether they are caused by the illness, by past or present treatment, or by concurrent illness. Investigations are then used either to test the hypothesis, a blood test to show hypercalcaemia for example, or to differentiate between possible causes, for example an X ray may show whether a patient has constipation or bowel obstruction.

Investigations are often not needed and in any case should be kept to a minimum, the potential benefits being carefully weighed against the cost to the patient.

Once a diagnosis has been reached, it should be discussed with the patient. The first step should always be to explore patients' knowledge of, and ideas, concerns and expectations about, their symptoms. They may have specific fears about the possible underlying causes, which may be an idea totally different from that of the doctor. These differences need to be addressed and understood at the outset or patients will not understand or be able to participate in further discussions. Thus, 'the doctor must line up the information he or she wishes to impart on the baseline of the patient's knowledge' (Buckman, 1992). The clinician then needs to explain clearly and simply, without using medical jargon, what the cause of the problem is believed to be and what treatment is being proposed. It is important to remember that treatments should always be individualized and that what seems appropriate for one patient, for example, morphine instead of acupuncture for pain relief, may be totally wrong for another. Deciding on the correct treatment for each patient, whatever its modality, is vital to the practice of effective holistic medicine.

The goals of treatment need to be discussed and should include a realistic examination of what can potentially be achieved. It may sometimes be necessary to agree a compromise between the benefits and the side-effects: some patients may be prepared to accept that they will still vomit once a day on their dose of medication to control nausea, rather than suffer more drowsiness with an increased dose of an antiemetic such as levomepromazine. Honesty in terms of what can potentially be achieved is important, but it is also vital to maintain a 'hook of hope'. The knowledge that someone cares and is trying to improve a symptom helps to sustain many patients even if the attempts are not always completely successful.

Situations change rapidly for patients, particularly in the terminal phase of their illness, so a regular evaluation of problems and flexibility of approach are vital. Treatment often needs changing from hour to hour. The clinical picture is always complex in these patients. Individual elements must be teased out in order to target treatments for rapid symptom control, and attention to detail is imperative.

The ability to listen and communicate effectively with patients, their families and other health-care professionals is fundamental to effective symptom control. There is increasing evidence that these 'bedside manners' (communication and psychosocial skills) of terminal care can be taught (Baile et al., 1999). Health-care professionals need to work as a team, each member bringing his or her own individual skills, so that patients and their families can receive maximum benefit.

IMPORTANT SYMPTOMS

NAUSEA AND VOMITING

The commonly encountered symptoms of nausea and vomiting affecting 40–70 per cent of patients (Turycross and Back, 1998), can be very distressing and may be difficult to control completely. The sensation of nausea, which is accompanied by autonomic symptoms such as cold sweats, pallor, salivation, tachycardia and diarrhoea, is often more unpleasant than actually vomiting and is frequently underreported by patients.

There are many causes of nausea and vomiting, and although some relate to the gastrointestinal tract, many are concerned with systemic disorders or external stimuli. Careful history-taking (Table 2.3) may point clearly to a cause. The patient who starts to feel nausea and vomits as soon as he starts strong opioid analgesia such as morphine, is, for example, likely to be reacting to the drug. The causes can be divided according to which area of the brain they stimulate to set off the efferent pathways that bring about nausea and vomiting (Table 2.4). It should in most cases be possible to formulate a potential cause for the nausea and vomiting from the patient's history and examination, and from clinical probability. This hypothesis may then be verified by investigation, for example a blood test to demonstrate hypercalcaemia or uraemia, or gastroscopy to confirm a peptic ulcer, although further investigation is in many cases not needed.

Once a diagnosis has been reached, the most appropriate treatment should be initiated. Simple 'non-drug' measures such as the avoidance of food smells or unpleasant odours, diversion, relaxation and acupuncture or acupressure may make a considerable difference to the symptoms. Specific treatments can be given for certain problems, for example antacids for gastritis, an H_2-receptor blocker

Table 2.3 Features to examine in history of patient with nausea and vomiting (Finlay, 1995)

- Concomitant nausea

- Nature of vomit

- Volume of vomit

- Timing of vomit

- Abdominal distension

- Constipation

- Urinary symptoms

- Headache on waking

- Dyspepsia

Table 2.4 Causes of nausea and vomiting

		Causes
Gastrointestinal		
	Upper	Sore tongue
		Candidal infection
		Difficulty expectorating
		Oesophagitis
		Carcinoma of the oesophagus
	Mid	Peptic ulcer
		Gastritis, e.g. steroids, non-steroidal anti-inflammatory agents
		Squashed stomach syndrome
		Carcinoma of the stomach
		Carcinoma of the pancreas
		Gall bladder disease
		Bowel obstruction
	Lower	Constipation
		Bowel obstruction
	Hepatic disease	
Chemical		Drugs, e.g. opioids, digoxin, antibiotics
		Biochemical, e.g. uraemia, hypercalcaemia
		Treatments: radiotherapy, chemotherapy
		Tumour toxins
		Infection
Cerebral		Anxiety
		Taste, smell
		Cerebral tumour
		Raised intracranial pressure
Vestibular		Vertigo
		Motion
		Acoustic neuroma

or proton pump inhibitor for peptic ulceration, or a bisphosphonate infusion for hypercalcaemia. Many patients however, have multiple, irreversible causes for their nausea and vomiting, and it is then important to find an effective antiemetic treatment. The form of this treatment – tablets, liquid, injection or via a syringe driver – must also be decided on according to the condition of the patient.

Vomiting is co-ordinated via two areas in the hindbrain – the chemoreceptor trigger zone, which lies outside the blood–brain barrier, and the vomiting centre or 'central pattern generator for emesis' (Figure 2.1). These two centres are linked by neural pathways. Afferent pathways carry stimuli to the centres from specific

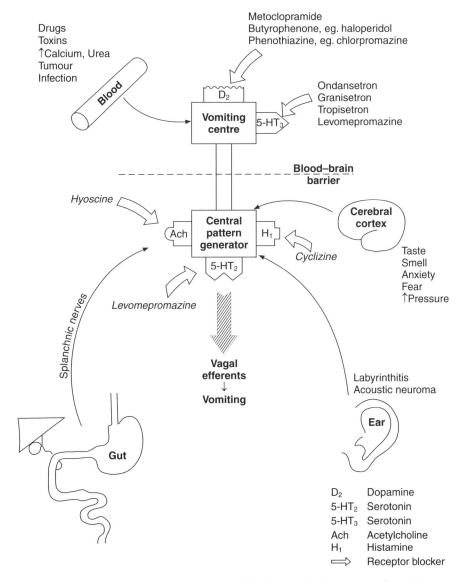

Figure 2.1 Central pathways, receptors and receptor blockers involved in nausea and vomiting

receptor sites. This triggers a complex series of reactions, which eventually stimulate efferent pathways and result in vomiting. Blocking the receptor sites therefore interrupts the incoming signals and prevents nausea and vomiting, which is how antiemetics work centrally.

As the chemoreceptor trigger zone lies outside the blood–brain barrier, chemicals in the systemic circulation, that is, drugs and toxins, as well as biochemical disturbances, act on this site. The main receptors here are for dopamine and serotonin, D_2 and $5-HT_3$ receptors respectively. Gastrointestinal impulses via the splanchnic nerves, vestibular impulses and cerebral impulses act on the

Table 2.5 Receptors and their main blocking agents

	Blocking agents
D_2	Phenothiazines, e.g. chlorpromazine, prochlorperazine, levomepromazine
	Butyrophenones, e.g. haloperidol
	Metoclopramide
	Domperidone (does not cross blood–brain barrier so there are no extrapyramidal effects)
$5\text{-}HT_3$	Ondansetron, granisetron, tropisetron
	Levomepromazine
	Metoclopramide (weak)
H_1	Cyclizine
	Levomepromazine (weak)
$5\text{-}HT_2$	Levomepromazine
Ach	Hyoscine
	Cyclizine (weak)
	Levomepromazine (weak)

vomiting centre. The main receptor sites here are histamine (H_1) and serotonin ($5\text{-}HT_2$), as well as cholinergic-muscarinic (Ach) receptors. Antiemetic drugs usually act predominantly on one type of receptor but may have weaker actions at other receptor sites (Table 2.5).

Peripherally, drugs are used to affect gastric motility and the secretion of fluids (Figure 2.2). Agents affecting motility, such as metoclopramide and domperidone, act on dopaminergic receptors in the proximal gastrointestinal tract. Stress, anxiety and nausea arising from any cause induce delayed gastric emptying via peripheral dopaminergic receptors, and these drugs therefore block this effect.

Ondansetron, granisetron and tropisetron act centrally but also work peripherally on $5\text{-}HT_3$ receptors in the gastrointestinal tract, which sensitize vagal afferents. Various stimuli, such as abdominal radiotherapy, chemotherapy and abdominal distension, cause the release of serotonin from enterochromaffin cells in the gut wall. These drugs thus block the emetogenic effect of these stimuli.

Octreotide is a somatostatin agonist that inhibits the secretion of insulin, glucagon, gastrin and other peptides to reduce splanchnic blood flow, portal blood flow, bowel motility and small bowel secretion. It is a useful agent in the management of intestinal obstruction (Twycross and Wilcock, 1998).

Dexamethasone and other corticosteroids are used as adjuvants in the treatment of nausea and vomiting. They may act by reducing the inflammation around tumours and thus reducing pressure symptoms. They probably also have a central effect in reducing the permeability of the blood–brain barrier to emetogenic stimuli and reducing the amount of gamma-amino butyric acid, an inhibitory peptide, in the brainstem.

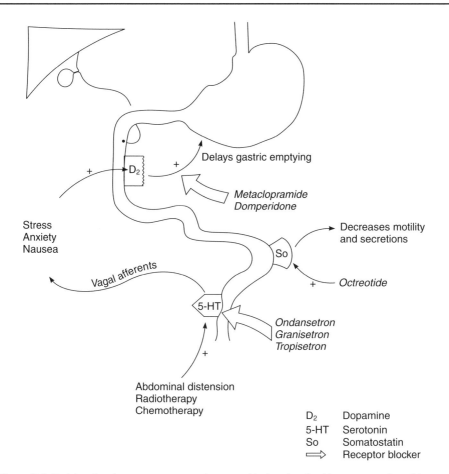

Figure 2.2 Peripheral pathways, receptors and receptor blockers involved in nausea and vomiting

Research continues to investigate the receptors involved in emetic pathways, neurokinin receptors having recently been identified. Antagonists to these are now being developed, which are thought to work both centrally and peripherally, are orally active and appear to be well tolerated (Navari et al., 1999). These will hopefully be the antiemetics of the future.

The situation can be very complex in some patients (Case study 2.1) and it may not be possible to establish a single cause for nausea and vomiting. In these cases, a simple management pathway based on the same concept as the World Health Organization pain ladder can be helpful (Table 2.6).

CONSTIPATION

Over half of all palliative care patients complain of constipation, which is defined as 'straining to pass hard stool'. Many factors contribute to this (Table 2.7): patients are often debilitated, their diet is poor, their food intake is decreased, and they are unable to take regular exercise. Many drugs, especially opioids and tricyclic antidepressants such as amitriptyline, also lead to constipa-

CASE STUDY 2.1

Joan, aged 55, was receiving chemotherapy for disseminated ovarian carcinoma. With each cycle of her chemotherapy, she developed profound nausea and regular vomiting. She was started on *metoclopramide* 10 mg four times daily in an attempt to improve gastric and small bowel motility and block some of the central effects of the chemotherapeutic agents at the 5-HT$_3$ receptors in the vomiting centre. There was only a slight improvement so the dose of *metoclopramide* was doubled to 20 mg four times daily. This did not alter Joan's symptoms and so she was started on *granisetron* 1 mg twice daily, given as a 3-day course after each chemotherapy session, which helped her nausea and most of her vomiting. Joan was then started on morphine slow-release tablets (MST) to help with increasing abdominal and pelvic pain, but her nausea returned almost immediately and became very severe. By this time, her chemotherapy had stopped, and she was started on *metoclopramide* again. This had no effect so the prescription was changed to *haloperidol* 1.5 mg at night, the assumption being that the symptoms were caused by the opiate and that haloperidol would help to counteract this at the chemoreceptor trigger zone.

Joan seemed to improve for a while but then started to develop crampy abdominal pain, intermittent severe constipation and increased nausea and vomiting. A clinical diagnosis of bowel obstruction was made. She was unable to tolerate oral medication because of the continuous vomiting so a syringe driver was set up with *haloperidol* 2.5 mg, *cyclizine* 150 mg and *hyoscine butylbromide* (buscopan) 40 mg in the syringe driver (see 'Intestinal obstruction', below). Fortunately, Joan's morphine had previously been changed to a fentanyl patch; otherwise, she might have required a second syringe driver for diamorphine.

Although this combination of treatments improved Joan's symptoms for several days, these then returned and increased in severity despite an increase in the dosage of haloperidol and hyoscine butylbromide. By now, Joan had entered the terminal phase of her illness, and the cyclizine was changed to *octreotide* 300 mg in the syringe driver. This was increased to 500 µg after 2 days, which kept her symptoms of nausea and vomiting under control for a further 3 days until her death.

Five different antiemetics were therefore used throughout the latter stages of Joan's illness for the same symptom of nausea and vomiting.

tion, as can concurrent medical problems such as hypercalcaemia and hypothyroidism. The complications of constipation include pain, intestinal obstruction, urinary retention or frequency, overflow diarrhoea, faecal incontinence and confusion or restlessness if the condition is severe.

Constipation can usually be diagnosed from a patient's history, although the situation in the patient with severe constipation who then develops 'overflow' diarrhoea (Figure 2.3 and Case study 2.2) can be misleading. An examination of the abdomen and rectum is usually sufficient to confirm the diagnosis, but an abdominal X-ray is occasionally required to help to differentiate between constipation and intestinal obstruction.

When carrying out a rectal examination, it is helpful to ascertain whether the stools are hard and pellet-like, or soft and difficult to expel as this will determine treatment. Hard stools need to be softened, whereas soft stools, which are

Table 2.6 The 'antiemetic ladder'

Step 1	Try a single agent according to the possible cause of nausea and vomiting, e.g. haloperidol, cyclizine or metoclopramide. (If a motility agent is required, domperidone acts as a motility agent at the oesophagogastric and gastroduodenal junctions but does not pass the blood–brain barrier and therefore does not have any central side-effects)
Step 2	If this is partially effective, increase the dose to maximum, optimizing the dose every 24 hours. If it is not effective, ask whether cause has been correctly identified and change the drug to one that will block other afferent stimuli, e.g. change haloperidol to cyclizine
Step 3	If there is no effect, add together two drugs that act on different receptor sites, e.g. haloperidol and cyclizine.* (About one-third of patients require more than one antiemetic for optimal control)
Step 4	If there is no effect, use a less specific antiemetic, e.g. levotrimeprazine, ondansetron, granisetron or tropisetron, or adjuvant drug, e.g. dexamethasone
Step 5	Reassess regularly as the cause of nausea and vomiting can change with time

*Do not use prokinetic drugs, i.e. metoclopramide and domperidone, with cyclizine as they antagonize each other's action.

Table 2.7 Common causes of constipation

	Causes
Patient	Poor diet or low fluid intake
	Lack of exercise
	General debility
	Immobility – paraplegia
	Depression
Gastrointestinal tract	Tumour, causing partial obstruction, stricture, adhesions and decreased motility
Metabolic	Hypercalcaemia
	Hypothyroidism
	Hypokalaemia
Drugs	Opioids
	Tricyclic antidepressants
	Antacids
	Phenothiazines
	Chemotherapy – some types

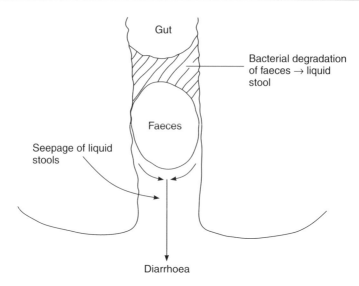

Figure 2.3 Faecal impaction causing diarrhoea

difficult to expel, require a stimulant to move them. The clinical picture is in reality often not so clear cut, patients often requiring both stimulants and softeners to help them to defaecate easily.

CASE STUDY 2.2

Bill was a 72-year-old retired farmer with disseminated prostate cancer. He had had long-standing problems with constipation. His medication was slow-release morphine (MST) 60 mg twice daily, diclofenac 75 mg twice daily and amitriptyline 25 mg once daily for neuropathic pain in his left leg. Bill's constipation became unbearable despite the use of two *senna* tablets at night and *lactulose* suspension 20–30 ml twice daily. The district nurse had attended on several occasions and given him a *phosphate* enema.

The first therapeutic manoeuvre was to change the MST to the less-constipating fentanyl patch 25 μg per hour. Bill's amitriptyline was changed to carbamazepine 200 mg twice daily. This improved his constipation to a tolerable level, and he was able to manage with lactulose, senna and the occasional *glycerine* suppository.

The constipation gradually started to return, and Bill's laxatives were changed to *co-danthramer forte*, two capsules at night (which contains a higher proportion of softener to stimulant than does co-danthramer). Three days later, Bill's wife phoned in a very distressed state saying that he had developed uncontrollable diarrhoea. Rectal examination revealed a hard rectal faecal mass. Diarrhoea resulting from faecal obstruction with overflow was diagnosed. The stools were softened with an *arachis oil enema* and then expelled with a phosphate enema. The amount of co-danthramer forte was then increased to 3–4 capsules daily.

Prior to Bill's death, a further episode of severe constipation was treated with *Movicol*, with good results.

Table 2.8 Types of laxative

	Examples
Softeners: oral	
Osmotic	Lactulose
	Magnesium hydroxide
	Movicol
Fibre	Fybogel
	Tryfyba
Stimulant: oral	Senna
	Bisacodyl
	Danthron
	Picolax
Stimulant: rectal	Glycerine suppositories
	Bisacodyl
	Phosphate enemas
Combinations	
Stimulant + softener	Co-danthramer* (dantron 25 mg + poloxamer 200 mg)
	Co-danthramer forte* (dantron 37.5 mg + poloxamer 500 mg)
	Co-danthrusate (dantron 50 mg + docusate 60 mg)

*1 co-danthramer forte capsule = approximately 3 co-danthramer capsules.

Once a diagnosis has been made, general measures should be proposed, that is, fluids encouraged, dietary fibre increased, mobility encouraged, privacy going to the toilet improved and medication altered if possible.

Laxatives can be divided into stool softeners and stimulants, and can be given both orally and rectally (Table 2.8). Oral measures should generally be attempted first, followed by rectal measures. Movicol should be used for resistant constipation (Ungar, 2000). It is always worth remembering that prevention is better than cure; in the case of opioid use, all patients should thus be started on a laxative as soon as the opioid is being given.

Although the treatment of constipation has not been changed for many years, research is continually trying to improve management. Interest has recently been concentrated on the use of opioid antagonists for the treatment of morphine-induced constipation. Studies so far have been small, but it seems clear that naloxone can counteract the gut-slowing effect of morphine while leaving its analgesic actions intact (Sykes, 1998).

DIARRHOEA

Diarrhoea can be defined as the frequent passage of loose stools and can have numerous causes, including constipation (Table 2.9 and see above). Investi-

Table 2.9 Common causes of diarrhoea

Caused by illness	Colonic tumour or polyp
	Carcinoid tumour
Caused by treatment	Chemotherapy
	Radiotherapy
	Antibiotics
	Non-steroidal anti-inflammatory drugs
Other causes	Infection
	Inflammatory bowel disease
	Diverticulitis
	Autonomic neuropathy
	Constipation. This is 'false' diarrhoea. There is faecal obstruction with bacterial degradation of the faeces proximal to this, producing a liquid that then seeps past the obstruction and causes 'diarrhoea'

gations include monitoring the urea and electrolyte levels to determine the level of hydration and the potassium concentration. Stool culture may be relevant, especially if patients are neutropenic or have received a large amount of antibiotics, which can predispose to *Clostridium difficile* infection.

Treatment includes the removal of any predisposing factors such as drugs, and specific therapies if appropriate, for example erythromycin for *Campylobacter* infection, surgery, radiotherapy and chemotherapy for tumours, and non-steroidal anti-inflammatory drugs for radiation-induced diarrhoea. If the patient is not already taking an opioid, codeine phosphate should be added. If this does not settle the problem, consider using either diphenoxylate or loperamide, which are non-analgesic opioids; loperamide may also have a direct effect on smooth muscle. Lomotil contains atropine as well as diphenoxylate.

If there is a large volume of diarrhoea, as with a fistula causing faecal incontinence, octreotide can be used to decrease fluid secretion, increase fluid absorption and decrease peristalsis.

INTESTINAL OBSTRUCTION

The overall incidence of intestinal obstruction in patients with advanced cancer is about 3 per cent, but certain cancers are associated with a much higher incidence of the condition, for example, ovarian cancer (25–40 per cent) and in any patient with abdominal or pelvic cancer. Obstruction can be mechanical, functional or both (Table 2.10) and may occur in more than one site.

Acute intestinal obstruction classically presents as a sudden-onset colicky abdominal pain, vomiting – the amount depending on the site of the obstruction – and absolute constipation, i.e. passing no faeces or flatus. In the palliative care

Table 2.10 Causes of intestinal obstruction

Caused by tumour	Extrinsic – tumour compression, omental mass
	Intrinsic – enlarging intraluminal tumour
	Functional – motility disorder resulting from tumour infiltration of the mesentery or bowel muscle
Caused by treatment	Adhesion formation post surgery
	Post-irradiation fibrosis
	Drugs, e.g. opioids, anticholinergic drugs and chemotherapeutic agents, particularly vincristine and Taxol
Other causes	Adhesions from previous surgery
	Volvulus
	Constipation/faecal impaction. This may precipitate obstruction if a lesion, particularly in the large bowel, limits the size of the lumen

setting, patients often present in a more insidious fashion, with far less distinct, and often fluctuating, symptoms.

It may be appropriate to investigate a patient with suspected intestinal obstruction with an abdominal X-ray, particularly if surgery is a possibility (Table 2.11). This should confirm the obstruction, indicate its site and differentiate it from constipation. Once a diagnosis has been reached, there are several treatment options to consider.

Palliative surgery
Surgery should be considered in all patients and the potential risk:benefit ratio assessed. Mortality is generally high (12–30 per cent) and survival low. Factors that suggest a worse prognosis are age over 70 years, poor medical condition, ascites, previous combination chemotherapy and multiple small bowel

Table 2.11 Steps in the management of bowel obstruction

- Clinical diagnosis of bowel obstruction

- X-ray if the cause may be constipation or surgery is contemplated

- If suitable, operate

- If unsuitable, consider pharmacological treatment – analgesic, antiemetic and antispasmodic medication

- If unresponsive, consider octreotide *or*

- Nasogastric/percutaneous venting *or*

- Consider a metallic stent, laser recanalization or percutaneous deflation

obstruction. The likelihood of a non-malignant cause for the obstruction is directly related to the length of time between definitive treatment of the primary tumour and the episode of obstruction (Wootfson et al., 1997).

Pharmacological control

Drugs can be used to decrease the symptoms. These are usually administered subcutaneously by continuous infusion pump, but the sublingual or rectal route can also be used. An opioid, usually diamorphine, in a dose equivalent to the previous oral dose, is mixed with an antiemetic, usually haloperidol and/or cyclizine, and the antispasmodic hyoscine butylbromide (see 'Nausea and vomiting' above). Metoclopramide can also be used as the antiemetic, although, because of its prokinetic potential, it may exacerbate the colicky pain of bowel obstruction. The doses are then adjusted according to the patient's symptoms of pain, vomiting and spasm.

Using this regime of drugs, abdominal pain can be controlled in up to 90 per cent of patients, as can colic and nausea. Vomiting can continue to present problems, but many patients are able to continue to eat small, often low-residue, meals for a considerable length of time.

If the symptoms continue, the somatostatin analogue octreotide can be added. This reduces secretions and motility, and increases the absorption of fluid by the gut. Octreotide can be administered via a syringe driver and can be mixed with other drugs.

Nasogastric suction

If, despite medication, vomiting remains a problem, nasogastric suction can be initiated, more frequently for a high obstruction. It can also be used in the period of preparation before surgery. If suction is to be used in the long term, a venting gastrotomy is more comfortable for patients and can be inserted under local anaesthetic.

Other options

Recent therapeutic manoeuvres include the insertion of expanding metallic stents, particularly in the colon and rectum, obviating the need for major abdominal surgery in patients with advanced disease, the laser recanalization of lesions near the entrance or exit of the gastrointestinal tract, and in patients too ill to be considered for surgery, the percutaneous puncture of loops of inflated, obstructed bowel, with the consequent release of flatus (P. Amsler and I. Finlay, personal communication, 2000).

Whether patients should be artificially hydrated during these treatments continues to be a subject for ethical debate and can only be decided on an individual basis for each patient.

For a case study, see 'Nausea and vomiting', above.

ORAL SYMPTOMS

This area of symptom control is often neglected among the other 'higher-profile' symptoms such as pain and vomiting, but problems are common and lead to

Table 2.12 Oral symptoms in palliative care (Jobbins et al., 1992)

	Percentage of patients
Xerostomia (dry mouth)	67
Oral mucosal disease	82
Oral candidiasis	85
Disturbance of taste	26
Dysphagia	37
Soreness	42
Denture problems	71

misery in many patients (Table 2.12). Poor oral health affects eating, speaking, laughing, singing and so on, and has an enormous effect on quality of life.

Patients are often immunocompromised, malnourished and generally debilitated. Their poor immune response and frequent use of antibiotics predisposes them to infection, a poor diet reduces the levels of vitamins and iron, and treatments such as chemotherapy and radiotherapy cause a severe dry mouth and ulceration. Disease may itself occur in the mouth, giving rise to pain and altering the local environment. Preventative measures are important for all patients and should include 12-hourly tooth-brushing, the overnight soaking and 12-hourly brushing of dentures, and the use of chlorhexidene or hexitidine mouthwashes.

If a patient complains of mouth problems, a full assessment should be made: is the mouth painful, dry, infected, dirty or ulcerated?

Infection
The most common infection is oral thrush, the white plaques of candidiasis seen in immunocompromised patients who have often taken antibiotics. Other common infections include herpes simplex virus (Table 2.13).

Dirty mouth
Dirty mouths give rise to an unpleasant taste and can be helped with proprietary mouthwashes, cider, soda water, sucking pineapple chunks and effervescent vitamin C tablets. Regular brushing with a soft baby toothbrush and fluoride toothpaste should be encouraged. If the tongue is still furry, it can be cleared in 2–3 days by chewing pineapple chunks.

Dry mouth
Dry mouth, or xerostomia, often occurs as a result of radiotherapy or drug treatment, for example with diuretics or tricyclic antidepressants. Dehydration, anxiety and mouth-breathing also cause this condition. A decreased amount of saliva leads to heavy plaque and food accumulation, causing tooth decay and

Table 2.13 Common oral infections and their treatment

	Treatment
Candidiasis	Nystatin suspension or pastilles
	Ketoconazole (a 5 day course for advanced disease)
	Fluconazole (as a single dose – equally effective but more expensive)
Viral infection, e.g. herpes simplex	Aciclovir (200 mg 4-hourly for 5 days)
	Valaciclovir (500 mg 12-hourly for 5 days)
Anaerobes	Metronidazole – orally, rectally or as a gel applied topically (often associated with malignant ulcers)
Aphthous ulcers	Topical corticosteroids or tetracycline mouthwash

gum disease. Saliva protects against cavities, cleansing tooth surfaces and neutralizing acid, so that people with dry mouths are very prone to cavities, especially on the roots of teeth.

Simple measures include sipping water regularly day and night, chewing sugar-free chewing gum, avoiding alcohol and tobacco, and carrying out oral hygiene regularly every couple of hours. Petroleum jelly on the lips may help to prevent cracking. Glycerine and lemon juice should be avoided as they increase dehydration. Specific drug therapy may have to be modified, for example tricyclic antidepressants charged.

Saliva substitutes are in many cases helpful to lubricate the mouth sufficiently for speech and improve chewing. These contain either carboxymethyl-cellulose or mucin, the latter having a longer duration of action. They should be sprayed beneath the tongue and between the buccal mucosa and the teeth, rather than in the back of the throat. If these measures do not help, pilocarpine has been shown to increase saliva production, especially after radiotherapy, but it is often poorly tolerated as it causes sweating and gastrointestinal side-effects.

Pain
A painful mouth can result from local tumour, ulceration and/or infection. An anaesthetic mouthwash such as benzydamine may help, as may a sucralfate mouthwash, carmellose paste or carbenoxalone.

It is important to remember that regular oral hygiene is essential for patient comfort and that in the terminal phase of life it is more effective at relieving thirst than is rehydration (Dunphy et al., 1995).

DEPRESSION AND ANXIETY

The incidence of clinical depression in patients with incurable illness is estimated to be 20–30 per cent. The diagnosis can be difficult and is often missed, the symptoms of depression often overlapping with those caused by the illness itself, or being attributed to a natural reaction to an incurable illness.

Certain factors may make depression more likely in a patient (P. McGuire, personal communication, 1998) and it is important to screen for these when taking a medical history:

- previous psychiatric illness;
- poorly controlled physical symptoms;
- personality traits hindering adjustment, e.g. rigidity, pessimism, or being a 'control freak';
- poor communication with staff – including the bad breaking of the news regarding the diagnosis.

Many of the physical symptoms relating to depression, for example difficulty sleeping, anorexia and fatigue are also found in patients with progressive, incurable illness. One clue to their aetiology is that they seem out of proportion to the illness and respond poorly to treatment.

It may also be more appropriate to look at psychological rather than physical symptoms. Although these may seem understandable, they are often different in severity, duration and quality from 'normal' distress. There is often a pervasive sense of hopelessness and nihilism, a great deal of guilt relating to being a burden to others and suicidal ideation (Casey, 1994; Block, 2000).

Different assessment tools, for example the Hospital Anxiety and Depression Scale and the Mini-mental Scale are used to try to improve on diagnostic power. These were designed for hospital-based patients so their results can be misleading (Lloyd-Williams, 1999). Recent work has suggested that one of the most sensitive and specific scales is the Edinburgh Postnatal Depression Scale. This is a 10-point scale used to detect depression in mothers during the postnatal period and has been found to have a sensitivity and specificity of greater than 80 per cent when looking at depression in palliative care patients (Lloyd-Williams et al., 2000). One study has suggested that simply asking patients if they are depressed will identify practically all dying people with a substantial mood disorder (Chochinov et al., 1997).

Treatment includes general measures such as providing an explanation about the illness in a supportive environment, allowing patients to express their feelings, support from a specialist nurse in palliative care, and the opportunity to visit a hospice day-care centre. Complementary therapies such as art, music therapy and aromatherapy massage may also help; these require 'patient participation' and may help patients to feel more in control of their lives. Drug therapy (Table 2.14) should be considered if a definite depressive syndrome is present or if an adjustment reaction fails to improve after 3–4 weeks.

Anxiety is often present with depression and is found in patients with similar risk factors. Patients are usually worried and apprehensive, have difficulty sleeping and concentrating, and are usually tired and restless, with trembling and jumpiness. They often complain of breathlessness, palpitations, nausea, sweats, diarrhoea and urinary frequency. Treatment includes beta-blockers to help

Table 2.14 Antidepressant drugs

	Examples
Tricyclic antidepressant *Effective in 80% of cases but are sedative and commonly* *cause constipation, dry mouth and blurred vision*	Amitriptyline Dothiepin Imipramine Lofepramine
Selective serotonin reuptake inhibitors *Equally effective as tricyclic agents but have fewer* *side-effects and are safer in overdose*	Paroxetine Fluoxetine Sertraline Lofepramine
Monoamine oxidase inhibitors*	
Lithium*	
Psychostimulants* *The drugs of choice for treating depression associated with* *advanced terminal disease because of their speed of action*	Dexamfetamine Methylphenidate
Electroconvulsive therapy*	

*These treatments should only be initiated after specialist assessment, and electroconvulsive therapy should be reserved for severely retarded patients.

somatic symptoms and the short-term use of benzodiazepines; in the longer term, low-dose neuroleptics such as haloperidol or thioridazine can be taken. Case study 2.3 shows the value of intervention with depression.

EMERGENCIES IN PALLIATIVE MEDICINE

With most situations in palliative medicine, there is time for a careful assessment and consideration of treatment options before any action is taken. There are, however, a few situations that require urgent treatment:

- spinal cord compression
- bone fracture
- superior vena caval obstruction
- haemorrhage
- stridor
- seizures.

The last three items commonly occur in the final 48 hours of life.

Spinal cord compression

All health professionals caring for palliative care patients should maintain a high index of suspicion for this pathology. Up to 5 per cent of patients may develop

CASE STUDY 2.3

Mike was diagnosed with stomach cancer at the age of 55. He was a gregarious, extrovert businessman who, prior to this, had hardly ever had a day off work from sickness. He coped well with his surgery and started to recover quickly, but he then found out that the tumour had not been completely removed and that he would need chemotherapy. After the second cycle of treatment, he became withdrawn and quiet. He did not want to see his friends and became irritable and tearful. His sleep pattern deteriorated, and his appetite, which was already poor, became even worse. Mike refused to acknowledge that he was depressed until he completely broke down one afternoon when talking to his hospice nurse and confessed to a continual desire to die and to suicidal intent. He agreed to start taking an antidepressant, although he still could not accept that it could do anything for him in this situation. Mike's general practitioner started him on *fluoxetine* 20 mg daily, taking into account its relatively good side-effect profile and safety in overdose, together with its motivational properties.

After 2 weeks, Mike became less tearful and more optimistic. He started to see a few friends again and wanted to go out. He completed his chemotherapy, showing a good response to this, and continued his fluoxetine for a further 2 months, giving a total of 6 months' treatment. He then had a relatively stable period until he developed headaches, a magnetic resonance imaging (MRI) scan showing multiple cerebral metastases. All Mike's previous symptoms recurred, and he was quite willing to restart his antidepressant. This once again helped his overall mood and enabled him to cope with cerebral radiotherapy.

Thus, although Mike's depression occurred in response to his situation and was 'understandable', he responded well to antidepressants. Despite his initial scepticism, these helped him to cope better with his difficult situation and improved his quality of life.

spinal cord compression, although this figure is higher with myeloma and prostate cancer, and approximately one-third of patients survive for over 1 year after symptoms have developed. The presentation is often insidious, the main symptoms of leg weakness and bowel and bladder disturbance often being attributed to general weakness and/or medication. The consequences are devastating as, once established, the resulting paraparesis is rarely reversible.

The most common site of spinal cord compression is the thoracic vertebrae, but it can occur anywhere in the cord. It can arise from an intradural metastasis but is more commonly extradural in origin. In 85 per cent of cases, it is caused by the extension of a vertebral body metastasis, but it can also result from the collapse of a vertebral body, the direct extension of tumour through the vertebral foramina or interruption of the vascular supply.

As mentioned above, the presentation of compression can be subtle. Patients have generally complained of backache for a while, this often being worse when lying down (compare this with mechanical back pain) and being exacerbated by coughing or straining. Patients then go on to develop leg weakness, with some altered sensation in their legs and sometimes hands depending on the level of the lesion (Table 2.15).

Table 2.15 Features on presentation of spinal cord compression (Back, 1997)

- 75% have weakness of the legs (arms and legs if cervical)
- 90% have pain
  - tenderness over the affected vertebrae
  - may be radicular pain only
- 50% have a sensory level on examination – this may be unilateral and difficult to elicit
- 40% have sphincter dysfunction – a very late sign, except with cauda equina compression

Urinary symptoms of retention and dribbling incontinence caused by overflow, or bowel problems with perianal numbness, are very late presentations, except with cauda equina compression. On examination, there may be a mixture of upper and lower motor neurone signs in the limbs, together with altered areas of sensation in the limbs or a definite sensory level. There may be a narrow band of increased sensation at this level with sensory loss below. The reflexes may be brisk or absent, and the plantar reflexes upgoing if present.

If the history and examination suggest spinal cord compression, treatment should be *immediate* (Case study 2.4). The patient should be started at once on dexamethasone 16 mg and an urgent referral made to a radiotherapy unit. There, the patient should be investigated by MRI scanning to confirm and

CASE STUDY 2.4

Christine, a 58-year-old lady with lung cancer, was deteriorating quite quickly. Her breathing was becoming more difficult, and she had absolutely no energy. One day she asked for a visit from her general practitioner, as she was unable to manage the stairs to her bedroom. A locum visited and, without examining her or taking a better history, told her that this was understandable 'with all her problems', recommending that she should move her bed downstairs. Within 48 hours, Christine had developed numbness in both feet and was virtually unable to move her legs. The general practitioner who came to see her suspected a spinal cord compression, particularly when Christine told him about her long-standing back pain, which had recently worsened, particularly at night. On examination, she had numbness from her feet to mid-calf level, with an increased area of sensation just above this. The power in her legs was minimal, and the plantar reflexes were absent.

Based on these findings, the doctor diagnosed spinal cord compression, gave Christine dexamethasone 16 mg immediately and phoned the local oncologist. Within 4 hours, Christine had had an MRI scan, which confirmed an area of spinal cord compression at the T12 level, and she had received her first dose of radiotherapy.

Sadly, although Christine's symptoms did not deteriorate further, neither did they improve, Christine never regaining the ability to walk independently. Greater professional vigilance might have prevented this.

define the site of the compressing lesion and assess whether there are any other sites of incipient compression. Treatment then usually consists of local radio-therapy and corticosteroids. Surgery may rarely be indicated if there is vertebral instability that requires fixation or if this is the primary presentation of the tumour and biopsy is required for diagnosis. Emergency chemotherapy may occasionally be appropriate, for example in lymphoma or if a patient is too debilitated to tolerate radiotherapy, in which case he or she should be treated with high doses of dexamethasone alone.

The neurological status at the start of treatment is the most important prognostic factor. If treatment is started within 24–48 hours of the onset of symptoms, the damage may be reversible. However, once paraplegia is established, fewer than 5 per cent of patients regain the ability to walk after treatment.

Bone fracture

Bone metastases are a common feature of advanced cancer, particularly of the lung, breast, prostate, kidney and thyroid. These predispose to fractures, often after minimal trauma. The long bones are generally fixed internally or externally, and metastases subsequently treated with radiotherapy to promote healing and prevent their further progression.

Bisphosphonates are increasingly being used in breast cancer and multiple myeloma to reduce bone pain and decrease morbidity caused by hypercalcaemia, vertebral fracture and the need for palliative radiotherapy (Heatley and Coleman, 1999).

Superior vena cava compression

This is associated mainly with bronchial carcinomas (75 per cent) and other tumours, for example lymphomas and secondary tumours, arising in the mediastinum. Although previously regarded as an acute emergency requiring urgent treatment, current management involves a period of full assessment, possibly including a tissue biopsy. The latter is particularly important if this symptom is the first presentation of a tumour (Table 2.16).

Table 2.16 Symptoms and signs of superior vena caval obstruction

Symptoms	Breathlessness
	Visual changes
	Swollen face, neck, hands and arms
	Headache
Signs	Rapid breathing
	Periorbital oedema
	Injected conjunctivae
	Cyanosis
	Non-pulsatile distension of the neck and arm veins
	Oedema of the face, hands and arms

High-dose corticosteroids, such as dexamethasone 16 mg, and rapid radio-therapy are the main treatments to relieve the patient's dyspnoea and 'sense of drowning'. Urgent chemotherapy may be appropriate for these with chemosensitive tumours such as lymphomas.

Superior vena caval stents can also be inserted, under local anaesthetic via a venous puncture. These have an immediate potency rate of 93 per cent, and over 90 per cent of patients die without any recurrence of their superior vena caval obstruction (Renwick, 1999). Complications occur in fewer than 5 per cent of cases including stent displacement and minor pulmonary displacement. The success of these stents mean that, in some centres, they are now being used as first-line treatment prior to radiotherapy (Nicholson et al., 1997).

Supportive pharmacological treatments such as opioids in low dosages and benzodiazepines, together with psychological support, may help the dyspnoea and associated anxiety.

Haemorrhage, stridor and seizures

These symptoms are often encountered in the final 48 hours of life and are frightening events for both patients and their families. The way in which the health-care professionals present handle them can have a significant effect on a family's distress and eventual bereavement. It is vital to give a full explanation about why something is happening and what is being done to help.

Major **haemorrhage** usually presents as haemoptysis, as haemetemesis or as the result of the erosion of a carotid vessel. Patients should be kept as warm and as quiet as possible. Dark towels should be used to mop up blood so that the visual impact of the bleeding is reduced. Benzodiazepines or opioids may be appropriate to lessen anxiety. If the patient is not in the terminal phase of the illness, an urgent decision is required regarding treatment, for example trans-fusion, surgery or radiotherapy.

Stridor occurs as a result of pressure on the large airways and is generally caused by an enlarging upper airway tumour. Further treatment may be appropriate, but opioids and benzodiazepines again form the basis of supportive treatment.

Seizures or fits are generally related to primary or secondary intracerebral tumours or metabolic disturbances. They require immediate management with benzodiazepines and then treatment with continued anticonvulsant medication and possibly dexamethasone if appropriate.

Weakness and fatigue

The generalized fatigue and weakness seen in patients with progressive, incurable illness can be extremely frustrating and demoralizing, and is often difficult to manage. Specific causes should be sought, but no obvious treatable cause may ultimately be found. These causes include:

- anaemia
- hypothyroidism
- hypercalcaemia
- spinal cord compression

- malnutrition
- depression
- infection
- electrolyte imbalance.

For these patients, supportive measures are important, including as full an explanation as possible about fatigue, the setting of reasonable, achievable goals for activity and support and encouragement.

If weakness is becoming a severe problem, often linked to anorexia, a trial of corticosteroids may be appropriate. A starting dose of dexamethasone 4–6 mg should produce a response within 5–7 days. If patients improve, they should be maintained at this level for a while before the dose is reduced. The response, however, is generally only maintained for about 4 weeks. If there is no response, the doses should be tailed off immediately.

If corticosteroids are contraindicated, as with previous peptic ulceration with haemetemesis, or if longer-term action is required, medroxyprogesterone or mege-strol acetate may be tried. Megestrol acetate has been shown in controlled trials to enhance appetite, improve the feeling of well-being, reduce fatigue and improve the quality of life. Drawbacks to the use of these hormones are their cost and their side-effects of oedema and thrombosis.

Hypercalcaemia

Hypercalcaemia can occur with any tumour but is most commonly seen with breast cancer, myeloma and non-small cell lung cancer. Bone metastases are often, but not invariably, present. The hypercalcaemia is thought to be caused by parathormone-related proteins, prostaglandins and local-action cytokines such as interleukin and tumour necrosis factor.

With mild hypercalcaemia – corrected calcium level of less than 3.0 mmol/l (Table 2.17) – observation only is required if the patient is asymptomatic. If the corrected calcium concentration is higher or the patient is symptomatic, treatment

Table 2.17 Symptoms of hypercalcaemia

	Symptoms
Mild (<3.0 mmol/l)	Slight nausea
	Anorexia
	Thirst
	Constipation
	Weakness
Severe (>3.0 mmol/l)	Dehydration
	Confusion
	Coma
	Cardiac arrhythmia

should be initiated. This can markedly improve a patient's quality of life and should be considered at all stages of the illness, even the end-stage.

Patients should be rehydrated with 1–2 l of normal saline and then given the bisphosphonate pamidronate 60–90 mg, by intravenous infusion in 0.5 l normal saline over 1.5 hours (Case study 2.5). The calcium level should correct over 3–5 days and the effect last for 3–4 weeks. The calcium level should be monitored and the infusion repeated if appropriate. Oral bisphonates such as sodium clodronate can be given, but they are less effective as they are poorly absorbed and only tend to delay, rather than prevent, the need for an infusion.

SKIN PROBLEMS

Pressure sores

Many patients are anorexic, cachectic and immobile, and therefore prone to pressure sores. Attention to regular turning and careful lifting can help to reduce the problem. Pressure areas should be inspected daily and specialist pressure surfaces or mattresses introduced early.

Comfortable dressings, usually colloid or gel dressings, adequate pain relief during dressing changes and for background pain relief, and the reduction of odour with oral, rectal or topical metronidazole are the goals of good symptom control. Appropriate hydration, high-protein and high-carbohydrate drinks, and vitamin C supplements encourage healing.

Malignant ulcers

The basic management is similar to that of pressure sores. Bleeding ulcers may also require radiotherapy, with topical sucralfate or tranexamic acid applied in

---

CASE STUDY 2.5

Sheila, aged 62, had metastatic breast cancer and was half way through a course of chemotherapy. Her husband phoned one Monday to say that he was rather concerned about her 'stomach bug', which had failed to settle over the weekend. On closer questioning, it seemed that Sheila had been vomiting for about 36 hours, had some abdominal pain and general aching, and was getting rather confused.

A visit confirmed this and also that Sheila was starting to become dehydrated. An emergency (corrected) calcium level was 3.6 mmol/l so she was admitted to hospital. Here she was rehydrated with intravenous saline, 1 l every 6 hours for 24 hours, and then given a *pamidronate* infusion 90 mg over 1.5 hours. Her confusion improved and she stopped being sick.

After 3 days, Sheila's calcium level was 2.6 mmol/l, and she was sent home. The level was rechecked after 2 weeks, when it was 2.9 mmol/l, but as Sheila was asymptomatic, she was not treated. At 6 weeks, her symptoms started to recur, and a further pamidronate infusion was given. Maintenance therapy was initiated to cope with these relapses, and Sheila was given a pamidronate infusion monthly until she died 4 months later.

the interim to control bleeding. If there is a residual distortion of body shape, cavity foam dressings can be used to restore some symmetry. Debridement can be achieved with polysaccharide, hydrocolloid or hydrogel dressings. Calcium alginate dressings absorb excessive exudates, and topical corticosteroids may reduce watery discharge. The pain from a malignant ulcer may improve with the use of topical morphine (Back and Finlay, 1995).

Body image can be severely affected by the erosion of body shape and odour, and attention must be paid to the effect that the fungating lesion is having on the social and psychological aspects of the patient's life.

Pruritus

Pruritus, with a prevalence of approximately 2 per cent in palliative medicine patients, is a skin sensation leading to a desire to scratch (Table 2.18). It can be a very debilitating problem, and it is estimated that one-third of patients with generalized pruritus may have depressive symptomatology. It is therefore important that a full physical, psychological and spiritual history should be taken before treatment.

The management of pruritus should consist of general measures, which can be topical or systemic, and more specific treatments for recognized conditions (Table 2.19).

URINARY SYMPTOMS

Very little is written about urinary symptoms in palliative care textbooks, yet the pain, spasm and incontinence seen with bladder and prostate tumours, and

Table 2.18 Causes of pruritus (Thoms and Edmonds, 2000)

	Causes
Skin rash absent	Cholestatic jaundice
	Opioids
	Iron deficiency anaemia
	Uraemia
	Thyroid disease
	Myeloma, lymphoma and polycythaemia rubra vera
	Diabetes
Skin rash present	Dermatitis
	Fungal infection
	Scabies
	Lichen planus
	Dermatitis herpetiformis
	Urticaria
	Bullous pemphigoid
	Metastatic infiltration

Table 2.19 Management of pruritus (Thoms and Edmonds, 2000)

General	Avoid overheating
	Avoid hot baths
	Use emulsifying ointment and aqueous cream instead of soap
Topical	Consider using menthol, camphor, zinc oxide, coal tar, Calamine, glycerine
	Newer agents:
	Topical doxiepin – a topical tricylic antidepressant with potent antihistaminergic effects
	Capsaicin – derived from hot chilli peppers; depletes substance P from the sensory nerves and blocks C-fibre conduction
	Transcutaneous electrical nerve stimulation
Systemic	Antihistamines
	5-HT$_3$ antagonists, e.g. granisetron
	Opioid antagonists, e.g. naloxone, for opioid-induced pruritus
Specific	Morphine induced – switch opioid, e.g. morphine to hydromorphone
	Biliary obstruction – surgery, cholestyramine, rifampicin, prednisolone, levotrimeprazine, cimetidine, phenobarbitone, heparin*
Complementary	Behaviour therapy
	Acupuncture
	Hypnotherapy

*The variety and number of treatments emphasizes the uncertain success of drugs and reinforces the importance of local measures.

other pelvic tumours that invade the bladder wall (Table 2.20), can be profoundly distressing to manage and difficult to help. These symptoms severely affect the quality of life of patients: smelling of urine and wearing incontinence appliances or pads can severely affect patients' body image and sex life. These issues need to be discussed and handled by health-care professionals in an open but sensitive manner (see Chapter 9).

Urinary infections should be treated with the appropriate antibiotics, and mist. pot. cit. may help dysuria. If catheterized, spasms may respond to a change to a smaller size of catheter, the balloon causing less irritation of the bladder neck. Oxybutynin and low-dose amitriptyline may also reduce bladder irritability. If spasm continues to be a problem, local anaesthetic bladder wash-outs using lignocaine or bupivicaine can be tried, caudal injections sometimes helping severe cases.

If it is caused by a tumour, haematuria can be improved with radiotherapy. Tranexamic acid can make clots harder and more difficult to evacuate so should not be used, but ethamsylate can reduce bleeding from any site along the renal tract. A bladder wash-out with a 1 per cent alum solution can reduce severe bleeding from the bladder.

Table 2.20 Symptoms and causes of urinary tract problems

	Causes
Dysuria	Infection
	Tumour infiltration of the bladder
	Radiotherapy cystitis
	Chemotherapy (cyclophosphamide)
Haematuria	Infection
	Tumour
	Calculi
	Other systemic causes, e.g. bleeding disorder
Spasms	Infection
	Tumour infiltration of the bladder or rectum
	Urinary catheter
	Radiation cystitis
Incontinence	Infection
	Retention with overflow incontinence
	Diuretics

Nocturnal incontinence can often be improved with a desmopressin spray or tablets.

ASCITES

Ascites is particularly associated with ovarian and colorectal tumours. It can be asymptomatic, but, as fluid collects, patients become increasingly uncomfortable and can develop nausea, vomiting, dyspnoea and leg oedema. Treatment consists of diuretics such as frusemide, spironalactone and metolazone, and paracentesis. This may have to be repeated on several occasions and can then lead to protein depletion. In such cases, if the patient is otherwise well and has a reasonable prognosis, a shunt can be inserted from the abdominal cavity to the venous system.

HICCUPS

Anything that irritates the neural pathways transmitting the reflex relevant can cause hiccups (Table 2.21). The treatment depends on the cause but is often empirical. It includes:

- rubbing the palate as far back as possible;
- decreasing gastric distension with, for example, peppermint water, Asilone or metoclopramide;
- relaxing the muscles with baclofen, nifedipine or midazolam;
- central inhibition, such as with haloperidol, chlorpromazine or sodium valproate.

Table 2.21 Causes of hiccup

Vagal irritation	Gastric distension
	Peritonitis
	Tumour
	Oesophageal obstruction
	Pneumonia
Phrenic nerve	Diaphragmatic tumour
	Mediastinal tumour
	Neck tumour
Central nervous system pathology	Intracranial tumours
	Brainstem lesions
	Uraemia
	Meningitis

TENESMUS

Tenesmus can arise from the bladder or rectum and is defined as 'ineffectual and painful straining at stool or in urinating'. It is usually associated with progressively enlarging pelvic tumours and can be aggravated by anything that increases pelvic pressure, for example sitting or constipation.

Treatment includes opiates, corticosteroids, calcium channel blocking agents such as nifedipine, radiotherapy, epidural anaesthesia and local anaesthetic enema.

SWEATING

Sweats can be related to a specific illness for example lymphoma or myeloma, but can also be associated with hormone manipulation (e.g. tamoxifen), chemotherapy, radiotherapy, a tumour often with hepatic secondaries, infection or drugs such as opioids. Specific causes should be treated. If non-specific sweats occur with a pyrexia, a non-steroidal anti-inflammatory agent should be used. If there is no pyrexia, consider thioridazine or propantheline.

TERMINAL RATTLE

In patients who are imminently dying, the breathing often becomes rattly or bubbly as a result of the collection of oral secretions, which cannot be cleared, at the back of the throat. This can be very distressing for carers, although it does not usually harm the patient. This should be explained to the family and carers. Only half of patients respond to treatment, earlier intervention usually being more successful. The patient should be repositioned and, if the rattle persists, given either hyoscine hydrobromide or glycopyrronium, the latter being far cheaper. The bed should if possible be tilted and suction used very gently if it is available.

CONCLUSION

Effective symptom control clearly requires an understanding of the causes of the symptoms and of their persistence. It also requires health-care professionals, to be able to communicate well with the patient, the family and other members of the health-care team. Recognizing when one's own knowledge is insufficient and further help is needed is also important for good patient care; it is essential to develop and maintain these skills.

The success or failure of palliative care as a speciality in its own right depends on the improvement in quality of life that we enable our patients to achieve and the legacy we leave their carers. The memories of a patient's last illness stay with the carers forever; if they are 'good' memories, they will call on us to help again. This is the challenge for today's palliative care.

REFERENCES

Back, I. 1997: *Palliative medicine handbook*, 2nd edn. Cadiff: Marie Curie Centre.

Back, I.N. and Finlay, I. 1995: Analgesic effect of topical opioids on painful skin ulcers. *Journal of Pain and Symptom Management* **10**(7), 493.

Baile, W.F., Kudelka, A.P., Beale, E.A. et al. 1999: Communication skills training in oncology. Description and preliminary outcomes of workshops on breaking bad news and managing patient reactions to illness. *Cancer* **86**, 887–97.

Billings, J.A. 2000: Recent advances: palliative care. *British Medical Journal* **7260**, 555–78.

Block, S.D. 2000: For the ACP-ASIM end of life care consensus panel. Assessing and managing depression in the terminally ill patient. *Annals of Internal Medicine* **132**, 209–18.

Buckman, R. 1992: *How to break bad news*. London: Papermac.

Casey, P. 1994: Depression in the dying – disorder or distress. *Progress in Palliative Care* **2**(1), 1–3.

Chochinov, H.M., Wilson, K.G., Enns, M. and Lander, S. 1997: Are you depressed? Screening for depression in the terminally ill. *American Journal of Psychiatry* **154**, 674–6.

Donnelly, S. and Walsh, D. 1995: The symptoms of advanced cancer. *Seminars in Oncology* **22**, 67–72.

Dunphy, K., Finlay, I., Rathbone, G., Gilbert, F. and Hicks, F. 1995: Rehydration in palliative and terminal care: if not – why not? *Palliative Medicine* **9**, 221–8.

Finlay, I. 1995: *Palliative care for people with cancer*, London: 2nd edn. Arnold.

Heatley, S. and Coleman, R. 1999: The use of bisphosphonates in the palliative care setting. *International Journal of Palliative Care Nursing* **5**(2), 74–80.

Jobbins, J., Bagg, J., Finlay, I.G. et al. 1992: Oral and dental disease in terminally ill patients. *British Medical Journal* **304**, 1612.

Lloyd-Williams, M. 1999: The assessment of depression in palliative care patients. *European Journal of Palliative Care* **6**(5), 150–3.

Lloyd-Williams, M., Friedman, T. and Rudd, N. 2000. The validation of the EPDS in patients with advanced metastatic cancer. *Journal of Pain and Symptom Management* **20**(4), 259–65.

Navari, R.M., Reinhardt, R.R., Gralla, R.J. et al. 1999: Reduction of cisplatin induced emesis by a selective neurokinin-1-receptor antagonist 754, 030. Antiemetic Trials Group. *New England Journal of Medicine* 340(3), 190–5.

Nicholson, A.A., Ettles, D.F., Arnold, A., Greenstone, M. and Dyet, J.F. 1997: Treatment of malignant superior vena cava obstruction: metal stents or radiation therapy? *Journal of Vascular and Interventional Radiology* 8, 781–8.

Renwick, I. 1999: Metallic stents in palliative care. *CME Bulletin of Palliative Medicine* 2, 41–4.

Sykes, N. 1998: The treatment of morphine-induced constipation. *European Journal of Palliative Care* 5(1), 12–15.

Thorns, A. and Edmonds, P. 2000: The management of pruritus in palliative care patients. *European Journal of Palliative Care* 7(1), 9–12.

Twycross, R. and Back, I. 1998: Nausea and vomiting in advanced cancer. *European Journal of Palliative Care* 5(2), 39–44.

Twycross, R., Wilcock, A. and Thorp, S. 1998: *Palliative care formulary*. Oxford: Radcliffe Medical Press.

Ungar, A. 2000: Movicol in treatment of constipation and faecal impaction. *British Journal of General Practice* 61(1), 37–40.

Woolfson, R.G. Jennings, K. and Whalen, G.F. 1997: Management of bowel obstruction in patients with abdominal cancer. *Archives of Surgery* 132, 1093–7.

FURTHER READING

Cooper, J. (ed.) 2000: *Stepping into palliative care*. Oxford: Radcliffe Medical Press.

Doyle, D., Hanks, G.W.C. and MacDonald, N. (eds) 1995: *Oxford textbook of palliative medicine*. Oxford: Oxford Medical Publications.

Fallon, M. and O'Neill, B. (eds) 1998: *ABC of palliative care*. London: BMJ Publishing Group.

Faull, C., Carter, Y. and Woof, R. 1998: *Handbook of palliative care*. Oxford: Blackwell Science.

Regnard, C. and Tempest, S. (eds) 1998: *A guide to symptom relief in advanced cancer*. Manchester: Haigh & Hochland.

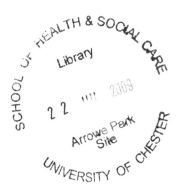

chapter 3

BREATHLESSNESS

Sam H. Ahmedzai and Vandana Vora

> Each person is born to one possession which outvalues all his others – his last breath.
> Mark Twain, *Following the Equator*, 1897

Breathlessness is one of the symptoms most commonly encountered in cancer and, for many patients (and professionals), the most feared. Alternatives terms for breathlessness include 'shortness of breath', 'difficulty in breathing' and 'dyspnoea'. The latter is derived from the Greek, and although it is the term used most frequently by doctors and is internationally recognized, it is not readily understood by the general public so is best avoided with patients. As with pain, there are many distinct words that people use to describe different types or levels of breathlessness, such as 'gasping', 'wheezing', 'feeling tight-chested', 'choking' and 'drowning'.

Partly because of the variety of ways in which people describe the sensation, it is hard to give a concise definition of breathlessness. Various descriptions have emphasized different aspects, such as the unpleasant sensation, the disproportion between the demands on the lungs and their ability to respond, and the lack of a consistent relationship between the sensation and its impact on the individual's physical activity (Ahmedzai, 1998). To try to encompass these different perspectives into a single definition is difficult, but we would propose the following:

> Breathlessness is the subjective sensation of difficulty or undue effort in breathing, which is not necessarily related to exercise and which compels the individual to increase ventilation or reduce activity.

This definition attempts to highlight the functional consequences of breathlessness, namely the pressing need to breathe harder or, if that is not possible, to reduce activity, with all the negative consequences that flow from becoming chair-, bed- or house-bound. The observed signs are therefore those of a patient who is either gasping or breathing more quickly (tachypnoea), or who is breathing normally but at the cost of reduced activity, independence and social interaction.

Why is it important to understand and describe breathlessness? First, the condition is very common, which means that a practitioner working in cancer care could encounter the symptom on an almost daily basis. It arises most frequently in primary lung cancer, which is the most common cancer of adult males across the world, and in some countries is also becoming the most common cancer in adult females. Breathlessness is present in 40 per cent of those with lung cancer at the time of presentation (Hopwood and Stephens, 1995). In general, the prevalence and severity of the breathlessness increase with the progression of the disease, unlike pain, which decreases over the same time course if the patient is in the care of specialists in palliative care (Higginson and McCarthy, 1989).

In addition, apart from primary lung cancer, the lungs and other thoracic organs can be involved in the later stages of cancers arising in other sites, notably the breast, bowel, kidney, larynx and lymphoma, by means of direct extension, pulmonary metastases or pleural effusions. The prevalence of breathlessness with advanced disease has been reported to be 50–80 per cent in different settings, regardless of the type of cancer (Davis, 1994; Vainio and Auvinen, 1996; Ahmedzai, 1998)

We should remember that breathlessness is a common symptom of many 'benign' chronic diseases, for example asthma, bronchitis and heart failure. These may exist as co-morbidity in cancer patients, especially in the elderly population, who may therefore show an increased risk of breathlessness not directly related to their malignant disease.

MECHANISMS OF BREATHLESSNESS

How do the sensation and physical signs of breathlessness arise? From the comments above, it will be clear that no single cause is relevant in all cancer patients. Many different causes may conspire to induce or aggravate breathlessness in a person who may already be limited by chronic obstructive pulmonary disease (COPD) or occupational lung disease. In such cases, it is important to tease out the new, cancer-related causes that are operating in the patient because that is the best way to direct appropriate therapies. Thus, merely asking a chronic asthmatic patient who now is struggling with increased shortness of breath caused by, for example, a mesothelioma to take more puffs of his bronchodilator inhaler is not likely to give rise to a helpful response.

It is necessary to understand some of the mechanisms that control normal breathing in order to understand how cancer can disturb them. Breathing is regulated every second of our lives by an interplay of chemical, neurological and musculoskeletal messages that pass between the lungs, chest wall, diaphragm and brain. Mercifully, we are not usually aware of these constant signals, although we can at any time consciously intervene and choose, for example, to hold our breath underwater, or conversely to make extra-large respiratory efforts, say to blow up a balloon.

The chemical factors that control breathing are the blood levels of oxygen and carbon dioxide, more precisely their levels in the tissues in the carotid bodies of the aorta (sensitive to oxygen) and in the respiratory centre, which lies in the medulla oblongata of the brainstem (sensitive to carbon dioxide). Of these two influences, it is the sensitivity to carbon dioxide that is the more important drive to respiration in normal conditions and in most disease states. Carbon dioxide dissolves in the blood and increases its acidity (i.e. lowers the pH of the blood). The chemoreceptors in the medulla are exquisitively sensitive to changes in pH, a fall leading into signals being passed to the chest to increase ventilation to get rid of more carbon dioxide. In contrast, the blood oxygen concentration can fall quite markedly before the carotid body receptors send equivalent signals to the brain, leading to increased ventilation. This is very important, as we shall see when we consider the role of supplemental oxygen as a therapy.

The chest wall muscles are obviously essential for the act of breathing, but they play an important part in its regulation, and also in the production of breathlessness. The diaphragm is another crucial part of the respiratory muscle group, its nerve supply also being intimately linked to the control of the normal cycle of breathing and its changes when lying down (when the chest wall is less able to move), during exertion and in disease states. There is a constant looping of messages from the brain, which is being influenced by the chemical receptors, down to the chest wall muscles and from them back to the brain, indicating whether the necessary change in ventilation can be produced or whether the muscles are failing. Many somatic changes occurring in cancer patients can adversely affect the respiratory muscles, these therefore impacting on how well the feedback loop can keep on circulating.

Two other physiological factors can influence whether a person feels breathless at a given level of exertion. One is the perfusion of the lungs, which is the ability of deoxygenated blood from the right side of the heart to flow efficiently round the ventilated parts of the lungs and to carry new oxygen back to the left side of the heart, ready for pumping round the systemic circulation. The balance between ventilation and perfusion is a delicate one; many disease processes interfere with it and thus cause inefficient lung function, which can be quickly perceived as breathlessness. This situation arises in pulmonary embolism, severe airflow obstruction, such as with chronic asthma or bronchitis, consolidation or collapse of the lungs.

Another factor is the ability of skin sensors around the mouth and nose to detect cool air flowing past the face. When stimulated by moving air, these sensors have an action that *reduces* the brain's perception of breathlessness (Wilcock, 1998). This explains the great benefit that patients obtain from sitting in front of an open window or from a gentle fan placed near the face. It may also explain some of the 'placebo effect' observed in many patients who apparently receive benefit from oxygen (or even compressed air) delivered by a face mask even though they are objectively not hypoxic.

CAUSES OF BREATHLESSNESS

Based on our understanding of the complex regulation of breathing, it is easy to see that there could be many causes of breathlessness in cancer patients. Table 3.1 summarises these causes, which fall into three main groups: those arising from the respiratory system, from the cardiovascular system and from other disease processes such as anaemia.

Table 3.1 Causes of breathlessness in cancer patients

Site of origin	Examples of causes
Thoracic	
Respiratory	Malignancy – bronchial/tracheal obstruction
	Pneumonia
	Pleural effusion
	Lymphangitis carcinomatosa
	Diaphragmatic weakness
	Superior vena caval obstruction
	Chronic lung disease
Cardiovascular	Heart failure
	Pericardial effusion
	Pulmonary embolism
Non-thoracic	Anaemia
	Ascites
	Drugs
	Radiotherapy
	Anxiety

RESPIRATORY CAUSES

Table 3.2 shows how breathlessness is a common final pathway for many cancers, especially lung, breast, colorectal, kidney and laryngeal primaries and lymphomas. There are four main *structural* types of cause:

1 bronchopulmonary (e.g. bronchial or tracheal obstruction, consolidation or collapse);
2 chest wall (e.g. tumour infiltration and pleural effusion);
3 cardiovascular (e.g. pericardial effusion or cardiac failure);
4 lymphatic (e.g. lymphangitis carcinomatosa and mediastinal lymphadenopathy).

Another useful way of looking at respiratory causes of breathing disorders is to divide them into their *physiological* mechanisms:

- problems of ventilating the lungs
- impaired perfusion of the lungs
- muscle fatigue
- pleural restriction.

Ventilation is most dramatically compromised when a cancer narrows the major upper airways, as seen with a laryngeal primary or a small cell lung cancer blocking the trachea; in such cases, patients have noticeably noisy wheezing

Table 3.2 How cancers cause breathlessness

Site of cancer	Mechanism			
	Pulmonary	Chest wall	Cardiovascular	Lymphatic
Primary lung cancer	+ +	+	+	+
Mesothelioma	–	+ +	+	–
Metastatic cancer				
Breast	+	+ +	+ +	+ +
Colorectal	+ +	+	+	+
Kidney	+ +	+	+	+
Larynx	+ +	–	–	+
Lymphoma	+	–	+	+ +

+ +, common; +, occasional; –, rare.

(stridor) and are very distressed. In most cases, however, the cancer lies in a smaller peripheral bronchus and may produce sufficient obstruction to lead to infection and consolidation in the affected lobe; alternatively, it may totally block a bronchus, causing part or the whole of one lung to collapse. It is important to remember that not all wheezing in lung cancer patients is malignant – chronic airflow limitation from asthma or bronchitis often plays a part too, particularly in smokers.

Some patients are found to have multiple metastases in their lungs on chest X-ray or computed tomography (CT) scanning. Even several discrete lesions, unless they are very large (occupying much of a lobe), do not themselves produce breathlessness unless they also occlude a bronchus or cause a ventilation–perfusion mismatch. Thus, if such a patient reports feeling breathless, it is important to look for other causes, such as heart failure, anaemia or COPD.

The perfusion of the lungs by the blood and lymphatic circulations is often compromised by cancer, this being a potent cause of breathlessness. The most common form of blood circulatory obstruction arises from pulmonary embolism. The large pulmonary embolus from a leg vein that causes sudden crushing chest pain, haemoptysis (coughing blood), fainting because of reduced blood flow back to the heart and rapid death if untreated is thankfully uncommon. The patient is more often found to have multiple smaller emboli that accumulate over days or weeks and cause progressive breathlessness, a scenario that is notoriously difficult to diagnose clinically. Many solid tumours can increase the clotting ability of the blood, which, combined with the tendency for patients with advancing cancer to remain in a sedentary position for prolonged times, predisposes them to form deep vein thromboses in the large leg veins.

The superior vena cava is the main blood vein returning blood to the heart from the systemic circulation of the head, arms and upper trunk. If this is blocked by tumour – or more probably by a combination of narrowing from the outside by tumour and lymph nodes and internally by local thrombosis – the situation described as superior vena caval obstruction (SVCO) arises. This is characterized by swelling and a dusky red discolouration of the face, with headache and oedema of the arms. It is unlikely that the reduced blood return to the heart itself causes breathlessness, but these patients are often limited because of the repeated emboli arising from the thrombus at the site of obstruction; in addition, the tumour is often so placed that it also obstructs a major airway or the trachea itself.

The lymphatic drainage of the lungs is often overlooked until it too is compromised by cancer. If a tumour is enlarging in the mediastinum, or gives rise to enlarged lymph nodes in the chest, the return of lymphatic fluid from the lungs to the main collecting ducts in the chest may become blocked. This situation is often seen in breast cancer that has metastasized to the chest. The resulting picture, lymphangitis carcinomatosa, is of congestion in the affected part of lung, which can present clinically and look on an X-ray like cardiac failure. The effect of lymphatic obstruction is to produce a stiff lung that is difficult to ventilate, and the patient becomes extremely breathless.

Cancer often causes the patient to lose appetite and weight, a situation called anorexia–cachexia syndrome (Woof, 1998). There are many factors in the generation of this syndrome, including the effects of the surgery, drugs and radiation used to treat the cancer itself. Even without these therapies, patients may, however, lose weight, often because of the effect of circulating cytokines, such as tumour necrosis factor and the interleukins (IL-1 and IL-6). Whatever the origin of the weight loss, the respiratory muscles are not spared. The result is progressive weakness of the chest wall and diaphragm, with a consequent reduction in ventilatory effort, at the same time as the patient is finding it more of a struggle to get up and walk or climb stairs as a result of the weakness of leg and other muscles.

Professionals looking after cancer patients should be aware that chest wall weakness can also arise with advanced COPD, motor neurone disease and chronic thoracic cage deformities. Furthermore, it is important to remember that drugs used in cancer treatments and palliative care can also affect the action of the chest wall muscles. This is especially true of corticosteroids, which can cause a measurable reduction in skeletal and respiratory muscle strength within a matter of weeks. Benzodiazepines such as lorazepam and midazolam, which are used to sedate patients and sometimes specifically to reduce muscle irritability, can also unavoidably cause a degree of respiratory muscle weakness.

Primary or secondary (metastatic) cancer within the lung may extend to the pleura and there stimulate the secretion of fluid, called a pleural effusion. If this is substantial, it may not only cause compression of the portion of the lung lying directly under the fluid, but also lead to a shift of the heart and other mediastinal structures over to the opposite side. The lung tissue is thus compromised on one or both sides, and the mediastinal shift is associated with central chest discomfort and cough. Mesothelioma frequently causes pleural effusions in the early stages but later makes the patient even more breathless by encasing the pleural space with thick tumour, which reduces the lung volume and makes the chest wall immobile.

Mesothelioma often extends to cover the diaphragmatic surface of the pleura. The diaphragm may also be 'splinted' or prevented from moving efficiently if there is a large effusion, tense ascites in the abdomen or even an enlarged liver. It can also be paralysed neurologically if a tumour in the mediastinum makes contact with and destroys the phrenic nerve as it passes from the cervical vertebrae down to the diaphragm muscle. All these give rise to inefficient ventilation of the affected side.

CARDIAC CAUSES

Cancer or lymphoma involving the central structures of the chest may directly invade the heart, but more often they infiltrate the pericardial lining of the heart. This can cause breathlessness via two mechanisms. First, the tumour can secrete fluid, just as with the lungs, the effusion in this situation being called a pericardial effusion. Second, tumour itself can encircle the heart and restrict its muscular activity, producing an effect like a restrictive pericarditis. In both scenarios, the patient rapidly becomes extremely breathless as the venous return to the heart, and thence to the lungs, is restricted. This condition is usually quickly fatal, but the treatment described below can give worthwhile palliation and may even prolong life for a short time, which could be valuable for some patients and carers.

A more common and fortunately more easily treated cardiac condition in cancer patients is the development of heart failure. The patient often has underlying ischaemic heart disease and may have had a myocardial infarction or angina before. Heart failure should be a rare occurrence nowadays, but certain drugs used to treat cancer, especially anthracycline cytotoxic agents, or high doses of radiotherapy applied over the centre of the chest, may aggravate a pre-existing heart failure or actually cause it.

ANAEMIA

Many other cancers that do not directly invade the chest may cause breathlessness by their tendency to make the patient anaemic. It is not possible to state exactly in every individual when a certain level of anaemia will cause breathlessness as this is related to the rate of decrease of the haemoglobin concentration and the person's activity level. Generally speaking, by the time the haemoglobin level has fallen below 9–10 g/dl, the oxygen-carrying capacity of the blood is reduced to the point at which most people will be breathless on exertion. Anaemia can arise in cancer patients through bleeding, for example from a gastric, colon or bladder carcinoma. Haemoptysis, although dramatic and frightening for patients and carers, is not usually severe or prolonged enough to lead to anaemia.

Even without overt bleeding, so-called secondary anaemia is common in cancer, being mediated by many factors including reduced blood formation in the bone marrow and the reduced intake and absorption of iron and vitamins because of anorexia–cachexia syndrome. Secondary anaemia can occur in most types of malignancy in adults and children so it should actively be sought in all areas of cancer care. Iatrogenic anaemia frequently follows the use of cytotoxic chemotherapy or radiotherapy to the bones involved in producing blood. All these types of anaemia can produce breathlessness by reducing the ability of blood to transport oxygen and eventually by precipitating heart failure.

ASSESSMENT

Although much of cancer care is now organized through multi-disciplinary teams, it is still often assumed that making diagnoses is the province of the doctor. It is however, not unreasonable to expect that experienced nurses (and others such as physiotherapists) who work with cancer patients should have a good background knowledge of breathing disorders and know how to make a skilled holistic assessment of the factors that may be operating in a particular patient (Thompson, 2000). This is in fact accepted with respect to the assessment of pain in cancer patients – in countries such as the UK, nurses who are trained and experienced are skilled at assessing pain and deducing whether the patient is suffering bone pain, or visceral colic, or the neuropathic complications of a vertebral metastasis. Such nurses are frequently 'in the front line', in regular, direct contact with patients in their homes, in hospitals or in hospice units, and it can speed up the time to the prescription of a suitable treatment for them to make this assessment and discuss it with their medical colleagues. It is not required (or even advisable) for nurses to make a formal *medical diagnosis*, but a structured *clinical assessment* is quite feasible and, within the context of a trusting multi-disciplinary team, will encourage the positive sharing of professional care.

Box 3.1 gives an outline of the steps in a structured clinical assessment of a patient who is breathless. The first items are history-taking and considering which investigations are relevant. In taking a thorough history of breathlessness, the practitioner should enquire how long the patient has had the symptom and whether it started suddenly or gradually. The previous medical history is also important here, especially enquiring whether the patient has had previous asthma or bronchitis, cardiac problems or anaemia, and whether he or she is a smoker or ex-smoker. The next important questions concern the severity of the breathing problem and whether it is variable (especially looking for the 'morning dip' of asthma, or the night-time awakening of cardiac failure, i.e. paroxysmal nocturnal dyspnoea). It is useful to ask about the provoking factors (such as movement and posture) and relieving factors (again, posture can be a clue: relief when sitting forwards in a chair or bed points, for example, to left ventricular failure or severe COPD).

BOX 3.1 ASSESSMENT OF THE BREATHLESS CANCER PATIENT: *IMPORTANT ELEMENTS OF THE HISTORY*

Onset

- Acute – pulmonary embolism, left ventricular failure, pneumonia (bacterial, viral, aspiration), pneumothorax, foreign body inhalation, upper airway obstruction, asthma
- Gradual – pleural effusion, chronic obstructive pulmonary disease, asthma, anaemia

Time course

Severity

Variability

Provoking factors – supine position (orthopnoea due to left ventricular failure, abdominal distension from any cause, respiratory muscles weakness), exertion, fear and anxiety

Relieving factors – e.g. upright posture in left ventricular failure

Associated symptoms

- *Pain* – angina, heartburn or indigestion from reflux oesophagitis or hiatus hernia, oesophageal rupture, pleuritic pain related to pulmonary embolism, pleurisy, rib fracture, chest wall or neuropathic pain in mesothelioma and Pancoast tumour
- *Cough and sputum* – purulent in bacterial pneumonia and lung abscess, frothy in pulmonary oedema
- *Haemoptysis* – endobronchial tumour, pulmonary embolism
- *Wheezing* – bilateral in asthma and chronic obstructive pulmonary disease, unilateral in large airway obstruction
- *Peripheral oedema*
- *Heart failure*
- *Anaemia*

Past medical history

- Chronic obstructive pulmonary disease, ischaemic heart disease, anaemia

Drug history

- Diuretics and bronchodilators
- Previous treatment with and response to corticosteroids
- Beta-blocker- (atenolol) or non-steroidal anti-inflammatory drug- (aspirin) induced wheezing

Patient's perception of the symptom

- Explore psychological concerns and any symptoms of anxiety or depression

The assessment should continue with questions about associated symptoms (such as cough and purulent sputum, indicating bronchial or pulmonary infection). There should then follow a thorough treatment history, concentrating on what drugs the patient has received and to what extent they have helped, or perhaps worsened, the problem. Last but not least, it is essential to explore the patient's own understanding and interpretation of the symptoms and their significance. Some patients with long-standing COPD may read little into their breathlessness compared with a non-smoker who has never had respiratory problems. Many will have a deep fear of choking, perhaps based on some early memories of watching a parent or other relative dying in great distress. At this time, it is helpful to make a general assessment of the patient's psychological state, particularly in terms of significant anxiety state or depression, as these may be specifically treated, which may help the patient to cope better with the physical symptoms.

There has in recent years been growing interest in the words used by patients to describe their breathlessness. Words that are emotionally laden, such as 'choking' or 'drowning', may indicate psychological or existential (spiritual) distress accompanying the physical symptom. A cancer dyspnoea scale has been developed that uses such words in order to separate the physical and psychological impact of breathlessness (Tanaka et al., 2000). Some researchers have tried to identify patterns of words that point to specific causes, but this is not reliable enough to make an accurate diagnosis.

For most patients who are breathless, it is helpful to consider some form of investigation. This should ideally be non-invasive, quick and easy for the patient to complete and cheap to perform, and should help to:

- confirm the clinical diagnosis;
- assess the severity;
- estimate implications for survival;
- identify any additional complicating factors that could interfere with the treatment plan;
- monitor progress after starting treatment.

'Routine' tests such as chest X-rays or blood counts cannot be justified, even though this is tempting when one is stuck for 'something to do', or even when the patient demands investigation. In the latter case, the proper response should be to explore why the patient (or often, the carer) feels that further tests are required – is he or she dissatisfied with the present care or anticipating worse problems; is there a gen eral reluctance to accept the advancing nature of the disease?

The tests that are helpful in elucidating the causes of breathlessness and in advising on rational treatments are shown in Table 3.3. The most useful and practical are chest X-rays, a full blood count (for the haemoglobin level) and pulse oximetry, which is a non-invasive way of checking peripheral blood oxygenation. The X-ray and haemoglobin concentration will help in determining any pulmonary, pleural and cardiac causes and will show or exclude anaemia as a contributing factor. Pulse oximetry is relatively underused in palliative care, and the cost of acquiring a portable instrument may be a problem for many services. It may however, be possible to gain access to one through a local pulmonary medicine department. The sensors are placed on the fingertip or ear

Table 3.3 Investigations that may be useful in assessing the breathless patient

- Full blood count

- Chest X-ray

- Pulse oximetry – a useful bedside non-invasive method for monitoring oxygen saturation. It is very valuable in both the hospice and the home setting, but its limitations should be borne in mind. It can be misleading in hypercapnic respiratory failure

- ECG

- Sputum culture

- Ultrasound scan of the thorax to differentiate collapse from effusion and to localize an effusion for aspiration

- Echocardiogram if a pericardial effusion is suspected

- Pulmonary functions tests – limited use in palliative care but may be of use in monitoring progress after treatment, such as radiotherapy. The peak flow rate is of value only in assessing asthma or bronchitis

- A high-resolution computed tomography scan may be useful in defining pulmonary pathology more accurately, e.g. to diagnose lymphangitis carcinomatosa

- Ventilation–perfusion scan – an important test for the diagnosis of pulmonary embolism

- Flexible bronchoscopy – useful in patients with haemoptysis or stridor

- Bronchoscopy and computed tomography scanning may be useful if considering an endobronchial stent or laser therapy

lobe and can give a continuous reading at rest or during activity. The benefit of pulse oximetry is twofold – a low oxygenation (<90 per cent saturation) indicates that oxygen treatment may be useful (see below), and the technique also gives patients immediate feedback and reassurance if the oxygen saturation is within normal limits.

TREATMENT

GENERAL PRINCIPLES

The principles of treating breathlessness are similar to those involved in any other symptom in palliative care:

- The treatment should wherever possible be based on a sound clinical diagnosis, backed up if appropriate by investigations.
- The ideal treatment is one that directly tackles the pathological cause of the symptom.

- The least invasive and potentially least 'toxic' treatment should be tried first, unless the severity of the situation demands aggressive intervention.
- The patient and usually the carers should be informed of the reasons behind the treatment plan.
- If there is a choice of methods to tackle the symptom the patient and, if appropriate, the carers should be involved in the final decision.

In the management of breathlessness, there has been a strong shift in recent years towards multi-disciplinary decision-making, the important role of nurses and physiotherapists having been highlighted (Bredin, 1999; Thompson, 2000). As discussed above, non-medical members of the team who are close to the patient and carers may form a better impression of the severity and impact of the symptom, and may be able to place this in the context of their overall needs, than may the doctors, who may sometimes see the problem in isolation. Working together, the best treatment decisions may be reached and offered to patients. The full range of approaches that can be helpful in reducing breathlessness in cancer patients are outlined in Box 3.2. These approaches will now be discussed in detail.

BOX 3.2 OVERVIEW OF TREATMENTS FOR BREATHLESSNESS IN CANCER PATIENTS

Anti-cancer therapy	Radiotherapy
	– external
	– endobronchial
	Chemotherapy
	Hormone manipulation
	Surgery
Physical methods	Pleural aspiration
	Pericardial drainage and window
	Airways stenting
	Superior vena caval obstruction stenting
Pharmacological	
• Drugs	Bronchodilators
	Diuretics
	Antibiotics
	Anticoagulants
	Sedatives
	Opioids
	Stimulants
	Steroids
	Saline

BOX 3.2 (*Continued*)

• Routes	Oral
	Inhaled
	Parenteral
Airflow	Fan
	Open window
	Air via a mask
Oxygen	Helium/oxygen
Breathing control and posture	
Psychological	Relaxation
	Massage
Complementary therapies	Acupuncture, etc.
Combination therapies	Multi-disciplinary teamwork
	Nurse-led clinic

CANCER-DIRECTED THERAPIES

Observing the principles above, it is crucial with cancer patients first to know whether the symptom is related to the malignant process or is the result of a co-existing condition or even the side-effect of a previous therapy. If the cause is believed to be cancer related, the best interventions are those aimed directly at this. There is ample evidence that, for lung cancer, radiotherapy can relieve respiratory symptoms such as cough, haemoptysis and dyspnoea, often with a single or two fractions of radiation, with minimal side-effects (Bisset, 1996; Hoskins and Makin, 1998). Both small cell and non-small cell types of lung cancer respond to such treatments, although the response is usually more dramatic with the former. Cancers from other primary sites should also be considered for radiotherapy to reduce respiratory symptoms.

Modern palliative regimes are designed to minimize the patient's need to attend the local radiotherapy centre, but some patients may even then not be fit enough or willing to travel for this option. Radiotherapy can be given conventionally by external beam or can in some centres be directed straight onto the tumour in the bronchus by means of a radioactive source placed into the lung via a bronchoscope. The latter technique is called brachytherapy; it can provide good relief from symptoms but is limited by the availability of the equipment and the patient's ability to tolerate bronchoscopy (Snape and Robinson, 1996). An alternative approach to brachytherapy is direct necrosis of the tumour by endobronchial laser therapy. This has fewer side-effects than radiation but is available in only a small number of centres.

For selected cancers, cytotoxic chemotherapy – given by intravenous injection – can be very effective in relieving respiratory symptoms (Hoskins and Makin, 1998). Small cell lung cancer is the most responsive to this approach, but recent studies show that even non-small cell lung cancer, which was previously thought to be 'chemoresistant', may respond to the newer agents such as gemcitabine (Anderson et al., 2000). Other malignancies that may respond well to chemotherapy include thoracic metastases from breast, colorectal and kidney cancers. However, chemotherapy carries a high burden of side-effects and the need to travel, and may, for cost reasons, be limited in availability.

Hormone therapy is effectively restricted to hormone-sensitive tumours, namely breast and prostate cancers. In both of these, there have been significant advances in recent years in the use of endocrine manipulations that can modify the progress of the disease (Hoskins and Makin, 1998). Hormonal therapies are generally slower to act than radiotherapy or chemotherapy but may be valuable in the relief of symptoms in hormone receptor-positive breast cancer. It should be noted that not all breast cancers are hormone sensitive, and the impact of hormone therapy becomes less as the disease advances. With prostate cancer, there may be a fairly rapid relief of some symptoms, such as bone pain, with hormone manipulations that reduce or eliminate testosterone. If the lungs are involved with metastatic prostate cancer, it is possible that endocrine therapy may be helpful in relieving the symptoms. However, as with breast cancer, not all prostate cancers are hormone sensitive, and any sensitivity reduces as the disease progresses.

SURGICAL AND PHYSICAL INTERVENTIONS

Effusions

Pleural effusions are usually dealt with by simple percutaneous drainage via a needle, placed between the lower ribs, and attached to a syringe. Larger effusions may be left to drain slowly by leaving in an indwelling intercostal catheter, connected externally to a drainage bottle. In some patients, the effusion recurs frequently over days or weeks. It is possible to inject drugs such as tetracycline or bleomycin into the pleural space after draining it, which usually stops further fluid production by causing the visceral and parietal pleurae to fibrose together.

In some cases however, even instilling interpleural drugs cannot prevent the fluid reaccumulating. In other cases, the effusion becomes loculated, which means that it is broken up into several compartments in the pleural space; it is not feasible, or kind to the patient, to drain all of these by multiple percutaneous needling. Surgery is not usually thought of as a palliative intervention, but it may be of value in these specific situations. Through a small thoracic incision, a surgeon can insert a thoracoscope and directly view the pleural space, break down the fibrous divisions between the loculated pockets and leave behind a larger intercostal drain. Although more invasive, this can be a more successful and ultimately more satisfactory procedure for the patient.

Surgery can also be invaluable in the rare condition of pericardial effusion. This is normally associated with extreme breathlessness, such that patients can hardly speak. With direct imaging via an echocardiograph or CT scan, a cardiologist or radiologist can drain a pericardial effusion via a needle and catheter externally. If however, the pericardial effusion recurs, it may be preferable, via a surgical approach, to cut a small 'window' in the pericardial wall so that the fluid can flow directly out into the pleural space, where the relatively small volume has less symptomatic effect.

Airways stenting

As mentioned above, the normal approach to reducing the effect of a tumour that is partially or totally blocking a bronchus or partially occluding the trachea itself is radiotherapy and, in certain tumour types, chemotherapy. These options are not available for some patients, for example in the presence of very poor lung function caused by smoking and bronchitis. Giving radiotherapy to such a patient might be beneficial for the tumour but could aggravate the existing lung bronchitic damage, and the resulting lung function could be worse, rather than better, than before treatment. Even after radiotherapy or chemotherapy, the tumour may regrow, and in most cases it is usually not possible to offer another dose of the same treatment, again because of the risk of damage to other tissues.

In these situations, endobronchial stenting is a very useful option. A stent is a metal or silicone device that fits into a hollow organ – usually a tubular structure – in the body and acts as an internal support to keep the tube open. Stents can be placed in many body sites, such as the gall bladder duct, the ureter or the airways. The usual indication for a stent is a partial or complete intrinsic obstruction by a tumour or external compression by lymph glands. In the airways, stents are called endobronchial if they are placed in the larger bronchi, and endotracheal if placed in the trachea. Stents have to be placed via a bronchoscope, so the patient must be fit and willing enough to undergo this procedure. The results can be dramatic: within hours the blocked airway is opened, the spring-loaded design of the metal stents allowing for more gradual opening over the following days.

One example of the successful use of a stent is that of a patient whose lung was collapsed by a tumour blocking the right main bronchus. The placement of a stent over the tumour lead to the total reopening of the airway and re-expansion of the lung 24 hours later. The patient experienced an immediate relief of severe breathlessness. The results may not always be so startling, the best results generally being obtained if the stent is placed early, preferably within days of the airway becoming blocked. The side-effects of having an endobronchial or endotracheal stent are surprisingly few apart from an irritable cough; this can be usually managed by an opioid cough suppressant such as codeine or low-dose morphine.

Vascular stenting

Stents can also be placed under radiographic imaging into various vascular structures, a potential site in the relief of breathlessness being the superior vena cava, which is occluded in SVCO syndrome, described above. If the occlusion does not respond to the standard treatment of radiotherapy or chemotherapy, a stent can help to open up the vascular channel and improve the blood flow back to the heart. This can have immediate benefit in terms of reducing the visible swelling of the face and upper limbs, but the breathlessness may not improve unless the patient is also anticoagulated to reduce the thrombus that has gathered in the sluggish flow of the occluded vein. Anticoagulation with oral aspirin may be adequate for some patients, but others may require heparin and warfarin.

PHARMACOLOGICAL APPROACHES

In the majority of cases, even if the anti-cancer and physical or surgical procedures described above are being used, the management of breathlessness depends largely on rational pharmacological treatment, using a combination of drugs acting on different mechanisms of the symptom production and experience. There are several drugs that can be helpful for the breathless cancer patient, summarised in Box 3.2 above. In overview, the approaches can be classified into the following categories of drug that work:

- on the airways
- on the lungs
- on the cardiovascular system
- on the perception of dyspnoea
- in non-specific or unknown ways.

Airways

Many of the patients with cancer – especially primary lung cancer – who are breathless because of thoracic disease may also have chronic airways disease. This can take the form of asthma or bronchitis. It is important to review the airways function of such patients and, if there is a reversible element to the airflow obstruction, to consider a bronchodilator. There are several types of bronchodilator, which are best explored in a respiratory medical text. The most commonly used are the beta-adrenergic stimulators (such as salbutamol) and the anticholinergic drugs (such as ipratropium), both of which are easily taken by most patients via inhalers or nebulizers.

Corticosteroids are also powerful bronchodilators in asthma and bronchitis. Drugs such as beclomethasone or budesonide can be taken by inhaler or nebulizer, and prednisolone or dexamethasone by mouth or injection. Because of the powerful adverse effects of steroids, they must be reserved for patients with asthma or bronchitis who fail to respond to the previous bronchodilators alone. One scenario in which a steroid could be prescribed in a non-asthmatic patient is acute severe stridor arising from a partial tracheal occlusion; in this situation a subcutaneous injection of dexamethasone could be extremely valuable while the patient is awaiting radiotherapy, chemotherapy or the placement of a tracheal stent. (Corticosteroids will be discussed again below in view of their widespread actions.)

A final type of bronchodilator is the aminophylline group of drugs, which are taken orally but can also be given intravenously in extreme situations, for example an allergic reaction with severe airways obstruction.

Diuretics

It is easy to overlook dyspnoea related to heart failure in the breathless cancer patient. This is particularly likely to arise in older patients and those who have a history of cardiac disease and then develop cancer. The management of cardiac failure is a complex topic, and the reader should refer to a cardiology text. Briefly, the most important drugs that can be beneficial in terms of reducing breathlessness are the diuretics. Low-dose bendrofluazide, followed by frusemide if the patient does not respond, may be very helpful in an older patient who has developed ankle swelling and increasing breathlessness. Some patients may become acutely breathless iatrogenically by inadvertent fluid overload from a blood transfusion, and in this case intravenous frusemide may be rapidly effective.

Anticoagulants

As described above, patients may become breathless if they have recurrent or large single pulmonary emboli, or if they develop SVCO with thrombosis in the superior vena cava or other blocked veins. Anticoagulation with aspirin may be sufficient to prevent further thrombosis forming in patients who have a stent placed in the superior vena cava. The decision of whether to start anticoagulant therapy with heparin and/or warfarin is very difficult in cancer patients. The risk of bleeding from overanticoagulation can be severe, particularly if the patient has a previous tendency towards haemoptysis. In older people, the danger of intracerebral bleeding also has to be weighed up. On the other hand, with careful regular blood checks and advice to patients and carers, anticoagulation may contribute to a reduction in breathlessness, especially when all other approaches have been tried.

Antibiotics

In a patient in the early stage of cancer, there can be little doubt that a pulmonary infection such as bronchitis or pneumonia should be treated with antibiotics. These help to reduce cough, sputum production, haemoptysis if the bronchial bleeding is related to an infective cough, and breathlessness. The situation is not, however, so clear in the advanced stage of the disease, especially when the patient is 'terminally ill'. It used to be said that pneumonia was 'the old man's friend', implying that a sick elderly person could slip away into unconsciousness and death fairly comfortably with a progressive pneumonia. Many now would challenge that view, which was probably coloured by the frustration of witnessing a person suffering pain and other unrelieved symptoms in the days before modern cancer symptom control.

There is debate over whether antibiotics given to a very ill person who is going to die anyway of advanced cancer will *ease* the suffering by reducing cough and breathless or *add to* the suffering by the requirement to take more medication and perhaps running the risk of prolonging the dying phase. This is as much a moral as a medical or pharmacological argument. Ideally, patients' own views should be respected as they may have experience of the benefits of previous antibiotic courses if they have had chronic lung disease, or they may make it clear that they do not wish further medical 'meddling'.

Opioids

This group of drugs is arguably the most useful, and also probably the least well understood, of those involved in the management of breathlessness. Those which occur naturally in the opium poppy include morphine and papaveretum, and are called *opiates*. All natural opiates, as well as the synthetic drugs such as diamorphine, codeine, dihydrocodeine, tramadol, fentanyl, hydromorphone and oxycodone, are referred to as *opioids*.

Opioids work by binding to the opioid receptors that are found in many parts of the body, especially the central nervous system and also the peripheral nerves. In these tissues, opioid receptors are intimately linked to the pathways for pain perception and modulation. They are also present in the intestinal tract and are probably responsible there for the constipating effect of the opioid drugs. Opioid receptors have been found in the lungs and the airways; it is not clear what their role is here, but there is no evidence that they are, in man, in any way related to the sensation of breathing (Ahmedzai, 1998). Opioid receptors are found in the medulla oblongata of the brain, in the 'respiratory centre'. Nearby, they are also found in the 'cough centre', which explains why opioids are useful in the suppression of cough.

It is the opioid receptors in the respiratory centre that are probably responsible for the important therapeutic benefits of opioids in the management of breathlessness. We previously emphasized the important role of the respiratory centre in the detection of small changes in the level of circulating carbon dioxide (or rather the acidity or pH of the blood). This is called the carbon dioxide drive to ventilation and is much more important in normal individuals than the oxygen drive. In any situation in which the respiratory system starts to fail (even after a voluntary breath-hold), less carbon dioxide is expired, which is immediately detected by the respiratory centre; the result is that the brain is aware of the need to take more breaths. If the respiratory centre could be rendered less sensitive, small increases in carbon dioxide could be tolerated without the individual feeling the need to breathe harder. This is the principle by which it is thought many drugs act to reduce the sensation of breathlessness.

Several types of drug can in fact reduce the carbon dioxide sensitivity of the respiratory centre (or, to put it another way, can diminish ventilatory drive). Sedatives such as benzodiazepines and barbiturates, the opioids and even alcohol reduce the ventilatory drive (Ahmedzai, 1998); this is why these drugs are dangerous in overdose. In therapeutics, we talk of 'respiratory depression' when any of these drugs inadvertently reduces the ventilatory drive to a worrying level. The propensity of opioids to reduce carbon dioxide sensitivity is the main reason why the old-fashioned teaching of doctors has for so long perpetuated the myth that morphine is dangerous for terminally ill patients. In reality, any of the stated classes of drug are potentially dangerous, but the answer is to use the drugs carefully and by titration rather than omiting them altogether and denying patients their potential benefits.

Opioids actually work in breathless patients by more than one mechanism. They can reduce carbon dioxide sensitivity, as just described. In addition, in acute left ventricular failure, they can help by temporarily reducing ('off-loading') the volume of blood returning to the failing heart. If the patient's breathing is compromised by pain, such as after thoracic surgery or with a chest wall tumour, the analgesic action of an opioid can remove that factor. Finally, and very importantly, the stronger opioids have a cerebral sedative effect and a calming (anxiolytic) action that helps to protect the patient from the fear of dyspnoea, even if the pathology remains unchanged.

Most research on the action of opioids on breathing has been conducted in COPD, and only in recent years has it been studied in cancer patients. To summarise the research, there is good evidence (Wilcock, 1998) that:

- codeine is of little value for breathlessness;
- dihydrocodeine can help patients with COPD breathlessness (but with considerable side-effects);
- morphine is of value in cancer patients but of dubious value in COPD;
- diamorphine has not been shown to be superior to morphine;
- hydromorphones is helpful in cancer.

There is a lack of evidence on the other opioids now used in cancer care for pain control, namely fentanyl, tramadol, oxycodone and methadone. These may well be helpful for relieving breathlessness, but there is at present no scientific basis for recommending them.

How should one use opioids in the management of breathlessness? The rules for this indication are not nearly as clear as those for pain control. It seems sensible, and safe, to use small doses (e.g. 5 mg) of morphine every 4 hours in patients who have not been exposed to strong opioids before. The timing could be 'as required' for patients who are breathless only intermittently, for example on exertion, or it could be regular for those who are breathless more or less continuously. For an elderly or a very small person, or if there is a history of respiratory disease and therefore a risk of respiratory depression, the starting dose should be 2.5 mg morphine. The drug is best given orally as a liquid or tablet in an 'immediate' or 'normal' release form.

Unless one is very familiar with using these drugs, there is a danger in starting a breathless patient straight away on a modified-release oral formulation, which can induce toxicity and respiratory depression if the chosen dose is too high. Similarly, it is unsafe to start a breathless patient on a transdermal fentanyl patch without having first titrated the dose upwards using normal-release morphine.

These comments are, of course, no different from the cautious approach to starting patients on morphine for pain control.

But what if the patient who becomes breathless is already taking morphine or a similar strong opioid for his or her pain? There is unfortunately, little research evidence to guide the practitioner here. It has been shown that increasing the 4-hourly morphine dose by 50 per cent can be effective and safe if the patient has previously been stable on morphine. For a patient on a modified-release, oral, strong opioid, or a transdermal fentanyl patch, it would seem prudent to start a new titration of normal-release morphine or an equivalent opioid, given 4-hourly or as required until the desired effect has been reached.

There is a delicate balance in using opioids for breathlessness, one that hangs between achieving the relief of this symptom and producing other adverse effects (especially sedation) and possibly respiratory depression. The latter should arise only in patients who have a known poor respiratory history or if the dose has been increased in a careless way. Many patients find that the extra burden of side-effects is not worth the trouble of taking a higher dose of morphine for breathlessness. Others may find it best to use the extra dose judiciously, when their breathing is most under pressure, for example when going for a walk or taking a bath.

There has been considerable interest in palliative care, as in respiratory medicine, in the role of nebulized drugs for the relief of breathlessness (Ahmedzai and Davis, 1997). Because of the huge absorptive area of the airways and their high permeability, drugs delivered by nebulizer enter the blood stream very quickly and act almost like a parenteral injection, which can be helpful for those who cannot reliably take oral medication.

Although early studies in COPD patients pointed to potentially powerful benefits from nebulized morphine, subsequent controlled and randomized trials have either failed to show any advantage of this route or demonstrated little discernible effect (Davis 1999). It was at first postulated that nebulized morphine could be working on the opioid receptors in the lung airways, but, as pointed out above, there is no experimental evidence that these are in fact involved in the sensation or modulation of breathlessness. Furthermore, most clinical experience suggests that when benefit is observed, it occurs when there is evidence of sedation and other signs to suggest that the drug is acting centrally, in the brain.

Some people, especially asthmatics, may respond badly to nebulized morphine because it can cause bronchospasm. For this reason, we recommend always giving a test dose of a nebulized opioid under supervision, with a bronchodilator, epinephrine and corticosteroids at hand. Fentanyl is a potent opioid that does not have the same intrinsic tendency to cause bronchospasm, so is our favoured drug. A starting dose of morphine in a patient not already receiving this drug orally is 25 mg, made up in 4–5 ml saline. With fentanyl, 25 μg in 4–5 ml saline is advised.

When is it reasonable to use nebulized opioids in palliative care? In our experience, few patients will need to use this route, but it can be very helpful for some.

It is better accepted by patients who are already familiar with nebulizer usage for the control of asthma. Patients who have paroxysmal episodes of dyspnoea, for example from suspected or known recurrent pulmonary emboli, or those prone to waking up panicking with pulmonary congestion, may find the rapid calming effect of morphine very useful. This is particularly important for patients at home, in a nursing home or in a small community hospital where medical help is not at hand and it may take time to summon trained nurses who can administer an injection of morphine.

At home, the presence of a carer who can fetch the drug and prepare the nebulizer is of course required. However, a positive effect of using this route is that carers and patients can feel more in control of the medication – and hence the symptom – and can learn to deal with occasional respiratory crises without calling for nursing or medical help. Even if they hardly ever use the nebulizer at home for delivering an opioid, it can be very reassuring to a family to have this technology sitting in the house.

Sedatives

Apart from the opioids, other drugs used in palliative care may be used to calm the psychological aspects of breathlessness. Thus, benzodiazepines such as lorazepam or diazepam may be used orally, although it is best to avoid the latter because of its long half-life and consequent risk of 'hangover'. Small doses of lorazepam (0.5–1.0 mg) may be given on an 'as required' basis or twice a day for patients who are frequently breathless. For dealing with the acute crises of respiratory panic, subcutaneous or intravenous midazolam is the drug of choice. In the terminal stage, midazolam is well suited to being given as a continuous subcutaneous infusion, as long as the dose is reviewed every day in relation to the patient's symptom relief and overall level of sedation.

Other drugs that may be useful for reducing anxiety related to dyspnoea include the phenothazines (e.g. low-dose levomepromazine) and haloperidol. There is no research evidence to support this usage, but these drugs are frequently employed by specialists in palliative care who are aware of their benefits and limitations.

As mentioned above, these non-opioid sedative drugs also have the ability to reduce carbon dioxide sensitivity and may therefore act like morphine in reducing the awareness of dyspnoea caused by failing ventilatory function. The disadvantage they then share with the opioids is that they may, in vulnerable individuals, run the risk of respiratory depression. This is particularly an issue when midazolam is being used in a syringe driver for general sedation in terminally ill patients: there is a delicate balance here between reducing anxiety and the awareness of suffering, and precipitating respiratory depression and accelerating death.

Nebulized saline

It may seem odd to mention nebulizing normal saline (0.9 per cent sodium chloride solution) in the context of potent drugs such as morphine and midazolam, but there is considerable clinical experience and some limited research evidence that nebulized saline can help the sensation of breathlessness. How this occurs is not understood, but it may work by:

- moistening the tracheal and bronchial mucosa and dried secretions, making it easier to expectorate the latter and clear the airways;
- encouraging the patient to slow down the breathing rate and concentrate on deeper breaths;
- the stimulation of receptors thought to reduce the perception of breathlessness by the flow of compressed air past the cheeks and nose when using a face mask.

It is worth trying to use nebulized saline for a patient who is breathless and also has trouble coughing as this technique may help both symptoms.

Oxygen

We have indicated above that a lack of oxygen is a relatively weak stimulus for breathing compared with an excess of carbon dioxide in the blood. In normal life, it is unusual to experience a significant lack of oxygen in the inspired air – except if one climbs very high mountains, when extra oxygen needs to be carried. Modern aeroplanes are pressurized and have sufficient oxygen in their air to be quite safe for most patients with cancer who become breathless on land.

In some diseases, the normally thin barrier between the air in the lung alveoli and the blood in the adjacent capillaries, which allows for the easy transfer of oxygen, may become thickened and present a barrier to diffusion. Such a barrier can arise when there is excess fluid in the lungs, as in heart failure or lymphangitis carcinomatosa. Thickening can also follow the inflammatory reaction to radiotherapy or with chemotherapy agents such as bleomycin. Infectious pneumonia also increases the diffusion barrier.

Oxygen transfer is also compromised in patients with advanced COPD and emphysema because of the extensive loss of lung tissue. In all these situations, there may be a genuine oxygen deficit in the blood (hypoxaemia), which can impinge on breathing control and manifest itself as dyspnoea. Patients are initially breathless only on exertion, but at a more advanced level, they are breathless at rest. A characteristic of such patients is that they become centrally cyanosed, that is, the mucosa of the mouth becomes blue. (This should not be confused with peripheral cyanosis, when the fingertips become blue, as this can arise in normally oxygenated people because of circulatory problems.)

It is relatively easy to monitor the level of blood oxygenation with pulse oximetry, as described above. Normal people have a resting oxygen saturation (SaO_2), measured through the skin, of over 95 per cent. When the SaO_2 dips below 90 per cent at rest or on exertion, most people will feel breathless. Some patients with chronic lung disease can however, tolerate a lower level, and with more advanced disease, there is in general a poor correlation between the oxygen saturation and the level of dyspnoea present.

Skin oximetry often reveals that patients who become genuinely breathless at rest or on exertion, and may even reveal peripheral cyanosis, do *not* desaturate their blood oxygen level. It is most helpful to tell this to the patient and carers, who often expect that oxygen therapy should be started. In such cases, another cause for the breathlessness must be found and conveyed to the patient.

Studies of cancer patients who are dyspnoeic at rest have shown that supplemental oxygen therapy can be helpful as long as there is significant desaturation (Wilcock, 1998). In patients who maintain a normal SaO_2 level of 95 per cent or above, there is evidence that giving the patient unlabelled compressed air to breathe can be just as helpful as giving oxygen. There are at least two reasons for this: first, there is undoubtedly a 'placebo' value in having a gas that the patient believes is oxygen and second, the increased gas flow around the face may give a true reduction in the sensation of dyspnoea.

We therefore recommend that, wherever possible, patients have their SaO_2 tested first breathing room air at rest and then on mild exertion such as walking at a normal pace for 5 minutes, both with and without oxygen. Only if there is observable desaturation that responds to oxygen should this gas be prescribed. If a pulse oximeter is not available, it is reasonable to give the patient a short clinical trial of oxygen while making a firm decision to review this within a few days.

Patients should be instructed to use the oxygen at first on an 'as required' basis rather than continuously. They and their carers should learn to place the oxygen mask on immediately the exertion comes to an end (unless there is a portable canister or long flexible piping for use during exertion around the house) and to take it off as soon as the breathing comes back to 'normal'. There is no evidence that, unless the patient is genuinely hypoxaemic, continuous oxygen therapy is of any advantage (as it may be, in contrast, with selected COPD patients).

The side-effects of oxygen therapy should not be overlooked. Apart from becoming psychologically dependent on the gas, the use of a face mask or mouth piece can impede conversation, prevent drinking and dry out the oral mucosa. Nasal prongs are better but may still dry the nose and become uncomfortable after a time. The cost of oxygen therapy should not be forgotten.

There is recent evidence that adding helium to the oxygen can result in a lighter gas that is easier for the chest to inhale (Ahmedzai, 1998). This can be very valuable for patients with severe airflow obstruction, such as in acute severe asthma attacks, and it may also be helpful for cancer patients who have endobronchial obstruction or tired, failing chest wall muscles. Further research is needed on helium/oxygen mixtures as well as on identifying better which patients can benefit from conventional oxygen or possibly compressed air therapy.

NON-MEDICAL MANAGEMENT

In the management of breathlessness, there is much scope for doing good without recourse to the medical interventions described above. Nurses, physiotherapists, psychologists and other non-medical members of the palliative care team should be empowered to make their professional contributions in such a way that each patient receives the package of care that suits him or her best. Non-medical approaches should be considered from the very beginning and should not be relegated to second- or third-line management when anti-cancer and drug therapies have failed. The patient and carers should ideally be involved in the decision-making process to determine the best combination of therapies, this being frequently reviewed.

Breathing control and posture

There is considerable experience in respiratory medicine and physiotherapy of the value of teaching patients with chronic lung disease the correct way to sit, stand and bend, and how to be in control of their breathing patterns in these positions. Such training is part of the pulmonary rehabilitation programme for patients with COPD. Nurses have in recent years adopted these techniques and applied them successfully also to cancer patients (Corner et al., 1996; Bredin, 1999). It is important to explain the action of the chest wall muscles and the diaphragm in moving the thorax, and then to show how certain positions can use these to best advantage. Patients with advanced COPD and emphysema, for example, who have hyperexpanded 'barrel-shaped' chests find it helpful to sit up, leaning forwards and, by resting the elbows on a table in front of them, to use the muscles of the shoulders to pull the chest up.

Some patients may indeed find it ideal to remain in a sitting or a semi-sitting position, especially if there is a history of episodes of pulmonary congestion resulting from heart failure. This may require that the patient be nursed in a reclining armchair rather than a bed. This is usually straightforward in hospital, but it may be problematic at home.

For the reasons discussed above, a patient who is breathless often finds it comforting to have cool air flow past the face, stimulating the facial and nasal receptors. This can be achieved by positioning the chair or bed by a window that can be opened, or by placing a fan on a table at the same height as the face. The speed and distance of the fan should be adjusted so that there is a gentle flow rather than a wind that can 'take the breath away' from very frail people!

Many patients find that bending causes an increase in breathlessness, this usually being related to temporary splinting of the diaphragm as a result of increased abdominal muscle tension. As the diaphragm is an important muscle for maintaining ventilation, this can cause too much limitation, even for a few seconds. It is helpful to provide aids to allow such people to reach for dropped items. Aids to help putting on socks and shoes will also help, especially if there is not always a carer at hand.

Other texts give further details of the specific breathing techniques that can help breathless patients to gain mastery over their chest movements and breathing patterns (Bredin, 1999). Although attempts have been made in COPD patients to improve breathing by yoga-based breathing control, there is no published experience with this in cancer.

Psychological and behavioural techniques

Interest has also been growing in the use of various psychological techniques in assisting patients who are breathless with either cancer or COPD. These methods vary from simple relaxation training to formal progressive muscle relaxation and more complex techniques (Bredin, 1999; Pan et al., 2000). The reader is again advised to consult specific texts for these approaches, which are essentially the same for the psychological and behavioural control of any psychosomatically influenced symptom.

Massage is another therapy that many patients find relaxing and comforting. There is no evidence that the use of specific aromatic oils, as in aromatherapy, has any advantage over massage with simple lubricants. The areas usually massaged are the feet, hands and shoulders. It is important to settle breathless patients into a comfortable position that will not compromise their breathing. If the chest wall muscles are weak, the shoulders should not be massaged in such a way as to restrict their contribution to breathing. If the patient has swollen ankles or legs, it is essential to exclude venous thrombosis before starting to massage them or the feet in case the added pressure could dislodge part of a thrombus and release it to the lungs.

It is important that practitioners should be aware of these approaches as patients are becoming increasingly sophisticated in finding out about them through various information sources, in particular the Internet. Some cancer patients may be tempted to pay for private counselling and psychological support, but such therapies should ideally be available in cancer centres and other units that treat cancer patients, for example hospices and day centres, and through home-care teams.

Complementary therapies

Some of the techniques mentioned above may be regarded as 'alternative' or 'complementary' therapies by strictly orthodox medical practitioners. It is important to distinguish between the two and to recognize when appropriate therapies that are not acknowledged by traditional medicine may play a part in easing patients' distress. There is no doubt that the public is increasingly interested in and availing itself of these approaches; sadly for patients, the cost of most of these has to be borne by those who may already have financial difficulties as a result of the illness.

Alternative therapies are those which stand quite separate from Western medicine and indeed may reject it, the patient often having to choose between one and the other (Whitlock, 1999). In the UK and many other developed countries, however, *complementary therapies* offer the public and patients the opportunity to continue with conventional, anti-cancer or other palliative treatments as well as to participate in non-conventional therapies. Thus complementary, but not alternative, therapies can be encouraged in cancer care.

A recent systematic review (Pan et al., 2000) of complementary therapies has found research-based evidence of benefit to cancer and/or COPD patients with breathlessness from several complementary therapies. Although some of the studies are small in comparison to those which are normally required to prove benefit with new drug therapies, there is merit in considering:

- acupuncture
- acupressure

- progressive muscle relaxation
- a nurse-facilitated programme of breathing re-training with counselling, relaxation and the teaching of coping strategies.

The last approach has excited considerable interest in the cancer field, as the study that demonstrated the benefit of the combined package was conducted using a conventional medical randomized controlled trial design (Bredin et al., 1999).

Multi-disciplinary teamwork

It seems almost unnecessary to state that the management of the breathless patient and his or her carers should be based on multi-disciplinary lines. Even with the advent of multi-disciplinary teams in cancer centres and clinics, it is however, likely that decisions about symptom control are still usually made by doctors or nurses in isolation. Ideally, as with palliative care teams, the patient's full history should be presented and discussed so that respiratory symptoms are seen in relation to other problems. Decisions to investigate or to start therapeutic trials of new approaches should be made jointly by team members and relayed promptly to patients so that their views are included before therapy begins.

The nurse-facilitated combined approach to the breathless cancer patient mentioned above has led to the development of specific clinics in the UK to which cancer patients are invited. This is clearly a step forward from the situation of cancer patients' needs being ignored. It is, however, important that the true multi-disciplinary nature of palliative care is not lost in the enthusiasm to set up these single-symptom clinics. It would be a pity to deprive patients of the potential benefits of some of the medical therapies discussed above by concentrating too heavily on a nurse-led approach. On the other hand, it is the duty of nurses and other non-medical clinicians to ensure that the medical approach does not dominate, to the detriment of holistic patient care.

MONITORING AND COMMUNITY CARE

Much of the preceding discussion has, by stressing the need for appropriate investigations and specific therapies, including anti-cancer treatments, focused on the 'acute' phase of the patient's illness and symptom management. Even with lung cancer, which sadly has a relatively short life expectancy, most patients will, however, spend the greatest part of their cancer illness at home. It is vital for good palliative care that investigations and hospital-based treatments are organized in such as way as to minimize the time spent away from the home and family.

Treatments started in acute settings, including palliative care units and hospices, need to be monitored once the patient goes home. Many services have outreach teams or liase with community-based services. The primary care team should of course be fully informed about investigations, new treatments and any changes in the current medication or doses. The community-based palliative care team could be the ideal route for conveying this information, but in some areas it is practical for hospital and hospice units to communicate directly with the primary care team.

Patients who are breathless frequently develop crises and may have panic attacks, which are often unpredictable. It is helpful if they have access to a 'hot-line', which could be the telephone number of the local cancer unit or hospice, or of the community palliative care team. In many urban areas, out-of-hours primary care services are regrettably less than ideally co-ordinated, and patients may demand a way to bypass this and seek help from those whom they consider to be the 'experts' in dealing with their problem.

As carers are essential in continuing the medical and other regimes when the patient is at home, it is also relevant to ensure that they too have access to information and support – both to enable them to care more effectively and to meet their own psychological and social needs.

TERMINAL CARE

By 'terminal care' we mean the palliative care of patients dying with cancer in the last few hours, days or weeks of their life. The management of breathlessness is in general terms the same during this stage as in the early phase of the cancer. Some specific points should however, be emphasised, these reflecting the physiological, psychosocial and existential needs of dying cancer patients and their families or friends.

It is often said that the preferred place of dying with cancer is the patient's own home, but this is in reality heavily influenced by the physical circumstances of the terminal illness, being breathless being one of the factors that may indicate the need to admit the patient to hospital or a hospice. It is extremely frightening for a patient to be gasping for breath or to have episodes of choking or drowning in secretions. This rebounds onto the carers, who may find it difficult to witness such distress. It should not be regarded as a failure if such a patient has to be admitted from home in the terminal stage of the illness.

Because of the fear of choking, a terminal patient with breathless attacks should ideally never be left alone or at least without some means of summoning help, such as a bell or buzzer. If the patient is at home, it is reassuring to have the telephone number of the community nursing staff, who can attend in a short time or give advice by telephone. Many caring general practitioners give such families their home or mobile telephone number so that they do not have to call the emergency services.

Nursing care is of paramount importance in this situation, and there should be special attention to the details already mentioned, such as:

- arranging the patient in the most comfortable position (often in a reclining chair);
- keeping a window open or having a fan on the table;
- regular saline nebulization to assist with expectoration and to keep the airways moist, especially if supplemental oxygen is being used;
- massage or other forms of personal contact that the patient finds comforting and relaxing.

If the patient is having frequent episodes of panicky breathless attacks, it is worth considering setting up a continuous subcutaneous infusion of midazolam and, if the patient is already receiving a strong opioid, adding morphine or diamorphine to this. In a normal-sized adult patient who has not previously had a benzodiazepine sedative, a reasonable starting dose of midazolam is 20 mg per 24 hours. For an elderly or cachectic person, or one who is at special risk of respiratory depression, this dose should be halved, and a test dose of midazolam 2.5 mg should ideally be given by subcutaneous injection to assess the response. The aim of this treatment is to allay anxiety and reduce the tendency to panic, and *not* to induce deliberate sedation and a loss of consciousness.

Family members, friends and others who are around the dying patient need to be informed of the purpose and probable effects of these measures. They may press for more urgent methods to relieve the distress, which they find unbearable to watch: the attending clinicians, have a however, duty to treat the patient with the safest and most ethical means, and to explain this and support the carers as they sit with the patient.

CONCLUSION

Breathlessness is a common and far-reaching symptom in palliative care. It arises in many cancers but is also caused by co-morbidity, i.e. concurrent diseases, especially COPD and cardiac disease. It is important to seek the anatomical or physiological causes, because these usually point to the most rational treatments; this can often be done with the minimum of investigations. Anti-cancer treatments should be considered if the patient is well enough, and invasive interventions may be needed for some complications of cancer, such as pleural or pericardial effusion. Pharmacological treatments form the mainstay of therapy for breathlessness: these include drugs which relieve concurrent conditions such as airflow obstruction and heart failure, as well as drugs which specifically palliate the distressing symptom. Opioids and benzodiazepines are the most reliable drugs used for palliation. Oxygen should be restricted to patients who have hypoxia but facial airflow from fans can give non-specific benefit. Non-pharmacological measures including breathing control, acupuncture and good nursing care are valuable alongside medical interventions. Ideally, the patient should be managed by a multi-disciplinary team which can offer several modalities of therapy.

REFERENCES

Ahmedzai, S. 1998: Palliation of respiratory symptoms. In: Doyle, D., Hanks, G.W.C. and MacDonald, N. (eds) *Oxford textbook of palliative medicine.* Oxford: Oxford University Press.

Ahmedzai, S. and Davis, C. 1997: Nebulised drugs in palliative care. *Thorax* 52 (supplement 2), S75–S77.

Anderson, H., Hopwood, P., Stephens, R.J., Thatcher, N. et al. 2000: Gemcitabine plus best supportive care (BSC) vs BSC in inoperable non-small cell lung cancer – a randomised trial with quality of life as the primary outcome. *British Journal of Cancer* 83, 447–53.

Bisset, M. 1996: Tumours of the lung. In: Tschudin, V. (ed.) *Nursing the patient with cancer*. Hemel Hempstead: Prentice Hall.

Bredin, M. 1999: Breathlessness. In: Aranda, S. and O'Connor, M. (eds) *Palliative care nursing: a guide to practice*. Melbourne: Ausmed.

Bredin, M., Corner, J., Krishnasamy, M., Plant, H., Bailey, C. and A'Hern, R. 1999: Multicentre randomised controlled trial of nursing intervention for breathlessness in patients with lung cancer. *British Medical Journal* 318, 901–4.

Corner, J., Plant, H., A'Hern, R. and Bailey, C. 1996: Non-pharmacological intervention for breathlessness in lung cancer. *Palliative Medicine* 10, 299–305.

Davis, C.L. 1994: The therapeutics of dyspnoea. In: Hanks, G.W. (ed.) *Cancer surveys. Palliative medicine: problem areas in pain and symptom management*. New York: Cold Spring Harbor Laboratory.

Davis, C.L. 1999: Nebulised opioids should not be prescribed outside a clinical trial. *American Journal of Hospice Palliative Care* 16, 543.

Higginson, I. and McCarthy, M. 1989: Measuring symptoms in terminal cancer: are pain and dyspnoea controlled? *Journal of the Royal Society of Medicine* 82, 264–7.

Hopwood, P. and Stephens, R.J. 1995: Symptoms at presentation for treatment in patients with lung cancer: implications for the evaluation of palliative treatment. *British Journal of Cancer* 71, 633–6.

Hoskins, P. and Makin, W. 1998: Lung cancer and mesothelioma. In: Hoskins, P. and Makin, W. (eds) *Oncology for palliative medicine*. Oxford: Oxford University Press.

Pan, C.X., Morrison, R.S., Ness, J. et al. 2000: Complementary and alternative medicine in the management of pain, dyspnea, and nausea and vomiting near the end of life: a systematic review. *Journal of Pain and Symptom Management* 20, 374–87.

Snape, D. and Robinson, A. 1996: Radiotherapy. In: Tschudin, V. (ed.) *Nursing the patient with cancer*. Hemel Hempstead: Prentice Hall.

Tanaka, K., Akechi, T., Okuyama, T., Nishiwaki, Y. and Uchitomi, Y. 2000: Development and validation of the Cancer Dyspnoea Scale: a multidimensional, brief, self-rating scale. *British Journal of Cancer* 82, 800–5.

Thompson, F. 2000: The role of the specialist nurse. In: Cooper, J. (ed.) *Stepping into palliative care*. Oxford: Radcliffe Medical Press.

Vainio, A. and Auvinen, A. 1996: Prevalence of symptoms among patients with advanced cancer: an international collaborative study. *Journal of Pain Symptom Management* 12, 3–10.

Whitlock, K. 1999: Complementary therapies. In: Aranda, S. and O'Connor, M. (eds) *Palliative care nursing: a guide to practice*. Melbourne: Ausmed.

Wilcock, A. 1998: The management of respiratory symptoms. In: Faull, C., Carter, Y. and Woof, R. (eds) *Handbook of palliative care*. Oxford: Blackwell.

Woof, R. 1998: Asthenia, cachexia and anorexia. In: Faull, C., Carter, Y. and Woof, R. (eds) *Handbook of palliative care*. Oxford: Blackwell.

chapter 4

OEDEMA IN PALLIATIVE CARE

Karen Jenns

I expect to pass through this world but once: any good thing therefore that I can do, or any kindness that I can show to any fellow creature, let me do it now: let me not defer or neglect it, for I shall not pass this way again.

Stephen Grenfell

Oedema has the potential to cause considerable physical and psychological distress. In advancing cancer, oedema is often compounded by other medical complications so treatment is rarely straightforward, and successful management often presents a real challenge to health-care professionals. This chapter will focus on the management of oedema encountered in advancing cancer.

OEDEMA IN ADVANCING CANCER

Oedema is a common symptom in advancing cancer, often exacerbated by several factors such as immobility and poor nutritional status. It is therefore not surprising that most people with advancing cancer are vulnerable to developing oedema at some stage. Often, in the palliative care setting it is a neglected symptom because neither the patient nor the healthcare professional perceives it as important when there are other issues such as pain to alleviate. Early recognition of oedema and those at risk can significantly reduce the distress caused when the symptom becomes troublesome.

OEDEMA

The pathogenesis of any type of oedema (tissue swelling) occurs as a result of an imbalance between the rate of interstitial fluid or lymph formation and the rate of lymphatic return (Johnston, 1985; Olszewski, 1991; Casley-Smith and Casley-Smith, 1997). Due to the difficulty in differentiating between the different types of oedemas generally acute oedema occurs rapidly and can subside rapidly after correction of medical problems such as heart or liver failure.

Persistent swelling i.e. over three months' duration is often termed 'chronic oedema'. Lymphoedema is only one type of chronic oedema that can be seen in advancing disease.

LYMPHOEDEMA

Lymphoedema has been defined by the International Society of Lymphology (ISL) as an abnormal collection of tissue proteins, oedema, chronic inflammation and fibrosis (Casley-Smith and Piller, 1985; Casley-Smith, 1992).

Lymphoedema occurs as a result of three mechanisms:

- a reduction in the transport capacity of the lymphatic system (e.g. by the surgical removal of lymph nodes). This is often referred to as true obstructive lymphoedema;
- an increase in capillary filtrate (e.g. in venous insufficiency). Over time, the transport capacity of the lymphatic system becomes reduced, with resulting lymphatic stasis. The primary cause lies outside the lymphatic system, this being termed lymphovenous oedema.
- a combination of reduced lymphatic flow and increased capillary filtration. An example of this is seen in patients who sit for long periods with little exercise who develop dependency oedema (Browse and Stewart, 1985; Olszewski, 1991; Föeldi, 1977).

Lymphoedema is classified as either primary or secondary (Keeley, 2000a):

- **Primary lymphoedema** occurs when there is a congenital lymphatic dysplasia, which may or may not be present at birth.
- **Secondary lymphoedema** occurs as a result of damage to the lymphatic system from a known cause, the most common of which are trauma, infection and inflammation.

SECONDARY LYMPHOEDEMA

Any disturbance to the lymphatic system has the potential to cause lymphoedema, so secondary lymphoedema is more prolific than primary lymphoedema. In the Western world, the most common cause of secondary lymphoedema is trauma resulting from cancer and/or its treatment (Mortimer, 1990; Brennan et al., 1996; Keeley, 1997).

Cancer related lymphoedema

There are some cancers that cause extensive damage to the lymphatic pathway either as a natural progression of the disease or because the treatment, for example surgery or radiotherapy, damages the lymphatic pathway. Common cancers causing lymph node, intrapelvic or retroperitoneal metastases are those of the bladder, prostate, ovary, uterus, cervix, rectum and breast (Souhami and Tobias, 1998).

In the UK, as in other developed countries, the most common cause of cancer related lymphoedema is breast cancer (Mortimer, 1990; Casley-Smith and Casley-Smith, 1997; Keeley, 1997; Szuba and Rockson, 1998). The incidence after breast cancer treated by surgery and radiotherapy is thought to be 30 per cent (Kissen et al., 1986; Markby et al., 1991; Logan, 1995). After radical hysterectomy, pelvic lymph node resection and radiotherapy for carcinoma of the cervix, the incidence is reported to be as high as 40 per cent (Werngren-Elgstrom and Lidman, 1994).

Oedema is a common symptom in advancing malignancy, often being exacerbated by factors such as immobility and poor nutritional status. It is therefore not surprising that most people with advancing cancer are vulnerable to developing oedema at some stage.

COMMON MEDICAL COMPLICATIONS THAT CAUSE OEDEMA

Systemic

- cardiac failure;
- hypoproteinaemia – malnutrition, renal failure and hepatic dysfunction;
- malignant ascites;
- drugs such as non-steroidal anti-inflammatory drugs and corticosteroids.

Local

- venous or arterial obstruction from compression by a tumour, superior or inferior vena caval obstruction or a deep vein thrombosis;
- infection;
- skin problems;
- immobility or paralysis;
- metastatic tumour progression (Keeley, 2000b).

SYMPTOMS

Symptoms common to all types of tissue swelling are:

- increasing tissue swelling leading to tissue tightness;
- a distortion of limb shape;
- skin problems such as lymphorrhoea, dryness, hyperkeratosis, lymphangiomas;
- reduced movement in the joints and muscles;
- pain or discomfort, for example heaviness and tissue tightness (Badger et al., 1988);
- infections;
- functional difficulties as the swelling becomes larger;
- psychological disturbances caused by alterations in body image, sexuality and social acceptance (Passik et al., 1993; Tobin et al., 1993; Woods, 1993; Woods et al., 1995).

In advancing disease, pain is exacerbated by nerve damage from tumour compression or other medical problems such as a deep vein thrombosis. There may also be further skin ulceration, often caused by skin tumour metastases or venous or arterial insufficiency. Lymphoedema, one type of oedema, may also be present or has the potential to develop over time.

Lymphoedema has a higher protein content than venous or cardiac oedema and is often referred to as a high-protein oedema (Stanton et al., 1996; Stanton, 2000). This high protein content causes fibrosis (hardening of the underlying tissues) (Daroczy, 1995). The specific changes that take place in the skin and subcutaneous layer differentiate lymphoedema from other types of chronic oedema. If left untreated, the lymphoedematous area can swell to huge proportions. Any area of the body can be affected, but it is commonly seen as limb swelling.

EVALUATION

It is vital to make an accurate diagnosis in order to optimize treatment effectiveness and plan realistic goals. Important considerations are whether the oedema is localized or generalized, symmetrical or asymmetrical, acute or chronic, and acquired or congenital. In most cases, evaluation involves taking an in-depth history and performing a physical examination, but in advancing disease, investigations should also include:

- a full blood count and electrolyte levels (for urea and creatinine);
- the plasma albumin concentration;
- disease evaluation, for example by computed tomography or magnetic resonance imaging;
- an assessment of venous complications.

In oedema of sudden onset, it is important to exclude any underlying pathology such as cardiac or renal failure.

Evaluation should be viewed as a cyclical process and should explore the experiences and expectations of the patients as well as the subjective aspects of the illness (Bates, 1995; Brown, 1995; Stewart et al., 1995). Factors affecting the outcome and goals of treatment can then be identified and treatment modified to facilitate the planning of optimal care. Over time, a shared understanding of the condition and how it affects the patient will develop.

GENERAL APPROACH TO CARE

Palliative care often begins when there is no longer a response to curative treatment and life expectancy is relatively short (Twycross, 1995). In patients with advancing disease, support is required from health-care professionals who are sensitive to the patients' specific physical and psychosocial needs, ideally in a palliative care enviroment. At this time, the focus of treatment becomes patient centred rather than disease driven. A patient-centred approach involves:

- exploring both the disease and the illness;
- understanding the whole person;
- finding common ground;
- incorporating prevention and health promotion;
- enhancing the relationship over time;
- realistic goal-setting (Loomis and Conco, 1991; Chin et al., 1998).

Central to the management of oedema is the prevention of complications and the development of the maximum possible level of independence. In advancing disease, the approach is always gentle, and the treatment should be modified according to changing health status and the patient's wishes. A multi-professional approach is desirable as it facilitates the incorporation of a number of skills and approaches. Education and access to a treatment centre, which will provide ongoing support and advice to minimize future problems, is paramount. Many palliative care centres in the UK have access to a lymphoedema service, which should be able to provide ongoing information and support (British Lymphology Society, 1995).

The British Lymphology Society (1997) considers the needs of people with chronic oedema in advancing disease in terms of two groups:

- those at risk of developing oedema;
- those with oedema in advancing disease.

THE 'AT-RISK' GROUP

Chronic oedema is a debilitating condition, but the physical and psychological morbidity suffered can be prevented or reduced if it is recognized and treated early on. Prevention is an essential concept in oedema management, one applicable to those at risk of developing or living with oedema.

In advancing disease, people are at most risk if they have one or more of the following:

- increasing immobility or a problem with the movement of a limb;
- cancer, which damages the drainage pathway (see below);
- cardiac, renal or liver failure;
- any underlying skin problem.

The at-risk group require information on why they are at risk, how they can minimize the risk and what they should do should swelling occur. Risks can be lessened by good skin care, the prevention of infection, elevation and gentle exercise. Early treatment intervention will help to minimize physical and psychological morbidity.

TREATMENT

Conservative therapy is the mainstay of treatment for any type of chronic oedema. In advanced cancer, the aim is to control the symptoms, reduce the effect of complications and improve the patient's quality of life. It is important also to correct any underlying medical condition such as hypoproteinaemia.

The two most common forms of conservative therapy used in the oedema of advancing malignancy are drugs and decongestive lymphoedema therapy.

DRUGS

Diuretics

Diuretics are often used as a first-line treatment in all forms of oedema; indeed, if there is a venous component to the oedema, diuretics are thought to be clinically indicated (Twycross, 2000). They have little place, however, in the management of true lymphostatic lymphoedema because lymphoedema is a failure of lymphatic drainage and is not caused by venous incompetence. Frusemide 20–40 mg for up to 1 week is initially advisable. A close monitoring of the response to the diuretic is required, the dose being adjusted to stabilize fluid loss.

Corticosteriods

Corticosteriods tend to be advocated when there is advancing disease causing or exacerbating the lymphoedema. By reducing tumour inflammation, the lymphatic obstruction may be reduced, allowing for an increase in lymph flow. Dexamethasone 4–8 mg once a day for 7 days, reducing to 2–4 mg, may considerably help the symptoms.

Oxerutins

Oxerutins are designed to enhance interstitial proteolysis by increasing macrophage activity. In the UK, oxerutins are licensed only for use in venous disease, but there have been reports of reduced limb swelling and fibrosis in people with lymphoedema. With advancing cancer however, the effect is too slow – several months – to be of any real benefit.

Analgesics

Analgesia is an important part of the management of those with advancing cancer and any form of oedema. Adequate analgesia can facilitate:

- the application or removal of any compression or support;
- gentle exercise and function;
- an improved quality of life.

DECONGESTIVE THERAPY

Decongestive therapy encompasses the elements of skin care, simple lymphatic drainage (massage), compression/support, exercise and compression pumps. An overview of treatment is presented in Table 4.1.

Table 4.1 Oedema management in palliative care

Treatment modality	Aim	Treatment
Skin care	Control and maintainance of good skin hydration Prevention of skin complications: • Lymphorrhoea • Ulceration, etc. Prevention and early recognition of acute inflammatory episodes, e.g. cellulitis	Daily inspection of all affected areas Gently wash and dry the affected areas Daily moisturising with appropriate oils or creams: • Well-hydrated skin – aqueous cream or other water-based emollient • For dry skin, use oil-based emollients, e.g. 50% soft white paraffin and 50% liquid paraffin Educate patients regarding • Avoiding trauma • Preventing and recognizing the signs and symptoms of acute inflammatory episodes. What to do if they occur (see text)
Simple lymphatic drainage massage	Reduction of congestion of oedema in the tissues Softening of underlying tissues and prevention of fibrosis Prevention of joint stiffness Promotion of comfort and psychological well-being Reduction of pain/discomfort from tissue tightness	***Principles*** • The pattern and direction of the lymphatic flow govern the movements • Gentle skin stretching – easing on, gentle pressure (skin stretching) and zero-pressure phase • Rhythmical movements (1 per second) • No reddening of the skin or discomfort • See Appendix 1 for details of the technique ***Avoiding areas affected by cancer*** Simple lymphatic drainage should ideally be performed daily either by the patient or by the family when appropriate. It may take several treatments for the patient to be comfortable with performing this technique him- or herself. Adaptations will need to be made as appropriate
Support compression	Prevention or control of the accumulation of fluid Prevention of tissue tightness Prevention of lymphorrhea Alleviation of discomfort/pain	If the patient is mobile, with no shape distortion, light-support hosiery, i.e. class 1 or 2, can be applied to the limb(s) In immobile patients – *shaped* (not tubular) Tubigrip can be used if it is comfortable In patients with distorted limb shape or very fragile skin – support bandages are indicated, applied daily over soft padding (see text)

Exercise	Prevention of joint stiffness	Gentle active and passive movements should be encouraged
	Increase in limb mobility (where appropriate)	Support the limb(s) when resting in the horizontal position
	Promotion of good posture	Use broad arm slings when mobilizing if the limb is heavy and painful. Patients should be encouraged to remove the sling as much as possible to try to prevent joint stiffness
	Familiarization of the patient with relaxation techniques	
		Encourage normal use where possible, avoiding static exercises
		Refer to an occupational therapist when mobility becomes reduced
		If dubious about advising patients on exercise, seek the help of a physiotherapist

Skin care

Skin care is arguably the most important concept in the management of chronic oedema, which predisposes to a variety of skin complications (Mallon and Ryan, 2000; Ryan, 1995). The aim of skin care is to maintain a good skin condition and to reduce the risk of skin problems (Veitch, 1993; Williams and Venables, 1996; Linnitt, 2000).

Daily skin care should involve inspection of the skin in all the affected areas, the treatment of any skin abnormality (e.g. fungal infections) and daily skin hygiene procedures, washing and patting the skin gently while drying the affected areas. The daily application of emollients is essential to maintain skin hydration. If the skin is well hydrated, use a bland emollient such as aqueous cream (Linnitt, 2000).

Common problems encountered in palliative care are acute inflammatory episodes, fragile skin, skin ulceration, cellulitis and lymphorrhoea (Table 4.2).

'Acute inflammatory episodes' is the term used to describe the attacks of infection that frequently occur in people with oedema and that are particularly common in lymphatic stasis because the cutaneous immune response is significantly impaired (Mallon et al., 1997). The clinical features are erythema, pain, increased swelling, influenza-like symptoms, fever, nausea and vomiting, the symptoms tending to occur quickly and often without warning. In many cases, it is, without systemic upset, difficult to distinguish between dermatitis, phlebitis and acute inflammatory episodes, although one or two clinical features are in some cases present (Mortimer, 2000). If acute inflammatory episodes are suspected, it is probably sensible to commence antibiotics as soon as possible to avoid a full-blown attack.

Treatment involves resting the limb, comfortably supported in elevation, and regular analgesia until the pain subsides. Any compression should be removed until the infection has resolved, and daily skin hygiene procedures should continue. In mild attacks without any systemic upset, phenoxymethylpenicillin or, if

Table 4.2 The specific management of skin problems

	Signs	Symptoms	Management
Fragile skin	Shiny over stretched skin Soft pitting oedema Shape distortion	Heaviness Limb swelling Pain/discomfort	Gentle compression with bandages for 48 hours. Then support bandages or shaped Tubigrip
Dry skin	Skin cracking – tiny or deep cracks Flakiness	Itchy skin Increased incidence of acute inflammatory episodes	Daily application of oil-based emollient, e.g. 50% soft white paraffin and 50% liquid paraffin or coconut oil Balneum plus bath oil
Lymphorrhoea	Leakage of lymph fluid through the tissues (mostly affects the peripheral areas)	Pooling of fluid Coldness of the sites affected	Prevent trauma to the limbs. Cover with dry dressings. Apply gentle compression bandaging for 48 hours until leakage has resolved. Then apply *shaped* Tubigrip only. Contact the local lymphoedema clinic for advice.

Ulceration	Superficial wounds on
	the skin's surface:
	• Tumour
	• Trauma
	• Dermatitis
	• Venous/arterial
	  insufficiency
	• acute inflammatory
	  episodes/wound
	  infection
	• Poorly applied
	  compression
		Pain and
		tenderness
		Exudate
		Strong odour
		
		Erythema
		Systemic upset
		from acute
		inflammatory
		episodes
			Active treatment with suitable
			non-adhesive and anti-odour
			dressing
			Avoid using adhesive
			tape on fragile skin
			Any dressing should be
			anchored to the limb
			using a cotton retaining
			bandage, i.e. Tubifast
			Consider prophylactic
			antibiotics

the patient is allergic to this, erythromycin 500 mg four times a day for 14 days is advisable. If the infection does not resolve, the antibiotics should be changed to flucloxacillin or, with allergy, cefradine 500 mg four times daily for 14 days. If this fails, a bacteriologist should be consulted.

With systemic upset, bed rest is essential, which sometimes means in-patient admission. Flucloxacillin 2 g intravenously four times a day or cefuroxime 1.5 g on the same dose schedule is advised. If the infection does not resolve, the antibiotic should be changed to clindamycin 450 mg intravenously four times daily.

Simple lymphatic drainage

Manual lymphatic drainage is a gentle non-intrusive, non-mechanical form of massage first developed by Emil Vodder in the 1930s (Wittlinger and Wittlinger, 1995). There are many studies reporting the effectiveness of skin massage in moving lymph (Leduc, 1988; Leduc et al., 1988; Wittlinger et al., 1995). Manual lymphatic drainage is contraindicated in active cancer, but a simplified form called simple lymphatic drainage can be beneficial in situations of advancing malignancy (British Lymphology Society, 1997). There are to date no research studies reporting the effectiveness of simple lymphatic drainage but a growing number of anecdotal reports from both patients and professionals have highlighted its benefits.

The aim of simple lymphatic drainage is to stimulate the contraction of the lymphangions, thereby increasing the movement of lymph along the pathway from the superficial vessels into the deep lymphatics. The sequence and direction of the massage is designed to stimulate lymphatic flow and drainage away from congested areas. This massage is very slow, gentle and rhythmical. The therapeutic benefits of simple lymphatic drainage are:

- improved lymphatic flow
- reduced tissue tension
- a reduction of pain
- relaxation – it can induce a deep sleep
- a general feeling of well-being.

There are several factors that effect the outcome of treatment, the first of which is the skill of the therapist performing the massage. The therapist should ideally undertake a course of training in simple or manual lymphatic drainage in order to perform the massage most effectively. In the palliative care setting, however, it is possible to perform simple lymphatic drainage on patients with advancing disease providing that the principles are adhered to. The patient's health status also influences the outcome, simple lymphatic drainage being contraindicated:

- in all areas of cutaneous cancer spread;
- with acute inflammatory episodes;
- if there are acute allergic reactions or skin problems;
- with severe cardiac failure;
- in superior vena caval obstruction;
- with deep vein thrombosis.

Simple lymphatic drainage should ideally be performed daily, if possible for 15–20 minutes – any more than this may leave the patient too exhausted. The patient, and when possible a partner or friend, should also be encouraged to perform the massage. Educating patients to develop the technique will help them to become skilled enough and perhaps motivated enough to carry on themselves.

Information on the technique of simple lymphatic drainage can be obtained in Appendix 1 to this chapter.

Compression and support

In lymphoedema, containment is applied in the form of multi-layer bandages that provide support, or compression garments (Föeldi et al., 1985; Casley-Smith and Casley-Smith, 1997):

- Support is used to provide retention and control without compression. The short stretch bandages used in lymphoedema management provide a low resting and a high working pressure. Variations of tissue pressure occur during periods of activity: in patients who are immobile, very little tissue pressure occurs.
- Compression is the application of direct pressure. In lymphoedema management, it is used to stimulate both lymphatic and venous flow.

In advanced cancer, the focus changes from actively reducing limb size, which is an unrealistic outcome at this stage, to controlling the swelling, reducing possible complications and promoting comfort and a good quality of life. It is for this reason that the pressures used in people with oedema in advanced cancer are very low, and treatment is regularly modified to take into consideration the patient's wishes and needs.

Bandages

Unlike elastic bandages, short stretch bandages apply an almost rigid casing when applied to a limb. These bandages exert a high working pressure with a low resting pressure. The pressures applied to the limb in advanced malignancy should be much lower because the focus is on easing the symptoms rather than reducing the oedema. The indications for using short stretches bandages are:

- large swollen limbs greater than 20 per cent excess volume with or without swelling of the digits;
- a distorted limb shape or skin folds;
- fragile skin;
- ulceration (not skin metastases);
- lymphorrhoea;
- fibrosis.

The contraindications are:

- infection (acute inflammatory episodes) as this can spread infection and increase discomfort and pain;
- severe cardiac failure as the raised venous pressure can cause cardiac overload;
- acute deep vein thrombosis (within 6 weeks);
- arterial insufficiency, which can cause tissue necrosis.

In advancing disease, further caution should be taken in the following situations:

1 patients who have increasing debility with impending cardiac or renal failure. A frequent evaluation of the current health status during bandaging is indicated to prevent complications;

2 patients with nerve damage, who may be unable to indicate whether the bandages are too tight, as tissue damage may result;
3 patients with fungating lesions at the root of the limb (particularly in breast cancer). Bandaging can also increase the amount of exudate, so patients should be warned and measures taken to change the dressings more often, but this should subside over time.

The bandages should not cause any discomfort or pain, numbness and tingling or discolouration of the digits; if this happens, *the bandages must be removed immediately.*

The principles of bandaging in advancing disease should be followed:

• Gentle pressure should be applied in patients with advanced cancer.
• Uniform pressure should be used along the limb.
• A regular inspection of progress should be made as rapid changes can occur.
• Patients should ideally be bandaged in a palliative care setting so that the monitoring of progress can take place.

The treatment should be carried out daily to deal with sudden changes in the patient's condition. Assessment should include changes in limb size, the presence or absence of truncal oedema, changes in shape, the appearance of the skin and the condition of the underlying tissues. Treatment is then adapted daily, more or less padding being applied for example, and should take into account how the patient is coping with the treatment. Once treatment finishes, a containment garment should be applied to control the oedema.

In advanced cancer, some patients may feel much more comfortable in support bandages' than in garments that exert compression on the limb. In such circumstances, the technique can be taught to the partner, relative or carer of the patient and the patient can remain in daily bandaging for long periods of time. In this situation, regular monitoring and follow-up are required to check on progress and avoid complications such as tissue damage.

Multi-layer bandages should be applied in layers (see Appendix 2 to this chapter):

• a cotton Tubifast bandage
• digit bandages – 4 cm wide
• padding or foam
• short stretch bandages. In advanced disease with extensive cutaneous metastases, crêpe can be used to offer light support.

NB: Short stretch bandages produce a high working pressure and a low resting pressure. Therefore, in an immobile patient the bandage pressure exerted will be low, however, on exercise it will be very high. Crêpe or a medium pressure bandage gently applied may also have the desired effect of containing the swelling. All bandages applied incorrectly can cause tissue damage, and extra vigilance and monitoring is needed when there is advancing disease.

Compression garments Compression garments promote both lymphatic and venous return (Brakkee and Kuiper, 1988; Bates et al., 1995), helping to maintain the reduction after bandaging and containing the limb swelling. Different compression classes are available via hospital supplies or directly from garment companies, continental compression class 1 or 2 being recommended for patients with advanced cancer. There are a wide variety of different types of garments available. Cosmetic acceptability is important but adherence to treatment may require compromise; the decision of which garment to use should thus be based on informed choice.

Compression garments are indicated if there is:

- a regular limb shape with no distortion;
- intact skin that is not fragile;
- Mild-to-moderate limb swelling, that is less than 20 per cent excess limb volume;
- and if the patient, partner, relative or carer is able to apply and remove the garments.

The contraindications are as follows:

- infection: the limb will swell as part of the inflammatory response so compression is not indicated until the symptoms subside. The patient will then need to be remeasured for the garments as the limb size will probably have changed;
- severe cardiac failure;
- arterial insufficiency;
- skin complications such as lymphorrhoea;
- shape distortion or skin folds;
- severe limb swelling.

Compression garments should ideally be applied in the morning and removed at bed time to allow for the skin care regime. The garments need to fit snugly around the limb, which makes them difficult to apply: in advancing cancer, with increasing weakness and lethargy, the task eventually becomes impossible. Shaped Tubigrip is an alternative to compression garments. It is important to keep compression or support on the limbs or the limbs may become more swollen. There should be no creases in the garments or shaped Tubigrip as this will cause skin damage and shape distortion. Compression bandaging may therefore be indicated if there is no one to help the patient to apply and remove the garments.

Compression garments are best used when the patient is mobile because exercise enhances their effect (Partsh, 1991; Rose et al., 1993; Hock, 1998). Patients who sit for long periods with their legs dependent should however also wear garments to control the oedema and prevent distal pooling and lymphorrhea.

Exercise programme

Movement and muscle contraction are important for venous return and helps with the uptake of lymph into the superficial lymphatics and the propulsion of lymph along its pathway. Exercises given to patients should aim to enhance lymphatic and venous flow while reducing arterial vasodilatation and flow. Gentle regular active and passive movements of the joints in the affected area will help to prevent joint stiffness and control the oedema (Hock, 1998). Exercise will also enhance the effect of any compression or support applied to the limb (Hughes, 2000). A programme of exercise during bandaging is not always appropriate in the palliative care setting.

Patients should be educated in terms of the following:

- Overvigorous activity, which can cause injury and further discomfort, should be avoided.
- They should wear well-fitting footwear when walking as oedema of the feet and ankles is liable to place patients at a higher risk of falls. Some patients cannot fit into their usual shoes and may require footwear several sizes larger. Training shoes are particularly good for safety and controlling the swelling.
- A discussion of lifestyle is important so that strategies for adaption without a reduction in the quality of life can be explored. Hobbies, for example, should be encouraged with some modification. Referral to an occupational therapist will help the patient to cope with functional problems while maximizing independence.

SUPPORT AND ELEVATION

Elevation and support will help to prevent joint strain and generalized discomfort from the weight of the limb. Between periods of gentle exercise, the limbs, should be supported along its entire length in the horizontal position. Raising the limb to this level helps to reduce arterial pressure in the capillaries, improving both venous and lymphatic flow to the heart (Hughes, 2000). This is most successfully achieved in a reclining chair or bed with end elevation. In advancing cancer, it is not necessary to elevate the limb to heart level as this may be uncomfortable.

If an upper limb is swollen, the arm should be placed on pillows, fully supported, the distal end of the limb being elevated slightly above the proximal end if possible. All patients should be educated in the importance of elevating and supporting the swollen limb, particularly when they become less mobile. This will help to control the swelling as leaving the limbs largely dependent will increase the oedema. Further elevation also helps to maintain the reduction gained from bandaging or wearing compression garments.

Intermittent pneumatic compression therapy

This type of treatment has been used for a variety of types of oedema since the 1980s. It is rarely used in lymphoedema as research has demonstrated that it does not affect protein reabsorption (Leduc, 1988). It does, however, increase blood velocity and the reabsorption of interstitial fluid. It also has a role in advanced disease as it helps to soften hard oedema and ease the discomfort arising from skin tightness.

Pneumatic compression therapy involves the use of an electric pump attached to a compressive air bag. When this is placed over the limb, a pressure of 20–40 mmHg should be exerted, although some models have the ability to exert a far greater pressure (up to 300 mmHg). There are two type of pump:

- segmental – several compartments, 3, 5, 10 apply compression in sequences;
- non-segmental, in which one air bag compresses and releases the limp.

In advancing disease, the segmental multi-chamber compression pump tends to be most effective at removing fluid from the distal to the proximal end of the limb (Bray and Barrett, 2000).

The indications for intermittent pneumatic compression therapy in advancing malignancy are:

- venous oedema
- dependency oedema (seen in immobile patients)
- venous insufficiency
- hypoproteinaemia.

The contraindications are:

- deep vein thrombosis;
- active cancer at the root of the limb;
- cardiac failure;
- renal failure;
- arterial disease is indicated when the ankle brachial pressure index (ABPI) is less than 0.8;
- oedema in the truncal areas, including the genital region.

Caution should be used in advancing disease the amount of compression to be used always being prescribed by a physician. A low pressure of 20–30 mmHg should be used at first, starting with 10 minutes and increasing to 30 minutes three times a day. The pressure can be increased to 40–60 mmHg if this is comfortable. Prior to treatment, the skin should be protected by a cotton cover such as Tubifast. Compression or support garments or bandages should be used between treatments to prevent the reaccumulation of fluid in the overstretched skin.

CLOTHING

Well-fitting shoes are vital for those who have swelling affecting the lower limb(s), and will help to control any swelling, encourage mobility and prevent falls. Shoes should be well fitting, comfortable and non-constrictive, preferably providing gentle, uniform pressure from the distal to the proximal end of each foot. Well-fitting footwear will limit foot swelling and prevent distortion so referral to an orthotist is recommended if standard-size shoes are unsuitable.

Clothes should be loose-fitting and non-constrictive. Bat-wing sleeves, or choosing plain-coloured clothes with a patterned neckline, can draw attention away from a swollen arm. Jewellery can be also used to dress up the neckline and draw the focus away from the swollen limb.

OUTCOME MEASURES

Evaluation of the treatment of effectiveness is a fundamental issue in today's health-care system (NHS, 1998). Outcomes of care should include a variety of different parameters, including patients' perceptions of treatment, levels of satisfaction (Erikson, 1987), quality of life and changes in shape, skin condition and joint mobility (Jenns, 2000). In adopting a multi-disciplinary approach to care, research into its effectiveness should also adopt a multi-disciplinary rather than a singular perspective (Sitzia, 1997; Piller, 1999).

Limb volume is commonly used as the main objective measurement because of its relative accessibility as a measurement tool (Badger, 1993; Woods, 1994; Sitzia, 1997). The most frequently used method of measurement in the UK is the calculation of limb volume using the formula:

$$\text{Volume per 4 cm} = \frac{(\text{Circumference}^2)}{\pi}$$

A reduction of limb size is often an unrealistic outcome measure in active malignancy so measurements of limb size are not indicated.

CONCLUSION

Uncontrolled limb swelling will lead to irreversible physical changes, an increased risk of infection and increasing disability so the perceived cost of non-treatment in terms of physical and psychological morbidity is high. The distress of patients with active malignancy is further compounded by complications, and it is therefore vital that their needs are met.

Conservative therapy considerably reduces the morbidity suffered by those who have or are at risk of developing chronic oedema in advanced cancer. The key to successful management involves developing an understanding of chronic oedema and its management, involving the patient in all aspects of care and setting realistic patient-centred goals. Listening, providing honest information, offering choices and adjusting the treatment accordingly will help to prevent much of the physical and psychological morbidity suffered by people with oedema in advancing malignancy.

ACKNOWLEDGEMENTS

The protocol for acute inflammatory episodes is that used in the Lymphoedema Service, Sir Michael Sobell House, Oxford, UK. The simple lymphatic drainage technique was developed at the Lymphoedema Service, Sir Michael Sobell House, by: Sara Bellhouse Vodder, trained manual lymphatic drainage therapist; Angela Williams, formally ICRF Research Sister; Karen Jenns, Clinical Nurse Specialist; and Karen Hughes, Senior Physiotherapist.

APPENDIX 1: SIMPLE LYMPHATIC DRAINAGE

PRINCIPLES OF SIMPLE LYMPHATIC DRAINAGE

- Proximal areas are treated before distal ones.
- Gentle skin stretching with very light pressure is used.
- The movements are very slow (1 per second).
- Massage should be rhythmical – always three times in each position.
- No pain, discomfort or redness of the skin should occur.
- Stationary circles are used, with the skin stretch on three-quarters of the circle. The last quarter of the circle accounts for the relaxation phase, the pressure returning to zero. This allows the vessels to fill and creates a suction movement along the lymphatic pathway.

The patient may be sitting or lying if you are working on the upper body, but should be *lying* if the oedema is in the legs. If the patient is lying down, it is preferable to ensure that the neck is free, that is, that there is no pillow beneath it. Whichever position is chosen, ensure that the patient is comfortable and warm. All garments should be removed from the areas to be massaged, but you need to accept the patient's preference on this.

It is also important that you are comfortable: ensure that you have the couch at the correct height for you, and ideally use an adjustable-height couch. Always position yourself so that you are comfortable, remembering to keep your back as straight as possible. If you are uncomfortable, the massage you give may not be as good as it could be.

Ensure that your fingernails are short, and remove any jewellery (although wedding rings can be worn as long as they are smooth). If your hands become sticky while you are massaging, lightly dust them with a non-scented talcum powder. Oils should not be used for this type of massage as skin stretching then becomes difficult.

Figure 4.1 outlines the principles of the massage technique.

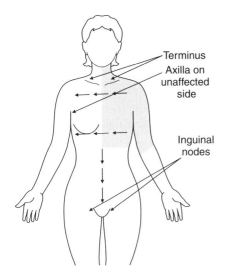

Terminus
Axilla on unaffected side

Inguinal nodes

- Shaded area denotes affected side
- Always start on unaffected side, moving lymph away from the affected side
- Arrows show direction of movement
- Always finish with deep breathing

Figure 4.1 Massage technique

NECK AND SHOULDERS (Figures 4.2 and 4.3)

Side of the neck (Figure 4.2 a–c)

- *First position.* Place your hands either side of the patient's neck with your fingers together and straight. Your index fingers should be just below the patient's ear lobes. Move your fingers in a stationary circle, taking the skin back and then down towards the shoulders. Release the light pressure and let the skin's elasticity return your hands to the starting position, thus completing the circle. **Repeat five times.**
- *Second position.* Move your hands down the neck to a second position approximately half way between the ears and the shoulders. Repeat the stationary circle as above. **Repeat five times.**

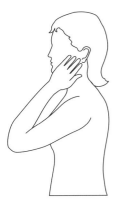

Figure 4.2a First position (both sides)

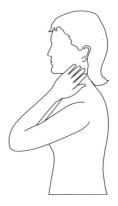

Figure 4.2b Second position (both sides)

- *Third position.* Move your hands further down the neck towards the shoulders, and repeat the stationary circle as above. **Repeat five times.**
- *Fourth position.* Place two or three fingers on the hollow area just above the clavicle, called the **terminus,** where the thoracic duct drains into the subclavian vein. Using the pads of the fingers, take the skin in towards the breastbone and slightly downward; then release the pressure, and let the skin return your fingers to the starting position. **Repeat five times.**

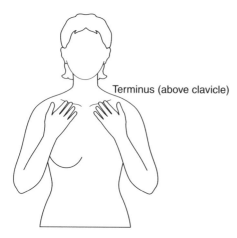

Terminus (above clavicle)

Figure 4.2c Fourth position

Repeat all of these positions three times.

Back of the neck (Figure 4.3)

- *First position.* Move your hands back to their original starting position but place them towards the back of the neck. Move the skin in a stationary circle towards the side of the neck and down towards the body. **Repeat five times.**
- *Second position.* Move your hands down so that they are approximately half way between the ears and the shoulders, repeating the stationary circle as above. **Repeat five times.**

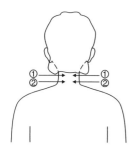

Figure 4.3 Back of the neck

- *Third position*. Place two or three fingers on the hollow area just above the clavicle, the terminus. Using the pads of the fingers, take the skin in towards the breastbone and slightly downwards, before releasing the pressure and letting the skin return your fingers to the starting position. **Repeat five times**. (See Figure 4.1 – Terminus.)

Repeat all of these positions three times.

Shoulders

- *First position*. Stand with your feet about 30 cm apart to give yourself a firm base. Cup your hands around the ball of the shoulders so that your fingers are lying on the patient's back. Move the skin forward towards the chest and in towards the neck. Then release the slight pressure, and let the skin take your hand back to the starting position. **Repeat five times**.
- *Second position*. With your fingers together and flat, place your hands on the shoulders at the border of the trapezius muscle. Bring the skin forward towards the chest and then release the pressure. A little more pressure can be applied here as you are working over the muscle. **Repeat five times**.
- *Third position*. Move your hands along the shoulders to a second position on the trapezius muscle. Bring the skin forwards and towards the chest, and then release the pressure. **Repeat five times**.
- *Fourth position*. Place two or three fingers on the terminus. Using the pads of your fingers, take the skin in towards the breastbone and slightly downwards; then release the pressure, and let the skin return your fingers to the starting position. **Repeat five times**.

Repeat all of these positions three times.

Side of the neck
Repeat once all the positions for the side of neck, as above (Figure 4.2 a–c).

UPPER LIMB

Neck and shoulders
Always start by massaging the neck and shoulders.

Axillary lymph nodes (Figure 4.4)
Stand on the affected side, just level with the patient's axilla, although you will be working on the unaffected side first.

- *First position*. Place one or both hands on the chest wall so that your fingers rest just below the axilla of the unaffected side. Ask the patient to relax the arm as a tense arm will stretch the nodes. Move your fingers in a stationary circle, taking the skin up towards the axilla and across towards the back. Then release the slight pressure, and let the skin return your fingers to the starting point. **Repeat five times**.

- *Second position.* Move your hands down the chest wall (approximately three finger widths) towards the waist. **Repeat the stationary circle as above five times.**

Repeat both of these positions three times.

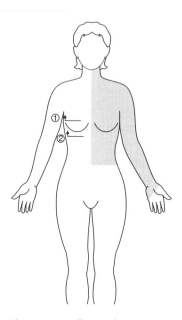

Figure 4.4 Axillary node massage

Groin lymph nodes (Figure 4.5)
It is better to massage one side at a time.

- *First position.* Place both hands on the thigh area slightly below the groin creases. Take the skin up towards the centre of the body and circle inwards towards the groin, releasing the slight pressure, and letting the skin return your hands to the starting position. **Repeat five times on each groin.**
- *Second position.* Place hands on the inner aspect of the thigh. Move skin downwards and upwards. Move down three finger widths and repeat movement. **Repeat whole sequence five times.**

Upper chest (Figure 4.6)
Place one or both of your hands on the front of the chest wall close to the unaffected axilla. Gently stretch the skin towards the unaffected axilla and circle slightly upwards. Then release the slight pressure, and let the skin return your hands to the starting position. **Repeat each movement five times in each position.**

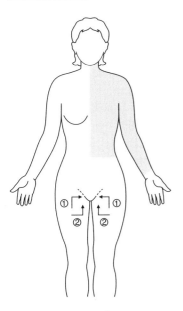

Figure 4.5 Groin node massage

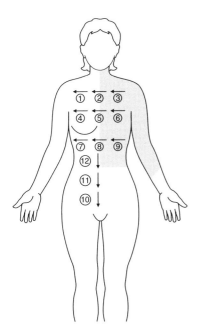

Figure 4.6 Upper chest massage

Slowly and gently work across the chest from the unaffected to the affected side, paying particular attention to the midline/watershed, which is over the sternum. **Repeat the movement 10 times at this point.**

Repeat the whole sequence three times.

Lower chest

This is only massaged if there is swelling below the breast or scar line.

Place your flat hands on the waistline or below any swelling on the affected side. Take the skin across towards the midline watershed and circle down towards the groin, then releasing the slight pressure and letting the skin return your hands to the starting position. **Repeat the movement five times in this position.**

Repeat this movement in as many positions as possible, working from the midline out towards the chest wall on the affected side. Reposition your hands on the midline slightly higher than the original starting point and repeat the sequence again, moving from the midline to the chest wall. **Do not work over the scar line.**

Shoulder area

Semi-circular movements can be used on the upper arm, starting at the shoulder and gradually working down the arm towards the elbow. Fibrosis can be broken down by using the pads of all eight fingers in a line. Gently indent the skin downwards and release the pressure. **Repeat this movement all over the fibrotic area.** If you work over the shoulder, you must clear the area by repeating the upper chest massage, as above.

Back (Figure 4.7)

Ask the patient to lie on the unaffected side. Place your flat hands level with the spine and waist. Take the skin towards the spine and circle to the buttocks, then releasing the slight pressure and letting your hands return to the starting position. **Repeat five times.**

Repeat this movement in as many positions as possible, working in lines from the spine towards the side of the chest wall and up to the axilla.

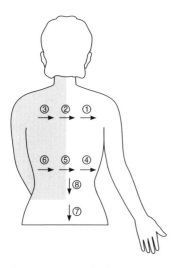

Figure 4.7 Upper back massage

Side of the neck
Finish the massage by carrying out one repeat of the sequence given above for the side of the neck.

Deep breathing
When you have finished the massage, ask the patient to lie on his or her back with the knees bent. Place your flat hand in the centre of the abdomen in order to offer slight resistance. Ask the patient to inhale (the abdomen should balloon out), thus pushing your hand away; then the patient should exhale, letting your hand sink. **Repeat three to five times, taking care not to let the patient become dizzy.**

LOWER LIMB

Neck and shoulders
Always start by massaging the neck and shoulders. Massage the shoulders on the first treatment, although for the second and subsequent treatments, it may be necessary to perform only sequences 1 and 2 (the side and the back of the neck).

Axillary lymph nodes
Stand on the affected side, just level with the patient's axilla, but remember that you will be working on the unaffected side.

- *First position.* Place one or both of your hands on the chest wall so that your fingers rest in the axilla of the unaffected side. Ask the patient to relax the arm; a tense arm will stretch the nodes. Move your fingers in a stationary circle, taking the skin up towards the axilla and across towards the back, release the slight pressure, and let the skin return your fingers to the starting point. **Repeat five times.**
- *Second position.* Move your hands down the chest wall (by approximately three finger widths) towards the waist. Repeat the stationary circle as above. **Repeat five times.**

Repeat both of these positions three times. (See Figure 4.4.)

Groin lymph nodes (Figure 4.8)
Stand on the unaffected side level with the thigh, facing towards the patient's head.

- *First position.* Place your flat hand on the unaffected side on the top of the thigh. Take the skin in towards the centre of the body and circle towards the groin; then release the slight pressure, and let the skin return your hands to the starting position. **Repeat five times.** Move hand down three finger widths, and repeat.

- *Second position.* Move the hands to the inner upper thigh and repeat the stationary circle as above. **Repeat five times.**

Repeat both of these positions three times.

Abdomen (Figure 4.8)

Stand on the affected side and place your flat hands on the unaffected side at the waistline. Take the skin towards the midline and up towards the axilla. Release the slight pressure, and let the hands return to the start point. **Repeat five times.**

Repeat this movement in as many positions as possible, working in lines from the midline out towards the side of the chest on the affected side. Complete this line and then begin a second line a little further down towards the groin. Work all the way down to the groin with the movements directing the fluid upward towards the draining lymph nodes.

Fluid can also be taken across the midline to the unaffected side moving fluid towards the axilla.

Repeat each line three times.

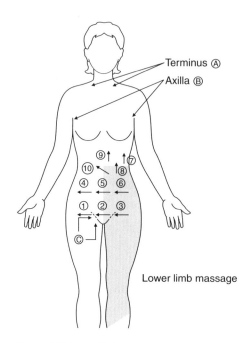

Figure 4.8 Lower limb massage

Thigh

Semi-circular movements can be used on the upper thigh. Start at the top of the thigh and gradually work down the side of the leg towards the knee. Fibrosis can be broken down by using the pads of all eight fingers in a line. Gently indent the skin downwards and release the pressure. **Repeat this movement all over the fibrotic area.** If you work over the thigh, you must clear the area by repeating the abdominal massage described above.

Back (Figure 4.9)

The same movement that is performed on the abdomen can be used on the back from the waistline to the buttocks, taking the fluid towards the axilla.

Side of the neck

Finish the massage with the sequence given earlier for the side of the neck, and clear the terminus.

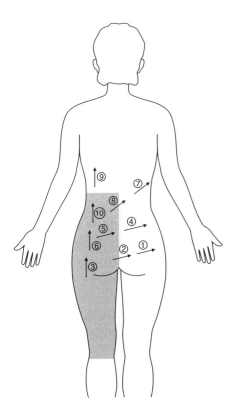

Figure 4.9 Lower back massage

Deep breathing

When you have finished, ask the patient to lie on his or her back with the knees bent or, if it is more comfortable, to sit up in a chair. Place your flat hand in the centre of the abdomen to offer resistance. Ask the patient to inhale into the abdomen, pushing your hand away (the abdomen should balloon out), and then exhale, letting your hand sink. **Repeat three to five times, taking care not to let the patient become dizzy.**

APPENDIX 2: BANDAGING

UPPER LIMB BANDAGING

Method

Application of the cotton tubular stockinette to protect the skin The stockinette should fit snugly from the base of fingers to the top of the arm, a hole being cut out for the thumb.

Applying digit bandages The initial turn of the bandage is applied around the wrist with no tension, the only tension applied being that on the fingers. The bandage is then taken across the dorsum of the hand to just below the finger-nail. Gentle tension is applied as the bandages are wrapped around each finger in turn from the distal to the proximal end. At the end of each finger, the bandage is taken loosely around the wrist and again across the dorsum of the hand. Check that all the bandages reach the base of the fingers, avoiding any gaps, and ensure that no discolouration or changes in sensation occur in the digits.

Applying padding or foam The aim of padding is to protect the bony prominences and create a cylindrical shape to aid uniform pressure. Skin folds should be padded out using pieces of foam or rolled-up soft padding. Padding can be double-folded to achieve a greater protection of the bony areas and an enhanced cylindrical shape.

Compression/support bandages The hand bandage begins at the wrist; a small (6 cm) bandage is used with gentle tension. The fingers should be splayed out firmly or finger movement will be restricted. Two wraps are made around the base of the fingers, the hand being covered in successive wraps, ensuring that there are no gaps. Gentle (not firm) tension is applied (30–50 per cent), and the remaining bandage is taken up the lower arm.

With the application of 30/50 per cent tension, apply the (8 cm) arm bandage from the wrist, overlapping it by two-thirds and covering the lower arm. The next (10 cm) bandage is started at the wrist and applied in a figure of eight up the arm to provide a rigid casing. Alternatively, it can be applied in the opposite direction in a spiral overlapping by two-thirds initially and by less towards the proximal end of the arm.

Tape Skin tape can be used on areas of floppy skin to ease the skin flat and create a more even shape. This will enhance the effect of the bandages and promote tissue contractility.

LOWER LIMB BANDAGING

Method

Application of the cotton tubular stockinette to protect the skin For the leg, the stockinette should lie from the base of the toes to where the bandage finishes, either below-knee or at the proximal end of the limb.

Digit bandaging The toe bandage starts from the base of the toes, with two turns around the dorsum of the foot and little or no tension to secure the bandage. Each toe is then individually wrapped from the distal to the proximal end. Because of the difficulty of obtaining small-width bandages, small toes are difficult to bandage, but the first three toes can usually be successfully dealt with.

Application of padding The aim of padding is to protect the bony prominences and create a cylindrical shape to aid uniform pressure. Skin folds should be padded out using pieces of foam or rolled-up soft padding. Padding can be double-folded in order to achieve a greater protection of bony areas and an enhanced cylindrical shape without the need for excessive padding. It is applied from the base of toes over the whole area to be bandaged. Foam pads can be used for areas that are particularly fibrotic, for example the malleolar region. Care should be taken to ensure patient comfort as these pads can create a very high tissue pressures. Retention bandages can be used to secure the padding in place.

Compression/support bandages The first 8 cm bandage starts at the base of toes. The foot should be positioned at 90 degrees, the bandage being wrapped around the foot and ankle. All soft padding should be covered and even gentle tension applied with the bandage at 30/50 per cent extension. Any extra bandage is wound up the lower limb. The next (10 cm) bandage is started at the ankle and, using a spiral movement, is taken up the leg, overlapping by two-thirds at each turn. The next (10–12 cm) bandage starts where this finishes until all the leg area to be bandaged has been covered.

Another layer is then applied to the whole leg from the distal (ankle) to the proximal (either below-knee or the top of the thigh) end. This bandage can be applied either in a figure of eight or as another spiral in the opposite direction to the first. Several (approximately 3–8) bandages must be used if the whole leg is to be covered.

REFERENCES

Badger, C. 1993: A guideline for the calculation of limb volume based on surface measurements. *British Lymphology Society Newsletter* **7**, 3–7.

Badger, C., Mortimer, P., Regnard, C. and Twycross, R. 1988: Pain in the chronically swollen limb. In: Partsch, H. (ed.) *Progress in lymphology XI*. Amsterdam: Elsevier.

Bates, B. 1995: *A guide to physical examination and history taking*, 6th edn. Philadelphia: J.B. Lippincott.

Bates, B., Stanton, A., Levick, J. and Mortimer, P. 1995: The effect of hosiery on interstitial fluid pressure and arm volume fluctuations in breast cancer related arm edema. *Phlebology* **10**, 46–50.

Bertelli, G., Venturini, M. and Forno, G. 1991: Conservative treatment of postmastectomy lymphoedema: a controlled, randomized trial. *Annals of Oncology* **2**, 575–8.

Brakkee, A. and Kuiper, J. 1988: The influence of compressive stockings on the haemodynamics in the lower extremities. *Phlebology* **3**, 147–53.

Bray, T. and Barrett, J. 2000: Pneumatic compression therapy. In: Twycross, R., Jenns, K. and Todd, J. (eds) *Lymphoedema*. Oxford: Radcliffe Medical Press.

Brennan, M.J., DePompolo, R.W. and Garden, F.H. 1996: Focused review: post mastectomy lymphoedema. *Archives of Physical Medicine and Rehabilitation* **52**, 449–52.

British Lymphology Society 1995: *Strategy for lymphoedema care*. Caterham: BLS.

British Lymphology Society 1997: *Definitions relating to the population and needs of people with or at risk of developing chronic oedema*. Caterham: BLS.

British Lymphology Society 1999: *Directory of treatment centres in the UK*. Caterham: BLS.

Brown, S. 1995: An interviewing style for nursing assessment. *Journal of Advanced Nursing* **21**, 340–3.

Browse, N. and Stewart, G. 1985: Lymphoedema: pathophysiology and classification. *Journal of Cardiovascular Surgery* **26**, 90–105.

Carroll, D. and Rose, K. 1992: Treatment leads to significant improvement. *Professional Nurse* **8**(1), 32–6.

Casley-Smith, J.R. 1992: Modern treatment of lymphoedema. *Modern Medicine Australia* **35**(5), 70–83.

Casley-Smith, J.R. and Casley-Smith, J.R. 1997: *Modern treatment for lymphoedema*, 5th edn. Lymphoedema Association of Australia.

Casley-Smith, J.R. and Piller, N.B. 1985: The incidence of high protein oedemas and lymphoedema. In *Progress in lymphology. Proceedings of the 10th International congress on Lymphology*. Adelaide: University of Adelaide Press.

Chin, P., Finocchiaro, D. and Rosebrough, A. 1998: *Rehabilitation nursing practice.* McGraw-Hill.

Daroczy, J. 1995: Pathology of lymphoedema. *Clinics in Dermatology* **13**, 433–44.

Dicken, S., Lerner, R., Klose G. and Cosimi, B. 1998: Effective treatment of lymphoedema of the extremities. *Archives Surgery* **133**(4), 452–7.

Economist 1999: Helping the poorest. *Economist* 14 August, pp. 11–12.

Erikson, L. 1987: Patient satisfaction: an indicator of nursing care quality? *Nursing Management* **18**(7), 31–5.

Föeldi, M. 1977: The lymphatic system. *Lymphologie* **1**, 16–19.

Föeldi, E. and Föeldi, M. 1991: Conservative treatment of lymphoedema. In: Olszewski, W.L. (ed.) *Lymph stasis: pathophysiology, diagnosis and treatment.* CRC Press.

Föeldi, E., Föeldi, M. and Weissleder, H. 1985: Conservative treatment of lymphoedema of the limbs. *Angiology* **3**, 171–9.

Hock, K. 1998: Lymphoedema and exercise. *Oncology Nursing Forum* **25**(8), 1310.

Hodkinson, M. 1992: Lymphoedema: applying physiology to treatment. *European Journal of Cancer Care* **1**(2), 19–23.

Hughes, K. 2000: Exercise and lymphoedema. In: Twycross, R., Jenns, K. and Todd, J. (ed.) *Lymphoedema.* Oxford: Radcliffe Medical Press.

International Society of Lymphology Executive Committee 1995: Consensus document: the diagnosis and treatment of peripheral lymphoedema. *Lymphology* **28**, 113–17.

Jeffs, E. 1992: Management of lymphoedema: putting treatment into context. *Journal of Tissue Viability* **2**(4), 127–31.

Jenns, K.E. 2000: *The Clinical Effectivness of Complex Decongestive Therapy in the Management of Unilateral Limb Lymphoedema.* Unpublished MSc thesis, School of Health Care, Oxford Brookes University, Oxford.

Johnston, M. 1985: *Experimental biology of the lymphatic circulation.* Amsterdam: Elsevier.

Keeley, V. 1997: The pathophysiology of lymphoedema associated with treatment for breast cancer – recent developments. *Progress in Palliative Care* **5**(3), 107–10.

Keeley, V. 2000a: Clinical features. In: Twycross, R., Jenns, K. and Todd, J. (eds) *Lymphoedema.* Oxford: Radcliffe Medical Press.

Keeley, V. 2000b: Oedema in advancing malignancy. In: Twycross, R., Jenns, K. and Todd, J. (eds) *Lymphoedema.* Oxford: Radcliffe Medical Press.

Kissen, M., Querci della Rovere, G., Easton, D. and Westbury, G. 1986: Risk of lymphoedema following the treatment of breast cancer. *British Journal of Surgery* **73**, 580–4.

Leduc, O. 1988: Manual lymphatic drainage: scintographic demonstration of its efficacy on colloidal protein reabsorbtion. In Partsh, M. (ed.) *Progress in lymphology IX.* Amsterdam: Elsevier.

Leduc, A. et al. 1988: Lymphatic re-absorption of proteins and pressotherapies. In: Partsch, H. (ed.) *Progress in lymphology X1* Amsterdam: Elsevier.

Linnitt, N. 2000: Skin management in lymphoedema. In: Twycross, R., Jenns, K. and Todd, J. 2000: *Lymphoedema.* Oxford: Radcliffe Medical Press.

Logan, V. 1995: Incidence and prevalence of lymphoedema: a literature review. *Journal of Clinical Nursing* **4**, 213–19.

Loomis, M. and Conco, D. 1991: Patients' perceptions of health, chronic illness, and nursing diagnosis. *Nursing Diagnosis* 2(4), 162–70.

Mallon, E. and Ryan, T. 2000: Lymphoedema and wound healing. *Clinics in Dermatology* 12, 89–93.

Mallon, E. et al. 1997: Evidence for altered cell mediated immunity in post mastectomy lymphoedema. *British Journal of Dermatology* 137, 928–33.

Markby, R., Baldwin, E. and Kerr, P. 1991: Incidence of lymphoedema in women with breast cancer. *Professional Nurse* 6, 502–8.

Mason, M. 1993: The treatment of lymphoedema by complex physical therapy. *Australian Physiotherapy* 39(1), 41–5.

Matthews, K. and Smith, J. 1996: The effectiveness of modified complex physical therapy for lymphoedema treatment. *Australian Physiotherapist* 42(4), 323–7.

Mirolo, B.R., Bunce, I.H. and Chapman, M. 1995: Psychosocial benefits of post mastectomy lymphoedema therapy. *Cancer Nursing* 18(3), 197–205.

Mortimer, P. 1990: Investigation and management of lymphoedema. *Vascular Medicine Review* 1, 1–20.

Mortimer, P. 2000: Acute inflammatory episodes. In: Twycross, R., Jenns, K. and Todd, J. (eds) *Lymphoedema*. Oxford: Radcliffe Medical Press.

NHS Executive 1998: *A first class service: quality in the new NHS*. NHS Executive. http://www.doh.gov.uk/newshs/qualsum.htm.

Olszewski, W. 1973: On the pathomechanism of the development of postsurgical lymphoedema. *Lymphology* 6, 35–51.

Olszewski, W.L. 1991: *Lymph stasis: pathophysiology, diagnosis and treatment*. CRC Press.

Partsch, H. 1991: Compression therapy of the legs. *Phlebology* 2, 799–805.

Passik, S., Newman, M. and Brennan, M.D. 1993: Psychiatric consultation for women undergoing rehabilitation for upper extremity lymphoedema following breast cancer treatment. *Journal of Pain and Symptom Management* 8(4), 226–33.

Piller, N.B. 1999: Gaining an accurate assessment of the stages of lymphoedema subsequent to cancer: the role of the objective and subjective information on when to make measurements and their optimal use. *European Journal of Lymphology* 7(25), 1–9.

Rose, K., Taylor, H. and Twycross, R. 1993: Volume reduction of arm lymphoedema. *Nursing Standard* 7(35), 29–32.

Ryan, T.J. 1995: Skin failure and lymphoedema. *Lymphology* 28, 171–3.

Sitzia, J. 1997: A review of outcome indicators in the treatment of chronic limb oedema. *Clinical Rehabilitation* 11, 181–91.

Souhhami, R. and Tobias, J. 1998: *Cancer and its management*. Oxford: Blackwell Science.

Stanton, A. 2000: How does tissue swelling occur? The pathophysiology and pathophysiology of interstitial fluid formation. In: Twycross, R., Jenns, K. and Todd, J. (eds) *Lymphoedema*. Oxford: Radcliffe Medical Press.

Stanton, A. et al. 1996: Current puzzles presented by postmastectomy oedema (breast cancer related lymphoedema). *Vascular Medicine* 1, 213–25.

Stewart, M., Brown, J., Weston, W., McWinney, I., McWilliam, C. and Freeman, T. 1995: *Patient centred medicine*. Mento Park: Sage.

Szuba, A. and Rockson, S. 1998: Lymphoedema: classification, diagnosis and therapy. *Vascular Medicine* 3, 145–56.

Tobin, M., Lacey, H., Meyer, L. and Mortimer, P. 1993: The psychological morbidity of breast cancer related lymphoedema. *Cancer* 72, 3248–52.

Twycross, R. 1995: *Symptom management in advanced cancer.* Oxford: Radcliffe Medical Press.

Twycross, R. 2000: Drug treatment for lymphoedema. In: Twycross, R., Jenns, K. and Todd, J. (eds) *Lymphoedema.* Oxford: Radcliffe Medical Press.

Veitch, J. 1993: Skin problems in lymphoedema. *Wound Management* 4(2), 42–5.

Werngren-Elgstrom, M. and Lidman, D. 1994: Lymphoedema of the lower extremities after surgery and radiotherapy for cancer of the cervix. *Scandinavian Journal of Plastic Reconstruction and Hand Surgery* 28, 289–93.

Williams, A. and Venables, J. 1996: Managing skin problems in uncomplicated lymphoedema. *Journal of Wound Care* 5(5), 224–6.

Wittlinger, G. and Wittlinger, H. 1995: *Textbook of Dr Vodder's manual lymphatic drainage. Vol. 1: Basic Course.* Brussels: Haug International.

Woods, M. 1993: Patients perceptions of breast-cancer related lymphoedema. *European Journal of Cancer Care* 2, 125–8.

Woods, M. 1994: An audit of swollen limb measurements. *Nursing Standard* 9(5), 24–26.

Woods, M., Tobin, M. and Mortimer, P. 1995: The psychosocial morbidity of breast cancer patients with lymphoedema. *Cancer Nursing* 18(6), 467–71.

World Health Organization 1998: Lymphatic filariasis.http://www.who.int/inffs/en/fact190.html.

USEFUL ADDRESSES

British Lymphology Society
PO Box 1059
Caterham
Surrey CR3 6ZU

Lymphoedema Support Network
St Luke's Crypt
Sydney Street
London SW3 6NH
(Patient support network)

MLD UK Ltd
PO Box 14491
Glenrothes
Fife KY6 3YE
(Manual lymphatic drainage courses)

Study Centre Manager
The Sobell House Study Centre
Sir Michael Sobell House
Churchill Hospital
Headington
Oxford OX3 7LJ
(Simple lymphatic drainage courses)

chapter 5

CONFUSIONAL STATES

Kathryn A. Mannix and Anne Pelham

All the physicians and authors in the world could not give a clear account of his madness. He is mad in patches, full of lucid intervals.

From *Don Quixote*, by Miguel Cervantes

WHAT IS CONFUSION?

'Confusion' is used to describe many different symptoms, such as difficulty with concentration, hallucinations or misinterpretations, or disorientation in time and place. Confusion is a description of muddled thought, which can present in different ways in different people.

Feeling muddled and being unable to make proper sense of one's surroundings can be very frightening. To help a patient who is confused, the professional carer must start to calm the patient's fear, try to find the threads of reality in the jumble, and help him or her to keep hold of reality as much as possible. At the same time, a cause for the confusion must be found. Confusion is not a diagnosis but only a symptom of illness, and we can hope fully to reverse the confusion only by identifying and treating the underlying physical illness.

SOME DEFINITIONS

When an illness is caused by physical damage in the body, it is described as an *organic* illness. Confusion is a psychological symptom of an organic illness; psychiatrists call this an *organic brain syndrome*. There are two recognized types of organic brain syndrome: acute (sudden and usually reversible) and chronic (slow and continuing). *Chronic organic brain syndrome* is caused by the death of nerve cells within the brain; it is of gradual onset and gets steadily worse. It is recognized as *dementia* and is almost always irreversible. *Acute organic brain syndrome* or *delirium* is the result of a physical illness in the body that prevents normal brain functioning. It is usually of fairly sudden onset and, instead of getting steadily worse, tends to fluctuate. It is always worth trying to find the physical cause of the delirium because treating this will often restore normal

Table 5.1 Differences between delirium and dementia

Delirium	Dementia
Often reversible	Irreversible
Clouding of consciousness	Clear consciousness
Misinterpretations	
Hallucinations, especially visual	Hallucinations rare
Release of emotion	Affect may be released or reduced
Fluctuating, often worse at night	Unchanging hour by hour, but a slow deterioration over months/years
Onset over hours or days	
Sleep disturbances (not enough or too much)	Normal amount of sleep but may sleep at the wrong time
Activity change (retarded or hyperactive)	No activity change
Global cognitive impairment	Often memory change before other changes

brain function. Even if the cause is not reversible, it is helpful to the family and caring team to understand it, and this may also help to predict the clinical course of the illness.

Table 5.1 shows the main characteristics of these two brain syndromes. Many patients with cancer are elderly, and hence some may also have dementia. The important point about delirium is that the person has changed over a short time. Thus, a demented patient may also become delirious: treatment of the cause of the delirium should restore cerebral functioning to its previous (albeit demented) norm.

Observing and listening to delirious patients shows that their mental processing of information (cognitive function) is affected in all its aspects; this is called a global impairment of cognitive function. The major aspects of psychological function are:

- consciousness
- attention
- perception
- thinking
- memory
- behaviour.

It will help to explain the changes seen in confused patients if each of these aspects is considered in turn.

CONSCIOUSNESS

This refers to how awake and alert a person is. A 'clouding of consciousness' (being less aware and alert) is the first, almost imperceptible, step on the slope from normal alertness down towards coma and death. It is different from sleep, which reflects normal, healthy brain function.

ATTENTION

Attention is the ability to select and concentrate on a particular stimulus, for example to listen to a conversation and ignore distracting noises. Confused patients often appear to be paying less attention than usual, even though they may in fact be paying more, but they cannot select a particular stimulus and their attention flits between, for example, their conversation, noises in the room, thoughts in their head and the colour of the carpet.

PERCEPTION

This is the process of becoming aware of the information being presented by the sensory nerves, such as a hard bed, the smell of burning toast, the sound of visitors' voices, feeling sick or being in pain. Perception can be altered by the circumstances in which the brain receives messages, which can lead to misinterpretations. Misinterpretations are more likely to arise in the following instances:

- *when the level of consciousness is reduced*: during sleep, for example, a person may dream about alarm bells ringing when he or she hears the alarm clock sounding;
- *when the attention is not focused on that sensory pathway*: while concentrating on typing (visual pathway), the sound of the radio (auditory pathway) may be misinterpreted as the telephone ringing. Darkness reduces a person's ability to attend to visual stimuli so visual misinterpretations are more common at night;
- *if a strong emotional state is present*: after reading ghost stories, a person may be frightened by the rustle of the curtains.

Thus in patients with delirium, whose conscious level is reduced, whose attention is difficult to focus and who are very often afraid, perceptions are often altered, conforming to their suspicions or fears (Case study 5.1).

By 'turning up the volume' of attention and emotion, people can alert themselves to perceive particular stimuli: a mother may sleep through the noise of traffic but will awaken instantly if her baby cries.

THINKING

People's thoughts can be recognized by their speech and behaviour. Thoughts are usually connected like links in a chain, so when a person thinks, the links into 'what is happening now', 'what happened in the past', 'how I feel inside',

CASE STUDY 5.1

Emily had a long history of agitated depression, so she surpised both herself and her family by how well she coped with the diagnosis of breast cancer at the age of 60 years. She did very well for 8 years, but when she was admitted to the hospice with bone pain, her family asked us not to tell her that her disease was advancing.

Emily did not settle well. She was shouting and fighting with the night nurses, although she remained withdrawn during the day. The night sister noticed that Emily kept referring to matches and accusing the night staff of trying to kill her. When she asked Emily whether she felt hot, Emily replied that anyone would feel hot if they had been set on fire! Emily's family told us that she had once been in hospital with depression when a schizophrenic patient set fire to the ward, and she had always been very afraid of fires at home after that.

Emily was found to have a high temperature, investigations revealing a urinary tract infection, which was treated with antibiotics. One of Emily's daughters came to sleep with her at the hospice for a few days. While her daughter was with her, we explored Emily's fear of burning to death, Emily told us she could feel that she was weaker and less well, and she thought that she might be dying. She was very afraid of losing control of herself if she became frightened during dying because she had experienced panic attacks in the past. She was told that when the time came, she was likely to lapse into a coma very gently; she found this so comforting that she told the story to all the patients who had become her friends at the hospice.

Emily went home for a further 6 months, returning to the hospice when she was dying, 'because you understand me here...'.

and 'how my friend seems to be feeling' can be separated out, and the person can make sense of a situation.

In delirium, the cross-linking becomes less easy to separate out and to follow, and sufferers have difficulty differentiating their internal and external worlds. They may misinterpret memories for present reality, and they speak more slowly, with long pauses as they try to focus their thoughts. Later, they lose their ability to reason, their ability to form abstract thoughts is impaired, and they display concrete thinking. They usually lose insight at the same time, not realizing that their thinking has changed in the way it has, although patients often have a vague feeling that all is not well, and many express a fear of madness.

MEMORY

The decreased ability to receive and process information accurately causes a disruption of memory. New information cannot be stored, and patients may require the same information to be repeated frequently, even though their memory for past events remains intact. When the episode of delirium is past, patients frequently have no memory of it at all or may remember only meaningless fragments.

BEHAVIOUR

As the control of normal behaviour is lost in their muddled mind, people may display signs of their illness by becoming noisy, hyperactive and irritable, which is seen in up to 20 per cent of delirious people. More commonly, however, they become slower and quieter. Their speech and spontaneous activity are reduced, and repetitive, purposeless movements are common. This perseveration of movements or speech seems to be caused by an inability to turn their attention away from a particular, fragmented thought. This can be very distressing for the patient and his or her family. Such hypoactive delirium happens in about 25 per cent of patients. Up to half of all delirious patients will show a mixture of these features.

LOOKING FOR A CAUSE FOR CONFUSION

Vulnerability to delirium is known to be increased by increasing age, serious physical illness, dehydration, poor eyesight or hearing, and a dependence on alcohol or sedative drugs. Many of these factors may affect cancer patients, increasing the likelihood of delirium if a further physical stress is added.

In cancer patients, it is important to determine as quickly as possible whether there is a treatable cause because the last period of a patient's life will be so much more comfortable, and comforting for his or her family, if the patient is lucid and peaceful. Table 5.2 lists some of the causes of delirium that are worth seeking in cancer patients. There are of course other causes, but those listed are the most common or, with rare causes, those which can be treated easily and effectively. In patients with advanced cancer, there may be several causes for delirium present at the same time.

Once the physical cause of delirium has been treated, it may take several days for the confusion to subside. During this time, it is important to continue to reassure the patient and family, and to keep assessing for signs of improvement. Because delirium is a fluctuating condition, there may be periods of complete normality followed again by confusion, which can reduce families to a state of emotional exhaustion as they celebrate 'recovery' only to be plunged once more back into despair. They need support and reassurance to cope with a beloved person who fails to recognize them or even blames them and accuses them of ill-treatment (Case study 5.2).

UNDERSTANDING THE CONFUSED PATIENT

Definitions and some understanding of what is happening to confused patients' bodies and brains may feel reassuring to the professional carer, but this is not a great deal of help when in the room of a frightened, confused patient whose relatives are looking to professional carers for help. It is necessary therefore to try to understand what is happening to the patients as people.

Table 5.2 Causes of delirium in patients with advanced cancer

	Examples
Drug	Any drugs acting on the central nervous system, particularly: • Antidepressants • Anticonvulsants • Sedative drugs Corticosteriods Opioids Anticholinergic agents Beta-blockers Diuretics Digitalis Remember drug withdrawal, especially: • Alcohol • Opioids • Benzodiazepines
Infection (*the patient may not be pyrexial, and very ill patients or those taking corticosteroids may even be hypothermic*)	Chest ⎫ Most common Urinary tract ⎭ in the elderly Diverticulitis Ears ⎫ Most common Throat ⎭ in children Pressure sores Necrotic tumours
Trauma	Head injury Subdural haematoma
Tumour	Cerebral primary, cerebral metastases 'Paraneoplastic' (malignant disease elsewhere) Anaemia caused by bleeding or bone marrow infiltration
Cardiovascular/respiratory disease (*cerebral hypoxia*)	Stroke(s) Myocardial infarction (classical symptoms and signs may be absent) Heart failure/hypotension/arrhythmias Deep venous thrombosis alone or with pulmonary embolism Respiratory failure
Biochemical/metabolic	Electrolyte disturbance (most commonly hyponatraemia, hypokalaemia, dehydration or hypercalcaemia) Uraemia Liver failure Hypoglycaemia/ketoacidosis Hypothyroidism

CASE STUDY 5.2

George visited his mother Hilda at the hospice every day. She was dying with bladder cancer, but she 'held court' and was queen of the four-bedded bay that she shared with two other patients.

Then George stopped visiting. No-one saw him for days. One of the nurses met him in town, and he angrily told her that his mother had accused him of spending all her money on parties and disreputable women. We asked Hilda directly about this, and she assured us that it was quite true and that George was only waiting for her to die to convert her house into a brothel.

Hilda's husband had left her when George was a little boy – she was now afraid that his father's traits were becoming evident in George and that he would go off the rails when she died. George did in fact have a girlfriend, but he had not told his mother in case she worried that he would leave home while she was ill.

We attributed Hilda's muddled thoughts to the corticosteroids she was taking for painful pressure on her pelvic nerves, and we explained this to George. We tried to discontinue the corticosteroids, but the pain came back. Gently probing her fears for George, Hilda wept to think of him living alone after her death. George was able to ask her how she would feel if he were to marry in the future, and she was overjoyed. Despite this, he did not risk bringing his girlfriend to meet her in case this was misconstrued. Hilda continued to ask uninhibited questions about his 'love life' from time to time, but George was able to understand that the origin of this thought was real concern for his future, and he continued to visit regularly until his mother died.

Start by looking at the mind of a normal healthy person – yourself, perhaps. The thoughts that are reaching your consciousness at this moment are arising from three main areas: from the environment (how warm the room is, how interesting your book is, whether there is a cup of coffee being poured for you); from your body (hunger, gritty eyes, the need to sneeze, respiratory movements, posture); and from your subconscious (memories of last weekend, hopes for your next holiday, remember to buy some milk today, wonder whether your child has got to school safely). If you pay attention to all these thoughts, you will get no work done, remember nothing of what you are reading and be too busy getting your coffee to reach for a tissue to catch your sneeze. The mind therefore has a selective filter that allows a person to concentrate on the job in hand and allows other thoughts into consciousness only if they are important. Figure 5.1 shows how the conscious mind is divided.

Figure 5.2 is a diagram of the consciousness of an awake, well person reading a book. The filter between the body and the subconscious is thick, but it allows relevant thoughts into consciousness (remembering a patient who illustrates the problem you are studying, getting a tissue in time for the sneeze). Note that the boundaries between the different areas of the mind are clear: you can easily separate which messages have come from your memory, your book, your nose.

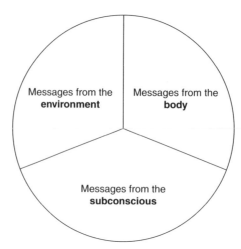

Figure 5.1 Input to the conscious mind

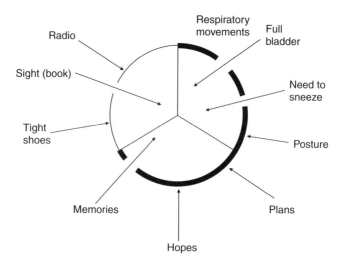

Figure 5.2 Thoughts reaching consciousness: awake, reacting

Figure 5.3 describes the consciousness of another healthy person, but one who is asleep. The boundaries of the three areas of the mind are less clearly demarcated. The environment is being filtered out; although some stimuli from the environment reach consciousness, they may be misinterpreted as part of a dream (the telephone ringing becomes a dream about fire-bells, for example). Similarly, the body is also being filtered out, but some stimuli still get through (pain, full bladder) and may be misinterpreted because the boundaries are unclear. Thus, a person may dream of being attacked because he or she has pain during sleep. The 'volume control' discussed earlier can be set to alert a person to particular stimuli, such as a full bladder, a baby crying or the post arriving.

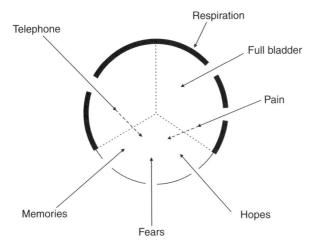

Figure 5.3 Thoughts reaching consciousness: sleep

From this model, it can be seen that all the thoughts in a person's consciousness have come from somewhere. They are all rooted in reality – real physical stimuli, real memories, hopes or fears, real feelings within a person's body. It is the same for the confused person, but it seems that the boundaries have broken down and that it is difficult for the person to work out where a thought has come from. The filter to the environment, however, is thick so that it is difficult for another person to reach the patient. This is illustrated in Figure 5.4.

With this model in mind, it becomes easier to understand why confused people have such bizarre experiences. Their 'volume control' is reset by their fear and anxiety, so stimuli they particularly fear or desire are perceived more

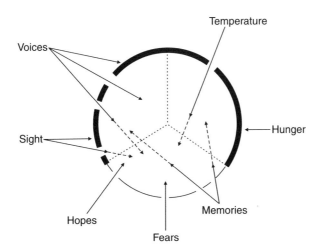

Figure 5.4 Thoughts reaching consciousness: delirium

readily. They may have difficulty in getting a grip on reality, or they may interpret reality as a dream. By trying to trace their (confused) thought back to its origin in reality, carers may be able to help to reduce the anxiety and thus to turn down the 'volume control' of their fears.

TREATMENT OF CONFUSED PATIENTS

It is easy to see why 'confusion' is such a common cause of admission to hospital (Box 5.1). Sometimes the patient's behaviour is too violent for him or her to remain at home, sometimes the family is too distressed to cope. It is also easy to see in retrospect where our management has gone wrong; it is getting it right as we go along that is the challenge.

Look back again to Figure 5.4. The aim of the health professional is to get the frightened, confused patient back in contact with reality. The carer is in the patient's environment, approaching the patient through his or her sight, hearing and touch, but the patient's filter is blocking out the professional carer. How can the carer reach the patient? If sedative drugs are given, the thickness of the filter in

---

BOX 5.1 RECIPE FOR CONFUSION

Ingredients:

- 1 confused patient
- 5 distressed family members
- 1 hospital room, with light switch
- 3 morning nurses, 2 afternoon nurses, 2 night nurses
- 1 ward doctor, 1 on-call doctor
- 2 large hospital porters
- 1 syringeful of chlorpromazine
- 1 green hypodermic needle
- 1 wardful of assorted sick patients

Method:

Remove the confused patient from his or her familiar bedroom at home and place in a cold hard bed in an unfamiliar hospital room. Ask family to leave. Ward doctor should examine patient. Change nurses regularly.

After 8 hours, switch lights off. Leave patient in dark room and disturb regularly to check that he or she is asleep. When he or she protests, send for on-call doctor.

Wait until patient becomes frightened. When he or she begins to rise over the edge of the bed, apply one large hospital porter to each arm. On-call doctor should give injection of chlorpromazine into patient's bottom while repeating the incantation 'This won't hurt' or 'This is for your own good.'

Agitate the whole ward for 4 hours and await ward round. Repeat chlorpromazine if patient shows any sign of waking up. Garnish with diazepam suppositories.

the direction of the environment is increased, and the internal divisions of consciousness are broken down even further. Sedating a patient will never improve his or her delirium, even though it may seem to improve the plight of the carers.

There are drugs available that help to redefine internal reality and thus reduce disordered thinking. These are antipsychotic psychotropic drugs and are not used in sedative doses. Sedation is sometimes really necessary, for example if, because of fear, patients become a danger to themselves or others, or if they are becoming exhausted. Psychotropic and sedative drugs are discussed later in this chapter.

Can a patient be reached via his or her body or subconscious? A gentle touch, holding the patient's hand, smiling – all these are messages of friendship and care that may get through the filter when spoken language is not helping. There is usually comfort from the presence of a trusted friend or relative.

The priorities for management from the patient's point of view are to:

1 stop or reduce the fear;
2 rationalize the underlying anxieties;
3 find and treat the cause of the delirium;
4 orientate to reality.

STOP OR REDUCE THE FEAR

There is fear of the situation in which the patient finds him- or herself, and the carer must help the patient to restore reality. Explain to patients that if they find they are muddled, it is because they are not well. Keep reassuring them and smiling. Keep assuming that they will understand at least some of what you say to them.

There is also a fear of madness: this is very common, but patients are often unable to express their fear. Patients and families need to be reassured that this muddled state is temporary and is caused by the physical illness. We do not think they will go mad; we do not think they are becoming senile.

Hallucinations may occasionally occur and are often visual. Colluding with patients is rarely helpful because their mental state is fluctuating; if you agree now that you can see the little pink frogs, then when the patient becomes more lucid later he or she may remember you 'went along with them' and stop trusting you – or even believe that you are mad for seeing those things! It is often helpful to acknowledge that the hallucination is real for the patient: 'Yes, I know you can see them and that they are very frightening. I can't see them, but you can. You want them to go away and I want to help you to make them go away.'

Misinterpretations are far more common but may be mistaken for hallucination unless a very careful history is taken. With misinterpretations, it is useful to explore the underlying thoughts: 'Did you wish I was your mother when I came in then? Tell me about her. Tell me what she would have done for you.' This should always be accompanied by reorientating that patient and explaining why he or she has become muddled: 'Your temperature is high, so you are

CASE STUDY 5.3

Paula was 33 with two young sons and a husband who worked shifts, so when she was dying of carcinoma of the ovary she was admitted to the hospice to try to keep the home 'normal' for the boys. She had a single room, and the whole family moved in at weekends. She slept well when they were with her, but during the week she slept badly and got increasingly tired and cross.

One afternoon Paula asked her Macmillan nurse, who was visiting, whether all the patients were discussed like this because it was stopping her from taking naps. Exploring this strange comment, we found that she could overhear voices in the patients' kitchen during the day. Although it was impossible to hear what was being said, Paula misinterpreted the voices as a discussion about her illness, as the onset of renal failure made her muddled and unable to separate her own thoughts and fears about her illness from the voices she was hearing. When the family was with her, she was too busy listening to her boys to perceive the sounds of voices in the kitchen.

She told us that the voices commented on her appearance and state of health. She had been a very attractive women before her weight loss, and she grieved for her lost looks. Paula's Macmillan nurse collected her make-up and some clothes from home. The ward nurses explained to her that although the voices were real, the words she heard came from inside Paula's head, and she was able to understand this. Once she knew she was not going mad, she decided to make friends with the voices. When she was dressed with her make-up on, the voices told her how nice she looked!

delirious like small children sometimes are'; 'You have a chest infection, so there is less oxygen than usual getting to your brain.'

Case study 5.3 describes the problem with misinterpretations. The message to the patient must be:

- you are safe here;
- this is not your fault;
- you are not going mad.

RATIONALIZE THE UNDERLYING ANXIETIES

Nightmares and misinterpretations are often clues to the fears residing in the patient's mind. If the carer can share the fear and help the patient to express it, the fear can often be reduced to more manageable proportions. During nightmares, the patient should be gently woken and re-orientated, the dream being explored there and then (Case study 5.4).

FIND AND TREAT THE CAUSE

Table 5.2 above shows some of the more common causes of delirium in cancer patients. Delirium is often multi-factorial. In patients who are physically very ill, unnecessary investigations may cause distress, and it is important to assess the patient with care, decide upon the most likely causes of confusion

CASE STUDY 5.4

Steve was a diver who worked for an oil company. He had a very rare cancer that was progressing slowly and had initially responded to surgery and chemotherapy. Now, however, he had lung deposits and damage to his pelvic nerves. Having spent long periods working away from home, Steve was unsure how to talk to his 9- and 12-year-old sons about his disease. He became angry if his doctor tried to discuss the future, saying that he had fought his cancer so far and would not allow it to beat him now.

The doctor noticed that Steve's wife was looking increasingly tired. She told the doctor that Steve was shouting in his sleep and waking everybody up, but the next morning he could not remember any of this. The doctor asked her to wake Steve up next time it happened and ask him about his dream.

When she did this, Steve woke up terrified and gasping, having dreamt that he was on a very deep dive repairing an oil pipe. Then he became aware of a difficulty in breathing and realized that his air supply was about to run out, but he could not attract the attention of his diving buddy. He knew he should not surface and leave his buddy alone, but he would suffocate if he did not surface. While he was deciding what to do, his air ran out.

Bravely, his wife asked him why he might have this dream. He told her that he thought it was about dying and that time was running out. He could not stay with her to bring up their children, and he felt guilty about leaving her. The next day they told the children how ill Steve was. Steve said he thought he might die but that he would never stop loving them. They all cried together. The dream never came back, and Steve died peacefully at home 2 months later.

and look for these quickly if they are treatable. If no cause is found, or if the cause is not reversible, this must be explained very carefully to the family, and to the patient if possible, care being directed towards managing the patient's distress.

ORIENTATE TO REALITY

Throughout the patient's confusion, it should be assumed that he or she understands what is being said. It will be easier for the patient to be orientated in time if the daily schedule is regular, with meals at predictable times, few changes of face (being nursed by the family and a few Macmillan nurses if possible) and lots of other cues, for example wearing a watch and having today's newspaper near the bed. Remind patients where they are, and ask them to try to remember this and how they came here. Keep the lights on. Remind patients of the date, world events and family news. Make sure their hearing and vision are as good as they can be and that hearing aids and spectacles are used appropriately and well maintained. Following a regular routine for daily activities and using a settling-to-sleep protocol without sedative drugs has been shown to reduce the number and duration of episodes of delirium in elderly people admitted to hospital.

Patients can also be re-orientated to reality by asking them questions that lead them to the correct conclusions, for example:

'What sort of place is this?'
'I'm not sure. . . Queer sort of place if you ask me. . . '
'Do you see all those beds here? And all these people in pyjamas? So what sort of a place do you think this is?'
'It looks like a hospital to me.'
'Yes, you're right, it is a hospital. We are at the Royal Infirmary. Do you remember coming here?'
'I don't know who sent me here. . . '
'You came with your son. What is your son's name?'
'Kevin.'
'Yes, Kevin brought you here. You had been staying at Kevin's house. Do you remember?'
'So this is a hospital, eh? And Kevin knows I'm here? How long am I staying?'
'You are welcome to stay until you are stronger. You have been very ill and things get muddled in your mind. You are improving. You will be home soon.'

Above all, the confused person needs constant reassurance by calm, sympathetic and familiar people that he or she is safe, sane and understood.

DRUG TREATMENT FOR CONFUSED PATIENTS

It occasionally becomes necessary to use drugs to manage patients with delirium (Table 5.3). There are several reasons why drugs may be necessary:

* uncontrollable terror, sometimes leading to dangerous behaviour;
* unreachable distress caused by muddled thinking;
* exhaustion resulting from hyperactivity.

With predominantly jumbled thinking, an antipsychotic drug is needed. This will help to rebuild the divisions within consciousness that are broken down in confusion. The problem is, however, that many of these drugs cause some sedation, which increases the barrier through which the carer is trying to reach the patient. The least sedative antipsychotic drugs are the butyrophenones, of which haloperidol is the drug of choice; risperidone is also a useful drug, but it is not available for parenteral use, which may be necessary if the patient is unable to swallow (e.g. end-of-life care).

With terror or dangerous behaviour, it may be necessary to sedate the patient. This means using a drug that is rapidly active and unlikely to cause serious side-effects. The best drugs in this category are the benzodiazepines, which are sedative but do not cause hypotension. Diazepam and midazolam are the drugs of choice. Many people use the phenothiazine chlorpromazine, but it can cause hypotension, which can in turn cause myocardial infarction or stroke in at-risk patients. In addition, phenothiazines lower the epileptic threshold and may thus

Table 5.3 Drug treatment for patients with delirium

Problem	Aim of treatment	Drug	
		First choice	Second choice
Fear caused by muddled thoughts or hallucinations Paranoid behaviour	Rationalize thoughts with minimal sedation so that patients can discuss their fears	Haloperidol 0.5–2.0 mg, repeated hourly if necessary (oral or subcutaneous)* *Watch for changes in muscle tone*	Risperidone 1–3 mg 12-hourly (oral)
Irreversible terror or distress Urgent behaviour control	Sedation	Midazolam 2.5–5.0 mg (subcutaneous or *slowly* intravenous) Repeat subcutaneous dose hourly as necessary to maintain sedation† *Watch for respiratory depression*	Levomepromazine 12.5–50.0 mg every 4–8 hours (subcutaneous or oral) *Watch for changes in muscle tone* *This drug can enhance any tendency to fitting*

*Maintenance dose of haloperidol: add up the dose required in the first 24 hours and give this subsequently as a single daily dose. Reduce this dose as quickly as possible, continuing to reduce it every day until the drug has been discontinued or the symptoms reappear.

†The maintenance dose of midazolam varies widely between individuals, with an approximate range of 20–150 mg per day. This must be titrated carefully for an individual patient and can be administered by subcutaneous infusion using a syringe driver.

increase the tendency towards fitting in patients who are more vulnerable to seizures because of their illness.

The use of drugs should be confined to the smallest effective dose for the shortest possible time. When possible, treatment for the cause of delirium should be carried out at the same time. Drugs should be given with the patient's permission and by mouth, although this is not always possible. If a patient is suspicious about medication, it is important to have the drug ready and then negotiate and give the tablets or elixir as soon as the patient agrees to take it: by the time you have gone to the drug cupboard, the patient may have forgotten or changed his or her mind.

The correct dosage of the drug should be established by starting with small doses, assessing the response and repeating as necessary. If the oral route is not possible, diazepam works quickly by rectum (diazepam injection *per rectum* via a 2 ml syringe can be used if no rectal solution or suppositories are available, but remember to take the needle off); both midazolam and haloperidol can be given by relatively pain-free subcutaneous injection.

CONCLUSION

Confusion is frightening for the patient and for the family. In previously lucid cancer patients, it is usually the result of an acute organic brain syndrome (delirium) so a treatable physical cause must be sought. It is usually possible to understand where the muddled thoughts are arising from and to allay patient's fears even though their thoughts may remain confused.

The priorities for treatment are to stop the patient's fear, rationalize the underlying anxieties, find and treat the physical cause of the confusion and help to re-orientate the patient to reality. This means enlisting the help of the family to maintain a calm, reassuring environment either at home or in hospital. The patient may need drug treatment, which should preferably be voluntary and by mouth.

Above all, it must always be assumed that the patient understands what is being said. The patient must be reassured that he or she is safe and is not insane, and that the carers are trying to understand. Confusion is often reversible, but even when it cannot be completely resolved, it can be understood and made manageable.

ACKNOWLEDGEMENTS

Thanks go to Dr Andrew Brittlebank and Mrs Jeanne Donaghy for their helpful criticisms and suggestions, Dr Averil Stedeford for diagrams upon which the figures are based, Heinemann Medical Books for their permission to use these and Mrs Andrea Green for typing the manuscript.

REFERENCES

American Psychiatric Association 1999: Practice guideline for the treatment of patients with delirium. *American Journal of Psychiatry* **156** (supplement), 1–20.

Anderson, F. and Williams, B. 1989: Practical management of the elderly. Oxford: Basil Blackwell.

Breitbart, W., Chochninov, H.M. and Passik, S. 1998: Psychiatric aspects of palliative care. In: Doyle, D., Hanks, G.W.C.D. and MacDonald, N. (eds) *Oxford textbook of palliative medicine*. Oxford: Oxford Medical Publications.

Breitbart, W., Marotta, R., Platt, M.M. et al. 1996: A double-blind trial of haloperidol, chlorpramazine, and lorazepam in the treatment of delirium in hospitalised AIDS patients. *American Journal of Psychiatry* **153**, 231–7.

Inouye, S.K., Van Dyck, C.H., Alessi, C.A. et al. 1990: Clarifying confusion: the confusion assessment method – a new method of detection of delirium. *Annals of Internal Medicine* **113**, 941–8.

Inouye, S.K., Viscoli, C.M., Horowitz, R.I. et al. 1993: A predictive model for delirium in hospitalised elderly medical patients based on admission characteristics. *Annals of Internal Medicine* **119**, 474–81.

Inouye, S.K., Bogardus, S.T., Charpeutier, P.A. et al. 1999: A multicomponent intervention to prevent delirium in hospitalised older patients. *New England Journal of Medicine* **340**(9), 669–76.

Lipowski, Z.J. 1992: Delirium and impaired consciousness. In: Grimley Evans, J. and Franklin Williams, T. (eds) *The Oxford textbook of geriatric medicine.* Oxford: Oxford University Press.

Regnard, C.F.B. and Tempest, S. 1998: *A guide to symptom relief in advanced cancer.* Manchester: Hochland & Hochland.

Stedeford, A. 1984: *Facing death. Patients, families and professionals.* Oxford: Heinemann.

Stedeford, A. and Regnard, C. 1995: Confusional states. In: Regnard, C. and Hockley, J. (eds) *Flow diagrams in advanced cancer and other diseases.* London: Edward Arnold.

chapter 6

DISEASE-MODIFYING TREATMENTS IN PALLIATIVE CARE

Mark Napier and Rajaguru Srinivasan

> Life is short, the art long, opportunity fleeting, experience treacherous, judgement difficult. The physician [nurse] must be ready not only to do his duty himself but also to secure the co-operation of the patient, of the attendants and of externals.
>
> *Corpus Hippocraticum*

A significant proportion of patients with cancer present in an advanced stage, and a further subset will relapse at distant times following their successful initial treatment. Curative treatments are not available for many of these patients, but oncologists will commonly prescribe treatments in this setting with palliative intent. These treatments may alter the natural course of the disease, leading to either longer survival or a reduction or resolution of symptoms, in some cases to both. These are known as disease-modifying treatments.

The treatments commonly affect cancer growth and spread by killing a proportion of the tumour cells, others acting by influencing the growth pattern directly rather than causing cell death, as is seen with the action of hormonal agents on growth factor receptors. The unifying theme is, however, that they act directly on the tumour rather than on the downstream effect that the particular cancer is having. By affecting the cancer directly, these therapies have the potential to reduce or eliminate the problems caused by it, which is why they are in common use. Rightly or wrongly, patients often focus upon these therapies to the detriment of others. Such treatments should not be considered in isolation but as another treatment in the armamentarium of those caring for cancer patients.

The decision to embark upon these palliative therapies is often complex, and the possible benefits must be weighed against the inevitable toxicities. An understanding of the cost:benefit ratio has to be conveyed to patients and their carers to allow an informed decision regarding treatment to be made. In some cases, the decision is relatively easy. Palliative short-course radiotherapy to a painful breast cancer bony metastasis can for example, usually be given with almost no short-term toxicity yet a high chance of producing reasonable pain control. In other instances, however, decision-making is extremely difficult: giving intensive chemotherapy to a patient with advanced sarcoma with only a small chance of effective symptom palliation is more problematic.

The decision to embark upon palliative chemotherapy is often not a question of 'if' but 'when'. With the intensive follow-up that usually follows cancer therapy, recurrences may be found that are asymptomatic. This is very common in diseases in which tumour marker elevation can predate clinical cancer recurrence by many months (for example, CA125 elevation in ovarian cancer and carcinoembryonic antigen elevation in colorectal cancer). In these patients, early intervention with further therapy will not palliate non-existent symptoms, but it may prolong life or delay the inevitable problems caused by the cancer. It has recently been shown (in colorectal cancer at least) that early intervention with chemotherapy, that is, intervention prior to the development of symptoms, is superior to delayed therapy in terms of survival and quality of life (Nordic Gastrointestinal Tumour Adjuvant Therapy Group, 1992). In patients considering second-, third- and in some case fourth-line therapies, with an inevitably smaller chance of success, the decision relating to the timing of therapy is more difficult, most oncologists favouring invoking palliative therapies only when the symptoms dictate.

Before becoming an accepted palliative therapy, most treatments will undergo a prolonged period of investigation in cancer clinical trials. The end-point or aim of these trials has until recently been the demonstration of efficacy in terms of clinical response, prolongation of life and disease-free interval. These end-points may not, however, be the most important in the palliative setting. More and more trials now include as one of their primary end-points the demonstration of an improved 'quality of life'. Indeed, some chemotherapy drugs have been licensed on this basis alone: gemcitabine was shown to be efficacious in advanced pancreatic cancer when it became clear that analgesic usage in the group given this drug decreased (Burris et al., 1997).

'Quality of life' is usually measured in clinical trials using an established questionnaire that is modified according to the cancer being treated. Some oncologists are unhappy using this alone so new scales often combine subjective, patient-centred questionnaires with more objective measures such as the disease free-interval and response rate.

At this point, it is worthwhile discussing in some detail the disease-modifying therapies used in palliative care. Such treatments can be broadly classified into the following categories:

- chemotherapy
- radiotherapy
- endocrine agents
- biological agents
- radiopharmaceuticals.

CHEMOTHERAPY

Systemic chemotherapy is the primary treatment available for disseminated malignant disease. Progress in drug therapy has resulted in the development of curative chemotherapy for many tumours, and it also has a significant role in palliation, often with improved survival, in a variety of other tumours. However, in several of the common solid tumours, chemotherapy has in general only modest activity (Table 6.1). All patients need a full assessment to document the extent of disease and the symptoms it causes. It is necessary to select the patients most likely to respond, this usually being decided by taking into

Table 6.1 Cancers in which chemotherapy is frequently used Examples

Cancers in which chemotherapy has a high efficacy or potential to cure	Acute lymphocytic leukaemia
	Acute myelogenous leukaemia
	Ewing's sarcoma
	Trophoblastic tumours
	Hodgkin's disease
	Non-Hodgkin's lymphoma
	Rhabdomyosarcoma
	Testicular carcinoma
	Wilm's tumour
Cancers in which chemotherapy has significant activity	Anal carcinoma
	Bladder cancer
	Breast carcinoma
	Cervix carcinoma
	Chronic lymphocytic leukaemia
	Chronic myelogenous leukaemia
	Endometrial carcinoma
	Head and neck tumours
	Small cell lung tumours
	Multiple myeloma
	Ovarian carcinoma
Cancers in which chemotherapy has only modest activity	Brain tumours
	Colorectal carcinoma
	Hepatocellular carcinoma
	Non-small cell lung tumours
	Melanoma
	Pancreatic cancer
	Prostate carcinoma
	Renal cell carcinoma
	Sarcomas

account the tumour type, previous treatments if any, the disease-free or progression-free interval after prior therapies and, importantly, the performance status of the patient.

Chemotherapeutic agents in general kill tumour cells by acting on a cellular process important for cell division. This generalization also explains their major drawback: they are usually indiscriminate in their activity, affecting all dividing cells equally. Luckily, tumour cells either divide more frequently or lack the capacity to repair any damage inflicted upon them so there is some inherent selectivity in their action. Normal tissues that have a high mitotic activity (e.g. bone marrow, gastrointestinal epithelium and gonadal and hair follicular tissue) are those in which most of the toxic side-effects are found. Despite these drawbacks, chemotherapeutic agents as a group frequently produce worthwhile improvements in those with advanced cancers.

Chemotherapy, whether given with curative or palliative intent, usually requires multiple cycles of treatment, and an assessment of the therapeutic efficacy prior to completing an entire course of treatment is desirable. This allows for the discontinuation of ineffective therapies, may allow the institution of other salvage regimes and, in the absence of other effective regimes, avoids unnecessary toxicity. The response to therapy can be measured by palpating superficial lesions or imaging internal ones, but in some cases, indirect assessment with tumour markers like carcinoembryonic antigen and CA125 is all that is possible. Uniform criteria for describing the response are widely accepted and enable a comparison of the efficacy of alternative treatments, but at the individual level, a subjective measurement such as the relief of pain or dyspnoea may be a worthwhile reason for carrying on. With each therapy, the decision to continue suggests that the efficacy of the therapy outweighs the morbidity associated with it.

Every chemotherapeutic regime will, if administered in an adequate dosage, produce some side-effects in the patient, myelosuppression being the most common unwanted effect of chemotherapy. In this, a reduction in the number of red blood cells, white blood cells and platelets can occur. The blood counts often reach their lowest point 7–14 days after treatment and usually recover within 21–28 days, allowing a further cycle of therapy. During this time, patients are at risk of infection and hemorrhagic complications. These complications can be life-threatening and are the prime reason for attenuating the dosage or dosage interval.

New approaches to the treatment or prevention of these problems include the use of prophylactic antibiotics and white cell and platelet growth factors. The anaemia associated with chemotherapy (and the attendant asthenia) is more difficult to control. Recent research has considered the efficacy of erythropoietin in this regard (this growth factor having had a major impact in the field of renal failure-associated anaemia). Currently, however, intermittent blood transfusions remain the easiest way to overcome this problem.

Nausea and vomiting are other major side-effects of chemotherapy. Significant progress has been made in the treatment of chemotherapy-induced nausea and vomiting, particularly with the advent of the histamine receptor antagonists such as ondansetron and granisetron. Individual chemotherapeutic agents are not equally emetogenic, drugs such as cisplatin, dacarbazine and doxorubicin consistently causing the most severe side-effects, whereas methotrexate and 5-fluoro-uracil may cause only minimal nausea.

The prevention of nausea and vomiting should be the primary goal. Antiemetic regimes should be given on a regular pre-emptive schedule, treatment on an 'as required' basis being inappropriate. These regimes should err on the side of being too aggressive rather than too weak as antiemetic failure can produce a syndrome of anticipatory nausea, which can be difficult to control. Despite the undoubted success of modern antiemetics, they are not without their own problems – in particular, the constipation associated with these new agents can be very troublesome.

Chemotherapy-induced hair loss (alopecia) is one of the distressing side-effects of treatment, being caused by a direct cytotoxic effect on the hair follicles. It is most severe in the scalp and may become noticeable 3–4 weeks after start of therapy. After cessation of the chemotherapy, hair regrowth begins and should eventually return to the pretreatment level. Drugs causing profound alopecia include cyclophosphamide, doxorubicin, paclitaxel and etoposide. Scalp-cooling devices that apparently decrease scalp perfusion have been employed, with mixed results.

Most chemotherapeutic agents have their own spectrum of side-effects, some unrelated to their cytotoxic activity. A thorough review is outside the scope of this chapter, but a fundamental grasp of the action and toxicity of these drugs is important when deciding upon the most appropriate therapy (Table 6.2).

Combination rather than single-agent chemotherapy regimes are now regularly used in the palliative setting, the positive aspect of combination therapy being a higher response rate. Drugs in combination are usually chosen to complement each other (i.e. with differing modes of action and a different spectrum of toxicities), with the aim of reducing the possibility of innate drug resistance. The downside is of course that the more drugs given, the greater the possibility of morbidity. Examples of common combination therapies include paclitaxel/carboplatin in ovarian cancer, and irinotecan/5-fluorouracil in colorectal cancer.

Table 6.1 above describes the cancers in which chemotherapy is commonly used and the chances of successful therapy, Table 6.2 outlining the most common chemotherapeutic agents grouped according to their class, mode of action, principle uses and major toxicities.

RADIOTHERAPY

Radiation therapy is used in the palliative management of many tumours. Irradiation of bony metastases reduces pain, and radiotherapy can also control problems such as bleeding, brain metastases and vital organ obstruction. Radiotherapy may be needed on an urgent basis to control, for example, spinal cord compression, airway obstruction and superior vena caval obstruction.

Table 6.2 Chemotherapeutic agents

Class/drug	Mechanism	Principle use	Toxicity
• Antimetabolites			
Methotrexate	*Dihydrofolate reductase* inhibitor	Breast, acute lymphocytic leukaemia, non-Hodgkin's lymphoma	Myelotoxicity Mucositis
Hydroxyurea	*Ribonucleotide reductase* inhibitor	Chronic myelogenous leukaemia	Myelotoxicity
5-Fluorouracil	*Thymidalate synthase* inhibitor	Colorectal, breast	Myelotoxicity Mucositis (gastrointestinal)
Cytarabine	Inhibits DNA replication	Acute lymphocytic leukaemia, non-Hodgkin's lymphoma	Myelotoxicity Mucositis (gastrointestinal)
• Plant alkaloids			
Vincristine Vinblastine	Inhibits microtubule assembly	Breast, testicular, Hodgkin's disease, non-Hodgkin's lymphoma	Myelotoxicity Neurotoxicity
Paclitaxel Docetaxel	Prevents microtubule disassembly	Ovarian, breast	Myelotoxicity Neurotoxicity
Etoposide	*Topoisomerase II* inhibitor	Lung, testicular, ovarian	Myelotoxicity
• Antibiotics			
Anthracyclines (doxorubicin, epirubicin)	DNA intercalating agents	Breast, bladder, lung	Cardiotoxicity Myelotoxicity
Bleomycin	DNA strand breaks	Hodgkin's disease, testicular	Pulmonary fibrosis
Mitomycin C	DNA cross-links	Gastrointestinal, lung	Delayed myelotoxicity

Table 6.2 (*Continued*)

Class/drug	Mechanism	Principle use	Toxicity
• Alkylating agents			
Cyclophosphamide	Inhibits DNA synthesis	Breast, lung, ovarian	Haemorrhagic cystitis
Ifosfamide	Inhibits DNA synthesis	Sarcoma, lymphoma, lung	Myelotoxic Urothelial damage
Cisplatin	Covalent DNA cross-links	Testicular, ovarian, lung, bladder	Nephrotoxicity
Carboplatin	Covalent DNA cross-links	Ovarian, testicular	Myelotoxicity
• *Topoisomerase* inhibitors			
Topotecan	*Topoisomerase I* inhibitor	Ovarian	Myelotoxicity
Irinotecan	*Topoisomerase I* inhibitor	Colorectal	Gastrointestinal toxicity

Radiotherapy is most commonly delivered using a linear accelerator that produces high-energy X-ray beams. A course of radiation therapy is usually preceded by simulation, with appropriate radiographic localization of the tumour. The treatment is delivered in multiple fractions over a period of time. This fractionation of radiotherapy allows a larger total dose to be given, may improve tumour control and reduces the effect on the surrounding normal tissues by allowing them a recovery period.

Radiation therapy is associated with both acute toxicity and long-term sequelae. The acute reactions are self-limiting and include skin reactions, gastrointestinal disturbances and myelosuppression. The long-term sequelae are dose-limiting and occur many months to years after completion of the radiotherapy. When the treatment is delivered with a palliative intent, the long-term complications of radiotherapy are rarely a constraint, but it is always good practice to limit the doses of radiation to below normal tissue tolerance.

ENDOCRINE THERAPIES

Endocrine treatments for hormone-responsive tumours have been utilized for many years. They generally lack the serious side-effects associated with cytotoxic chemotherapy and can be administered as an out-patient treatment. Endocrine therapies can act selectively against tumour cells, and it is often possible to predict which patient will respond based upon the presence or absence of a particular receptor. Many belong to the steroid family, binding to specific receptors and regulating the expression of the gene(s) necessary for initiating or promoting cell division.

The following is a selection of the commonly used endocrine therapies.

CORTICOSTEROIDS

These agents have activity against leukaemias and lymphomas. They act by binding to specific steroid receptors and inducing programmed cell death (apoptosis). Agents frequently used are prednisolone and dexamethasone. Corticosteroids have some useful side-effects in the palliative setting: their ability to improve appetite and elevate mood has for example, made them a useful adjunct in the treatment of many cancers.

ANTI-OESTROGENS

Tamoxifen is the most well-known member of this group, being used mainly in breast cancer. Those patients whose tumours are positive for oestrogen and progesterone receptors benefit most, tamoxifen binding to oestrogen receptors and functioning as a weak antagonist/agonist. Treatment is simple and can in general be given with few worrisome side-effects. The use of this single agent has dramatically improved the lot of patients with advanced breast cancer.

AROMATASE INHIBITORS

The enzyme aromatase converts androgens to oestrogens. Anastrazole is the commonly used agent in this group. It is useful in the palliative treatment of metastatic breast carcinoma in postmenopausal women and can be useful in those patients in whom tamoxifen therapy is no longer effective.

GONADOTROPHIN-RELEASING HORMONE AGONISTS

The gonadotrophin-releasing hormone agonist leuprorelin (Zoladex) is used in treatment of metastatic prostatic carcinoma. It acts by suppressing the release of follicle-stimulating hormone and luteinizing hormone from the pituitary gland, leading to a suppression of testosterone secretion. In the initial few weeks of treatment, the levels of leuteinizing hormone and follicle-stimulating hormone may rise, leading to a transient increase in testosterone level. This should be counteracted with drugs such as flutamide, which directly block the action of testosterone.

PROGESTINS

Progestational agents such as medroxyprogesterone and megestrol are used in the treatment of endometrial and breast carcinoma. Their mechanism of action is unclear, but they may be directly cytotoxic to tumour cells. They also alter the expression of oestrogen receptors and interfere with the hypothalamic-pituitary-gonadal axis. Common side-effects include fluid retention, thromboembolic events and menstrual disturbances.

SOMATOSTATIN ANALOGUES

The long-acting somatostatin analogue octreotide is useful in treatment of carcinoid tumours producing carcinoid syndrome. An improvement in the diarrhoea, flushing and hypoglycaemia seen with this condition can be expected.

BIOLOGICAL THERAPIES

The term 'biological response modifiers' is used to suggest that these agents act by altering the patient's response to cancer rather than by a direct cytotoxic effect on the tumour cells. The role of such agents is currently limited, but its expansion is to be expected.

MONOCLONAL ANTIBODIES

Monoclonal antibodies are some of the newer agents that are available for the treatment of cancer. First, one has to identify the specific tumour antigen expressed mainly by the tumour cells. Monoclonal antibodies are then raised against these antigens using hybridoma technology (the fusion of an antibody with a murine myeloma cell line to produce a clone of specific antibodies). The antibodies produced are administered to the patient to act against the tumour, for example inducing the host to set up an immune reaction against the tumour. These effects tend to occur specifically against the tumour deposit so side-effects are rare.

Rituximab is a unconjugated antibody against the CD20 antigen, which is commonly found in B-cell lymphomas. It is a useful agent in relapsed and resistant low-grade lymphomas and follicular lymphomas that are CD20 antigen positive. Herceptin is a monoclonal antibody used in treatment of breast cancer, blocking the receptor for the HER2/Neu protein and interfering with the growth of the cancer cells. Patients with tumours that express an excess level of the HER2/Neu protein benefit from this treatment.

CYTOKINES

Cytokines are intra- and extracellular messenger proteins that have a key role in immunoregulatory functions. Interferons are an important member of this family of proteins, interferon being licensed in the treatment of hairy cell leukaemia, chronic myelogenous leukaemia, low-grade non-Hodgkin's lymphoma, multiple myeloma, melanoma and Kaposi's sarcoma. Interleukins are cytokines that function mainly as leukocyte messengers; they can produce responses in melanoma and renal cell carcinoma. These agents, although effective, have a wide range of side-effects that have limited their use.

RADIOPHARMACEUTICAL PRODUCTS

These are medicinal products that have a radioactive component attached to them. Following their administration to a patient, they will follow defined metabolic pathways. The properties of a particular radiopharmaceutical agent may allow a high and specific tumour uptake, with at best its prolonged retention in the tumour. Radiopharmaceutical agents usually give out alpha or beta emissions and have a long half-life. A few examples of such substances are given below.

^{131}I is an isotope of iodine that emits beta and gamma radiation. It is selectively taken up by functioning thyroid tissue, leading to selective damage to the thyroid. Hence it is useful in the treatment of papillary carcinoma of the thyroid. Similarly, the ^{32}P isotope of phosphorus is used to treat polycythaemia and bone metastases. ^{131}I-labelled MIBG is used in the palliative treatment of carcinoid tumours and phaeochromocytomas.

All these have implications for radiation protection, and patients may need to be isolated for a short time following the administration of such treatment. Although they can be specific and very effective therapies, their use is limited by the irradiation of the patient's bone marrow while the radiopharmaceutical agent is circulating prior to tumour uptake.

RECENT DEVELOPMENTS IN DISEASE-MODIFYING AGENTS FOR CANCER

Cytotoxic drug development has come a long way since the development of the first alkylating agents in the late 1940s. Despite this, the major impact has been seen with the less common cancers, and there is still a great deal of improvement needed in the therapy of the common solid malignancies. All too often, new agents continue to have the same limitations and side-effects that were seen in their parent compounds so recent research has focused on developing agents with novel and non-cross-reacting mechanisms of action. These tend to focus on the mechanisms whereby cancers develop and metastasize and tend to be cytostatic rather than cytotoxic.

Major work has focused on tumour vasculature. Cancers require blood vessels to supply them with nutrients to grow and will induce new vessel growth by secreting cytokines such as vascular endothelial growth factor. This fact allows cancer researchers to target drugs or antibodies to disrupt this pattern. Similarly, new agents are being developed against the enzymes required by cancers to invade new tissue and metastasize (matrix metalloproteinases).

This explosion in our basic knowledge of cancer development and growth has led to the development of many new agents, which are now reaching clinical practice. Our hope is that, because of their innate selectivity, they will have fewer of the side-effects of the older agents and may thus be more useful in palliating cancer symptoms.

ETHICAL AND OTHER DILEMMAS IN THE PROVISION OF PALLIATIVE CHEMOTHERAPY

CLINICAL TRIALS

> Clinical research is an obligation...
> Sir William Osler

New agents in development as anti-cancer therapies require testing in patients, usually in the context of a clinical trial (Table 6.3). The earliest testing is often carried out on patients with advanced cancers in whom conventional treatment has ceased to be useful or effective. It is in this group of patients that chemotherapy is in general the least effective.

Thus, a major dilemma exists. In our thirst for knowledge and our laudable aim to improve treatment for future generations of cancer patients, we often expose patients to treatments of unknown toxicity, with little chance of actually helping them in any meaningful way. Patients, however, often welcome the possibility of further therapy and inclusion into early-phase trials. This is often related to the close medical and nursing supervision that goes with trial entry rather to than a realistic improvement related to the experimental therapy itself.

OVEREXPECTATION OR UNREALISM?

Patients are constantly bombarded with television and newspaper articles concerning cancer and its treatment, many focusing on new (often experimental and/or untried) therapies. The word 'breakthrough' tends to be mentioned. Good news makes good press, and patients often believe the fight against cancer to be nearly won, but with most of the common solid malignancies, we are in fact some way from possessing truly effective therapies. Although it is true that

Table 6.3 Clinical trials in cancer therapy

Phase of trial	Objectives	Patient population
I	Maximum tolerated dose	Advanced malignancy
	Pharmacokinetic parameters	Not amenable to conventional therapies
II	Anti-tumour activity	Advanced malignancy
	Side-effects	Less heavily pre-treated
		Good performance status and preserved organ function
III	Comparison with standard treatments	Chemotherapy-naive
		Good performance status

great advances have been made and new therapies are changing the outlook for many people with cancer, most new treatments have led to an improvement in progression-free and overall survival that is measured only in weeks or months.

Irinotecan, for example, is a relatively new anti-cancer agent that is now used commonly in patients with advanced colorectal cancer. The initial trials suggested that this agent was superior to 'best supportive care' in patients failing the standard therapy with 5-fluorouracil (Cunningham et al., 1998), the improvement in survival being 2–3 months. A similar improvement in survival was seen in patients treated as a first line with irinotecan combined with 5-fluorouracil compared with 5-fluoruracil alone (Douillard et al., 2000). Although quality of life data supported the use of irinotecan, the irinotecan-containing regimes were in both trials more toxic. Although these trials showed this drug to be a valuable and worthwhile addition to the treatment for this difficult condition, the improvements were hardly earth-shattering. Similar improvements in survival statistics have been seen with new agents for the other common cancers.

Small improvements in life expectancy are often considered to be very valuable to the individual patient, but, in statistical terms, patients, more often than not, derive no benefit from these therapies when they are used as other than first-line treatment. In addition, in those who do, much of the extra life expectancy will be spent receiving treatment (with regular visits to hospital and chemotherapy suites) rather than with their families and loved ones.

COST AND POSTCODE PRESCRIBING

The development of a new cytotoxic agent is not cheap: many millions of pounds need to be invested in development and trial costs before a new drug is licensed and the company involved can charge for its use and recoup its investment. To do this before a patent runs out, drug companies require a high cost to be levied on new agents. For example, a six-cycle treatment with a taxane drug (paclitaxel or docetaxel), which is an effective agent in breast and ovarian cancer (among others), costs in the region of £6000–9000. This level of expenditure is difficult for many health authorities to bear given that new agents tend to be given in addition to, rather than in place of, more established treatments.

In the UK, at least, this has given rise to what is known as 'postcode prescribing', some health authorities allowing the use of expensive new agents and others not, and patients rightly feel aggrieved that they may be denied useful treatment by virtue of their address. The press has of course made much of this, headlines such as 'Patients denied life-saving cancer drug' being commonplace. For those oncologists practising in areas with restrictions, the already strained doctor–patient relationship can reach breaking point. Decisions on prescribing issues that are truly national may go some way towards improving this situation.

THE INTERNET

The increasing ease of gaining access to the Internet and its seemingly limitless supply of information has radically altered some patients' approaches to therapy.

Patients often arrive armed with information that previously fell only into the domain of physicians reading medical journals. The advent of specific cancer discussion groups also allows patients directly to compare and contrast their treatments and outcomes. Although a well-informed patient is usually a blessing, any misinterpretation of the information they uncover can hinder their progress.

The phrase 'We have little left to offer you' is often uttered when the treating oncologist holds the considered opinion that the risk of expected toxicity from the therapies available outweighs their potential benefits expected rather than because there really is nothing left to offer. Patients are clearly now able to determine that further treatments are available, and many wish to have access to them. What this means is that many patients are now having three, four or even five lines of palliative therapy. The benefits of treatments at this late stage are, however, largely unproven, and it is impossible to extrapolate results from early trials in younger, good performance status patients into wider practice.

Information technology can also have its downside. Cancer patients searching for web-based information on their disease and its treatment are often the target of unsolicited and often salacious mail shots. These may imply that 'mainstream' practitioners are not only withholding life-saving treatments, but also prescribing ones that are at best damaging. Further reading often will lead to the attempted sale of largely unproven, and often disproved, agents such as laetrile or shark cartilage. These will often come from countries without (through no fault of their own) the legislation to stop this illegal advertising.

CONCLUSION

The main aims of treatment with disease-modifying agents for patients with advanced cancer are an improvement in the quality of life and, to a lesser extent, a prolongation of survival. The decision to start treatment must be made with these goals in mind, and an assessment with a view to continuing treatment should be made after measuring the extent to which these goals have been achieved. Many patients will derive no benefit from treatment with these agents, and the diagnosis itself is not the only indication to start treatment.

New treatments, some with potentially few morbid side-effects, are changing the way in which we treat patients with advanced cancer. There are, however, ethical and other non-medical issues that influence the provision of what are essentially palliative therapies.

REFERENCES

Burris, H.A., Moore, M.J., Andersen, J. et al. 1997: Improvements in survival and clinical benefit with gemcitabine as first-line therapy in patients with advanced pancreatic cancer: a randomised trial. *Journal of Clinical Oncology* 15, 2403–13.

Cunningham, D., Pyrhonen, S., James, R.D. et al. 1998: Randomised trial of irinotecan plus supportive care versus supportive care alone after fluorouracil failure in patients with metastatic colorectal cancer. *Lancet* **352**, 1413–18.

Douilard, J.Y., Cunningham, D., Roth, A.D. et al. 2000: Irinotecan combined with fluorouracil compared with fluorouracil alone as first-line treatment for metastatic colorectal cancer: a multicentre randomised trial. *Lancet* **355**, 1041–7.

Nordic Gastrointestinal Tumour Adjuvant Therapy Group. 1992: Phase III trial of chemotherapy at detection of advanced disease versus delaying chemotherapy until development of symptoms in asymptomatic advanced colorectal cancer. *Journal of Clinical Oncology* **10**, 904–11.

FURTHER READING

Doyle, D., Hanks, G.W. and MacDonald, N. (eds) 1993: *Oxford Textbook of Palliative Medicine*. Oxford: Oxford University Press.

Smith, I.E. 1983: Measuring response in incurable cancer. In: Stoll B.A. (ed.) *Cancer Treatment: End-point Evaluation*. London: John Wiley.

Walsh, T.D. 1994: Palliative care: management of the patient with advanced cancer. *Seminars in Oncology* **21**, 100–6.

Wyatt, J.C. 2000: Knowledge and the Internet. *Journal of the Royal Society of Medicine* **93**, 565–70.

OTHER SOURCES OF INFORMATION

Cancer BACUP
3 Rivington Place
London EC2A 3JR
UK

EORTC Quality of Life Study Group
Avenue Mounier
83 B11
1200 Brussels
Belgium

US National Cancer Institute
www.nci.nih.gov

Part 2

MEETING NEEDS: ART AND SCIENCE

chapter 7

EMOTIONAL PAIN AND ELICITING CONCERNS

Maggie Fisher

There's a man in my bed I used to love him
His kisses used to take my breath away
There's a man in my bed I hardly know him
As I wipe his face and hold his hand
And watch him as he slowly fades away

He fades away, not like leaves that fall in autumn
Turning gold against the grey, he fades away
Like the blood stains on the pillowcase I wash every day
He fades away.
From a song by Alistair Hulett as recorded on
Andy Irvine's album *Rain on the Roof*

When I recently asked a woman what she felt she needed from me she said, 'to provide a cradle for my emotions'. When offering support in palliative care, much of our work is about offering an emotional cradle – something of ourselves, our willingness to walk the road, providing a presence together with the skills and structures to hold the kind of pain spoken of above.

A PSYCHOSOCIAL CARE CULTURE

In order to set the scene for these skills and structures, I wish to begin by defining and exploring psychosocial care:

> Psycho-social care is concerned with the psychological and emotional well-being of the patient and their family/carers, including issues of self esteem, insight into and adaptation to illness and its consequences, communication, social functioning, and relationships.
>
> National Council for Hospices and Specialist Palliative Care Services (1997)

Psychosocial care is concerned with health as well as pathology and forms part of our holistic spectrum of symptom management expertise. The most common model of psychosocial provision in health care is often what Nichols (1993) calls 'the psychological casualty model'. This is a crisis intervention model, the assumption being that people are basically fine unless they appear to be otherwise. When they appear not to be fine, a so-called 'expert' is brought in, or the problem may be suppressed by drugs. Within this model, the person needs the ticket of significant psychological distress before he or she can receive care.

An extensive literature exists on the experience of adjusting to dying, much of it focusing on observational studies of dying people's responses; the best known of these is probably that describing Kübler-Ross's stage theory. This has come to be viewed as normative rather than descriptive (Kübler-Ross, 1970).

While being concerned not to overuse labels that pathologize, we need to bear in mind an awareness of the most common 'psychiatric' problems in palliative care. These are mood disorders, for example depression and anxiety states (Dean, 1987; Fallowfield et al., 1990; Pinder et al., 1993), mania, delirium, panic and paranoid states (Fainsinger et al., 1993). Foley (1985) found that pain, depression and delirium all increased in relation to an increasing level of physical debilitation and advanced disease. In one study, depression was estimated to affect 77 per cent of people with advanced disease (Bukberg et al., 1984). Another report (Power et al., 1993) found the figure to be 26 per cent, compared with 11–26 per cent for the general medical in-patient population (Rodim and Vershort 1986) and 2 per cent for the general population (Meltzer et al., 1995). It is, however, worth noting that general physicians have been estimated to recognize depression in only 25–50 per cent of medically ill patients.

To act only using a crisis model tends to pathologize distress and disturbed behaviour. What we need to have is a culture of psychosocial care, not just 'experts' who respond to expressed need. This culture model would include a 'casualty' model, that is, one in which a crisis response is available, but only as part of what happens.

A psychosocial care culture could include the following:

- the acknowledgement of suffering and the careful use of labels to describe emotional experience;
- 'culture carriers': clinical staff who have a particular responsibility to carry the culture of psychosocial care in their day-to-day practice and have ideally had extra training or regular supervision to be able to do so;
- assessment skills;
- responding skills;
- specialist and crisis intervention skills;
- counselling skills/case supervision and support for clinical staff;
- individual and organizational frameworks that both contain and influence psychosocial practice.

We will now explore each of these proposed cultural elements separately, focusing particularly on skills.

THE ACKNOWLEDGEMENT OF SUFFERING AND THE CAREFUL USE OF LABELS TO DESCRIBE EMOTIONAL EXPERIENCE

We tend to think of palliative care as being concerned with the relief of suffering; probably it is, however, often about engaging with people who are experiencing suffering. To talk of 'suffering' and 'soul pain' is often more helpful than using pathologizing labels to describe psychosocial distress as this can hold the possibility of a human as well as a medical response and can enable us to start with compassion, meaning 'suffering with'.

Michael Kearney (1996) speaks of soul pain as 'the experience of an individual who has become disconnected and alienated from the deepest and most fundamental aspects of him or herself'. Suffering can rupture a person's sense of wholeness, fracturing his sense of himself. The novelist D.H. Lawrence said:

> I am not a mechanism, an assembly of various sections. And it is not because the mechanism is working wrongly that I am ill. I am ill because of wounds to the soul, to the deep emotional self.

Surprisingly little comment has been made about any relationship between the physical deterioration of people with life-threatening illness and their psychological response. In health care generally, and even in specialist palliative care, we tend to behave as if a 'normal' response to illness is to express no distress, to display no disturbed behaviour, and indeed we tend to behave as if it is 'abnormal' to be distressed or disturbed. But surely being distressed or disturbed is 'normal'? And so too is denial – it may represent the beginning of adjusting.

Kaye's (1996) model of emotional adjustment holds this to be true. He considers the common emotional responses to be fear, anger, sadness, dependency and hopelessness. Kaye feels that, within each of the emotional responses, there can be a closed or an open response; those who are fearful may be denying or facing their fears, those angry be blaming or full of fighting spirit, those sad being in misery or grieving, those dependent feeling helpless or participative, those hopeless being despairing or seeking a sense of meaning. Oscillating between feelings and closed and open responses is common. All of these feelings and responses are normal and very painful.

'CULTURE CARRIERS'

These are clinical staff who have counselling skills and an ongoing clinical presence, and have a particular responsibility to carry the culture of psychosocial care in their day-to-day practice. They will ideally have extra training and regular supervision. Presence transcends the self and represents a willingness to share the journey and come alongside the other person.

In order to fulfil this role effectively, additional skills training is helpful and could include the following:

- assessing and responding skills;
- an exploration of counselling models and specific skill development in the therapeutic use of metaphor and image;

- experiential group work in music, art and creative writing in order to raise an awareness of these tools so that appropriate referral can be made to specialist therapists and 'culture carriers' who can use these tools in everyday practice;
- case supervision and presentation;
- ongoing training and counselling skills/case supervision.

The importance of training and supervision in assessment and counselling skills is emphasized by a study of hospice nurses (Heaven and MacGuire, 1997) describing how patients were highly selective about what they disclosed and showed a strong bias towards disclosing physical symptoms. Over 60 per cent of their concerns remained, however, hidden, concerns about the future, appearance and loss of independence being withheld more than 80 per cent of the time. In addition, patients who were more anxious or depressed were less likely to disclose their worries. The nurses only registered 40 per cent of the concerns disclosed to them, and fewer than 20 per cent of patients' worries were appropriately identified.

ASSESSMENT SKILLS

There is no accepted model for the routine assessment of psychosocial need in palliative care, although a number of short standardized assessment scales can be used, the most popular of which is perhaps the Hospital Anxiety and Depression Scale. Although this will confirm the diagnosis, especially as it was designed with physical illness in mind, it will not discriminate between adjustment and depression. If we are to understand his or her journey, each person's needs must be assessed.

The areas that can be helpful to include in an assessment are as follows:

People's description of themselves
How do they describe themselves as a person? How do they see themselves?

Personal history
This can include significant life events, what or who has been important, what has been difficult and what has brought happiness.

Mood and 'coping' history
This is a history of how individuals tend currently to feel, how they view their current situation and how they have coped with difficulties in the past. What or who has hindered or helped them? Have they needed psychological help in the past, and if so, in what circumstances? Do they want or need specific specialist psychological help at present; if so, from whom? What previous experience have they had of death and dying? What impact does this currently have on them?

Concerns/things that matter
Both practical and existential concerns are included here. What things matter most to this person to sort out?

Only two studies, one American, the other British, have addressed people's perceptions of their own needs. Green and Mor (1983), in the USA, found that patients needed three things: supportive friends, religion and to be needed themselves. The British study found two central and interrelated themes: needing to be in control and to complete unfinished business, blocking information from time to time, and having faith in God (Fisher, 1995).

What is important to individual patients? Do they have a belief system that helps them? Are they struggling with their faith? Are there things they particularly want to do? Are there things that they particularly want to have control over, if they can? Are there things or people they particularly want or do not want around? Do they have questions needing to be answered? It is perhaps easy to focus only on problems or to make assumptions about what is most important or needs sorting out.

Genogram

The health-care professional should complete the family tree and also ask about the family of choice. It can also be helpful to use a 'network diagram' comprising concentric circles with the patient at the centre and the names or details of people close to him or her around this, with those closest being near the centre of the diagram; this can enable us to take account of their 'family of choice'.

It is often also useful to bear in mind the concept of the 'symptom-bearer' that is used in family therapy; these are people who are presented, or present themselves, as carrying much of the family's emotion or problems. Such a person may have taken on or been given this role by the family. We are often told, 'Well, Bill – he is the emotional one of all of us.' Perhaps Bill carries the family's emotions, and if they were more shared out, Bill would have less to carry. This could be very important in the context of the family's grief. If other members of the family were encouraged to express their feelings, Bill's load of grief could be lightened.

Although the above list focuses on patients, their family, including their family of choice, should be assessed on a similar basis. In relation to coping, their experience of death, dying and loss should also be explored in order to assess how they may cope with bereavement and to anticipate the support they may need then as well as now.

All of these aspects can all help us to gain both a subjective and an objective picture of patients, those close to them and the support they may need. Without this type of assessment, we often make assumptions about who people are, how they cope and what they need from us.

RESPONDING SKILLS – SKILLED COMPANIONSHIP

In order to offer skilled companionship, we need to be practically and emotionally available and consistent, and to create a safe and holding space in which people's individuality is honoured and they have the opportunity to express and explore their needs and feelings. We need to develop focused skills to take account of the fact that patients' energy levels are low. We need to be able to share, to touch, to hear their pain, vulnerability and suffering, to develop a listening ear.

Skills from counselling that are particularly useful include listening, drawing out, holding strong feelings, reflecting back or echoing, paraphrasing, summarising, clarifying and the use of questions. Skills in breaking bad news and handling difficult questions are also helpful.

Drawing out

Drawing-out skills are mainly non-verbal ways of demonstrating that you are listening and willing to be there with the person: nodding, smiling, saying 'Mm' or 'Ahaa'. Although these can help, using them too much can be irritating and rather patronizing.

Holding strong feelings

We often attach moral values to feelings and describe emotions as either positive or negative. It is easier to block out strong feelings in ourselves and others than to experience them and sit with patients. People who dying and those who are soon to be bereaved are both grieving so strong emotion will tend to be present; indeed, we should probably be concerned if it is not. Being present with anger and sadness is demanding, and these emotions call for our full attention. Anger is a life-giving energy, and when it is not expressed, we can became depressed and cut off from ourselves and others.

Symptoms such as fatigue and severe breathlessness can make sadness and anger difficult and sometimes impossible to express. Physical pain can become a person's total experience and block emotional expression or be used to defend against emotional experience. Some people are unable to communicate because of their disease process, others perhaps because they never have discussed their feelings. Expressing sadness can be cleansing and releasing. Having materials around for drawing, writing and other creative work such as collage, and having plasticine, clay, music and musical instruments easily available, can help to create opportunities for the expression of ideas, thoughts and feelings that words may not allow.

People need to have their feelings acknowledged and accepted, to be given the choice of whether or not they are touched or left alone. The following pointers aim to offer thoughts on how to stay with anger and sadness and facilitate emotional expression.

For staying with anger:

- try to recognize that it relates to the situation, and try not to take it personally;
- acknowledge it, for example, 'You seem very angry';
- validate it: 'I can understand you feeling angry about…';
- don't try to rationalize people's anger with them;
- do try to enable them to express their feelings;
- try to resist calming them down before they have expressed everything as this can make them feel unheard and even angrier;

- people who are angry tend to speak quickly so try to talk calmly at their speed;
- check that they have said everything they need to before you then take each issue and focus on it;
- explain what you are going to do, and check that this would be helpful.

For staying with sadness:

- you may that find this will evoke your own sadness – acknowledge this to yourself, trying to put it to one side and giving yourself space to reflect on it later;
- acknowledge it, for example, 'You sound/look full of sadness';
- validate it, for example, 'It's sad that Anne is dying and begining to leave you';
- don't try to produce tissues quickly as this can feel as if you are telling the patient not to cry.

For facilitating emotional expression:

- have drawing and writing materials, music and instruments, and plasticine or clay readily available;
- emphasize that expression can be helpful;
- if this is difficult, explore what the patient is scared of;
- offer a choice of medium, stating that it is not the end-product that matters but rather the expression involved in doing the drawing, the writing, the playing of or listening to the music or the moulding of the clay.

Case study 7.1 shows how such therapy can be of value.

CASE STUDY 7.1

Matt was in his 70s and had cancer of his tongue, most of his oral cavity being affected. He was frustrated and angry and in a great deal of psychic pain. Matt was offered a number of mediums to express his feelings, but he rejected them all. It wasn't until he saw the drums that things changed: his face lit up, he stared and stared at them, and then he banged and banged and banged. Matt then began to write about his feelings. When he was dying, he asked for the drums to be placed beside him.

Using the responding skills that follow may also enable the expression of grief.

Reflecting back

This is a very important skill. It is about reflecting back or echoing the person's words, for example 'So you feel very angry.' This sort of reflection will usually encourage a further expression of feeling. You can also reflect what you are picking up: 'You sound...', 'You appear to me to be...'. This can really allow patients to feel as if you are there with them and willing to enter into and share their experience.

Paraphrasing

This is about trying to précis what people have said in your own words; it can reflect the fact that you are helping them to hold all the aspects of their experience.

Clarifying

If you are not clear or feel uncertain whether you have understood, ask for clarification. Demonstrate your wish to understand by asking, for example, 'Am I correct in...?', 'Can I just make sure that I have understood...?' 'Do you mean that...?'or perhaps 'Let me go over this and make sure that I have heard what you said...'.

Focusing/prioritizing

If many concerns have been raised, energy and time are limited and physical symptoms are getting in the way, it can be important to focus and prioritize, saying, for example, 'Given your low energy, out of all the things you are concerned about which stands out/feels the most important/causes you the most distress/anxiety?'

Confronting

This can sound rather like attacking, but it is more to do with noticing and gently commenting on discrepancies, for example 'You say you are not sad, but I am noticing that your eyes are full of tears.'

The use of questions

Questions need to used with thought and care – we need to ask ourselves why and for whom we need to know: providing supportive companionship is not a fact-finding mission. We sometimes feel as if we have done a good job when we have gleaned much information, but when we are with someone in their woundedness and distress, we need to balance our questioning carefully against sitting quietly with them in the midst of their sadness without being intrusive.

Questions can be open or closed, closed questions allowing only a 'yes' or 'no' answer. Open questions offer the person freedom of expression: 'What/how are you feeling?', 'What are your thoughts about that?', 'What do you imagine will happen?'

Listening and silence

The key skill we have to offer is listening. This can sound very simple, but it is actually a very complex area. Listening is active and requires both attention and commitment. It is about standing attentively at the interface of the person's conscious and unconscious worlds. We can tend to feel pressure to talk and feel uncomfortable in silence, but silence enables reflection, and breaking into it too soon can disrupt this process. Silence is a response if, in it, we continue to listen to the atmosphere.

In ordinary listening, we tend to listen only to the content of the person's story and often try to relate it to our own experience, thinking of interesting responses and trying to have a conversation. When we are listening therapeutically, however, we listen to the content as a potential symptom of the experience with which the person is struggling, and we tend to pay attention not to our own experience but to how we experience the person when we are together. Our focus is not on having a conversation but on using skills that enable self-reflection and exploration. In therapeutic listening, we need to empty ourselves of all the clutter we carry so that the time we spend with others can be truly their time.

McKay et al. (1983) describe 12 blocks to listening:

- *comparing* – for example, 'When my mother died, I coped much better';
- *mind-reading* – trying to figure out what the other person is really thinking and feeling without asking;
- *rehearsing* – giving attention to the preparation and delivery of our responses;
- *filtering* – listening to some things and not others: we often filter out things we do not wish to hear or cannot bear;
- *judging* – not listening to what is being said because you have already decided what the problem is;
- *dreaming* – only half-listening to what the person is saying, when, for example, what they have said has triggered off some of your own associations;
- *identifying* – referring everything the person says to your own experience;
- *advising* – being the great problem-solver or rescuer;
- *sparring* – getting into a debate;
- *being right* – going to any lengths to avoid being wrong;
- *derailing* – changing the train of conversation when you are bored or uncomfortable;
- *placating* – not really tuning in but just trying to be nice.

Try to be aware of your specialist blocks and work on them, monitoring yourself and catch yourself early in the blocking process. It can be helpful to be aware of your breathing. We can tend to brace ourselves in preparation for and during weighty conversations so try to breath in and out gently and regularly. This can help you stay more fully present and connected to the person.

Key things to listen for are:

- their story;
- their words or use of metaphor;
- their images;
- their questions and need for information;
- their feelings or mood;
- their body;
- their family and social context;
- their untellable story – the gaps;
- where their struggle, stuckness, emotional pain or woundedness lies.

Their story Listening to others' stories honours their life and living as well as their dying because their dying is part of their life story. Incompleteness is often a fear for those who are dying: they need to finish their story. What is it that they are saying they need to talk about? Why now? What has happened to make this important today? What effect does the story have on them? What effect does it have on you – emotionally and physically? It can be very useful to notice what you think about, feel or find yourself needing to do both when and after you have spent time with someone. Do you feel agitated? Feel like jumping up and down? Need to scream? Is this about you, or is this an aspect of their lived experience?

When we are acting as a cradle for someone's emotions, we are containers for various aspects of their experiences. Although no one can truly feel others' pain, we can allow it to resonate in our thinking and feeling to enable us to experience their world. It can be helpful to notice what we experience when or after we have been with them and reflect it back to them. This sort of resonance relates to allowing the person's thoughts and feelings to echo in your head, your heart and your body. Reflecting your experience of being with them can enable them to feel very understood and understandable at an often confusing and isolating time.

Their words or use of metaphor How do they describe their experiences? How do they sound? Are they able to describe their world – emotionally, physically, spiritually? Might they need specialist help to explore their thoughts and feelings?

Some metaphors provide us with a very strong sense of how someone feels. If you really listen to the statement 'I feel as if I am drowning' in an open-hearted way and let it resonate with you, it sounds very frightening, so acknowledge and explore such images with patients. Let them know you have really heard: 'That is a very powerful image', 'You sound as if you must be very scared', 'What do you feel so engulfed/overwhelmed by?' or perhaps 'Is there anything that you could do/I can help you with that would help you to feel less...?'

Their images Images can include many things: the visual image we conjured up from their story, a dream, a picture they draw in a literal sense, movements they make. All of these also tell a tale.

It is all too easy to assume that nightmares and similar disturbing pictures are caused by the drugs used in palliative care. It is obviously important to review medication, but it is also important to hold the image as a representation of that person's inner world and explore it gently together. Such images often hold a message from the unconscious that needs attention: 'Negative and disturbing images are vital stimulants for healing in that the toxin is the antitoxin' (McNiff, 1994).

We need to treat the world of the person's dream or drawing as a world in its own right and, together with the person, befriend the dream or drawing and get to know it. Working with dreams and drawings is a specialist area of practice, but it is important to hold the dream or picture with the person. Encourage patients to tell the story of the drawing: when they drew it, what it represents to them, what it may remind them of...be curious about it with them. This sort of work concerns not interpretation but exploration. Work in the same way with dreams: encourage patients to tell the story of the dream and wonder about it with them.

Case studies 7.2a and b powerfully illustrate that simple, straightforward interventions can elicit a great deal and facilitate the process of the toxin becoming the antitoxin.

CASE STUDY 7.2

7.2a A woman was having a recurring dream about fishing, which she found very 'disturbing' and which often woke her. I asked her to tell me a bit about her experience of fishing, which she had always enjoyed. I asked her if there was anything she found disturbing about fishing. She thought and suddenly said, 'When you kill the fish on the side of the bank.' She then broke down in tears and began to talk for the first time about dying.

7.2b A man kept having dreams that he could not remember and woke feeling disorientated. When I asked him if anything else was feeling disorientating, he said, 'The idea of not existing any more.'

Their questions and need for information What do patients want to know? What do you feel they need to know but do not ask? It is often helpful to offer a specific opportunity for the person to ask questions or check things out. An explicit demonstration of the carer's willingness to answer questions or explore concerns sometimes makes all the difference. Can you explore these issues, or do you know of someone else who can? Could you say, 'I am puzzled that you seem to have no questions/thought/views about. . .'?

Some questions are difficult to answer, and others 'When will I die?', 'Why me?' – may have no answers at all. Bad news is news that we cannot change or soften so it is important to pace it. If it is broken too abruptly, it may disorganize the person psychologically and hinder their adaptation. When handling difficult questions,

- reflect the question back, so that 'When will I die?' leads to 'When do you imagine. . .?';
- ask what has triggered the question;
- if the patient's perception is correct, confirm their view and check how they feel;
- if they do not have an appropriate perception about what is happening, begin to break the news.

Kaye (1996) suggests 10 steps for breaking bad news:

1 *Preparation*: know all the facts and ensure privacy.
2 *What does the person know?*: ask for the story of what has happened.
3 *Does he or she want more information?*: ask, 'Would you like me to explain a bit more?'
4 *Give a warning shot*: 'I'm sorry, it's more complicated than you have thought.'
5 *Allow denial*: allow the person to control the amount of information, and remember that denial is a response.

6 *Explain*: narrow the information gap step by step.
7 *Listen to concerns*: 'What are your main concerns now?'
8 *Encourage the expression of feelings*.
9 *Summarise and plan*: decide the next step.
10 *Offer to be available*: for further conversations.

Their feelings or mood These can often emerge through the way in which things are said: for example, the tone of the person's voice may be flat, or you may sense a suppressed panic. If feelings appear to be absent, try to imagine what might be felt and gently reflect the absence of feeling and what you have been imagining the individual might be feeling; although you may not get this right, what you will do is demonstrate your willingness to imagine their world and share in it.

Might patients benefit from antianxiolytic or antidepressant medication alongside psychological support?

Their body Listen to patients' body language. Remembering to take account of their physical disease, the apparent 'dis-ease' in their body, for example their breathing pattern, can also be very revealing. By breathing at the patients' rate and depth or shallowness, you may be able to pick up where they are holding themselves and explore this with them. Do they feel tense all over? Do they feel as if they have a volcano rumbling away? Is their face taut and frozen? Notice discrepancies between what they say and how they seem in their body. When do you see any change? Perhaps when the topic being discussed is more painful or when a particular person arrives. Gently reflecting your experience of being with their body as well as their words can enable patients to feel more able to express their concerns and feelings: 'I notice when you spoke of... you almost held your breath as if you needed to protect yourself from the feelings you experience when you think...'. Our bodies are a rich storehouse of memories and experiences.

Their family and social context From your assessment, you will have constructed a family tree and the concentric circle diagram illustrating patients' relationships and family of choice. Ask them to give you a sense of what it is like for them to be in their family, both now and in the past.

Their untellable story – the gaps Try to pinpoint what is never talked about or what always gets skirted around. When someone is clearly restless and agitated, it may be important to ask directly about what it is that seems to be unmentionable. Acknowledge the fear or other feelings you may sense in relation to this and ask whether patients would feel able to talk with you or someone else about this to try to address it.

Where their struggle, stuckness, emotional pain or woundedness lies What do you sense or imagine their distress relates to? Are there thoughts, feeling, ideas and situations that appear to be confusing, distressing, puzzling? Reflect these confusions back to explore them together: for example, 'I find myself wondering...' or 'I feel a bit confused by...'

We sometimes find ourselves feeling inadequate and struggling; indeed, we may well be struggling. It is worth wondering at these times whether what we are experiencing is part of the patient's lived experience. It can then be useful to say something like, 'I get a sense/feeling that...'.

When we feel we have gone as far as our skills allow us to journey with others, we should discuss this with them in a positive and open way, for example 'We reflected/talked/discussed a lot about...and I feel it would be helpful for you to look at/explore this area with...as s/he has...What do you think?' Referral is a skill rather than a failure as recognizing the contribution and specialist skills of others is part of team-working and high-quality holistic palliative care.

We tend to think that supporting children and young people is a specialist area, and although this is to some extent true, we often feel inadequate around children and young people as we have a strong sense of their vulnerability. Thus, additional training is useful to build up skills and insights in this area. With each person, however young or old, offering skilled companionship is about being willing to be present and trying to understand their experience of the world, clarifying and offering information that may be helpful.

SPECIALIST AND CRISIS INTERVENTION SKILLS

Specialists who can help include social workers, counsellors, art and music therapists, activity co-ordinators, bereavement visitors and counsellors, patient welfare officers, chaplains, staff counsellors, clinical psychologists and/or a psychiatrists.

Counsellors or social workers can deal with those who need ongoing, in-depth work or need specialist intervention at a time of crisis. Music therapy can be particularly helpful for people whose clinical condition makes verbal communication difficult, as in motor neurone disease or dysphasia caused by a cerebral tumour. Engaging people in spontaneous musical improvisation can enable emotional expression and effective communication independent of words. Equally, some people who have the capacity to talk may find that expression through music deepens their capacity to let their feelings out or enables them to express thoughts and feelings that are beyond words. Art therapy can do this too, both feelings and situations being symbolized through the use of materials such as paints and clay. Images can expand communication and offer insights beyond the reasoning mind. Offering activities can also facilitate creative expression and a sense of fun.

Welfare officers or other staff members who carry responsibility for this area can ease distress related to aspects such as finances, housing and wills. Having bereavement visitors, usually volunteers with specific training in the use of counselling skills, and bereavement counsellors, who are also often volunteers, can be helpful in providing different levels of supportive intervention.

It may be of benefit for a psychiatrist and/or psychologist to be available on a sessional basis, one who shares the ethos of palliative care and can provide support and expertise in specific situations. If someone is not responding to antidepressant or antipsychotic medication, for example, an expert psychiatric review of the person and the medication may be helpful. If the patient has a previous psychiatric condition that appears to be causing a problem, the psychiatrist can reassess their needs. Involving a psychologist can be particularly helpful with those suffering behaviour or thought disturbances as they work in a focused way with these processes. As professionals working in psychologically related fields tend to have a range of types of training and areas of special interest, getting to understand their individual expertise is valuable.

COUNSELLING SKILLS/CASE SUPERVISION AND SUPPORT FOR CLINICAL STAFF

Supervision can enable professional development and support, ensuring a high standard of clinical practice. It is an exchange between practising professionals with the intention of developing their professional skills (Butterworth and Faugier, 1992) and can be viewed as having three functions (Proctor, 1986):

1 *an educative or 'formative function'*: developing skills, understanding and abilities by reflecting on and exploring the person's work experience;
2 *a supportive or 'restorative function'*: providing support to enable the person to deal with what has happened and move on;
3 a managerial or 'normative function': providing quality control.

Supervision and learning are strongly connected through the process of reflecting. Learning involves three stages (Burnard, 1985) the first of which is personal experience – the fact of something happening. The second stage is reflection, or looking back on experience. This stage may be passed over as the event may not be noticed or may not be thought to be significant. The third stage is the transformation of knowledge, leading to new insights.

In palliative care, we are continuously faced with dying, death and bereavement. Worden (1983) suggests that working with bereavement may touch us in at least three ways; it may:

• make us painfully aware of our own losses;
• contribute to our apprehension of our potential or feared losses;
• arouse existential anxiety in terms of our personal death awareness.

People who are dying may also touch us in these ways. In palliative care, we can 'experience professional bereavement' (Fisher, 1996) as we are continuously forming and ending, often deep, relationships. Raphael (1980) considers that working with those who are dying and those who are bereaved heightens mutual empathy and identification as the experience of loss is universal. The opportunity to reflect and the supportive restorative function of supervision are therefore perhaps particularly relevant in palliative care: people who are grieving reflect on their memories, their feelings and thoughts about the person's death and the future (Nerken, 1993).

CASE STUDY 7.3

I was encouraged to explore my responses to issues that had caused specific problems. As the group process developed, I found that sharing these feelings often gave me a tremendous understanding of my own and others' emotional reactions. It was and is a safe, contained environment in which I can take risks.

I drew some pictures and when I showed my pictures to the group, there was a long silence, during which I became aware that the horror didn't belong to me alone. It was shared by all of us, had belonged to each of us at different times with different people. Eventually, someone asked, 'Where are *you* in these pictures?' In some way, I feel that I *am* these images. Although they each tell a story about the deaths of particular patients, they are containers for all my own pain and fear about the awfulness of dying in this way.

Supervision offers a specific opportunity to reflect and build on skills with a named person who facilitates the process and usually comes from outside the organization. Supervision can take the form of one-to-one interaction with someone with a high level of skill, or involve a peer or group. Group supervision is often the most cost-effective way of approaching this area. Whatever the framework, the boundaries of time and confidentiality need to be clear from the outset.

Judith, an experienced staff nurse in palliative care, describes in Case study 7.3 one of her experiences of supervision.

The following poem was written by Judith to give words to one of her incredibly powerful pictures.

For three long nights you stared into me.
Eyes filled with terror, lungs full of fluid.
Your need for succour overwhelmed me – you seemed
A starving, greedy child, desperate to be held and comforted.
Each night you roamed sleepless and breathless
Until totally exhausted you stopped and stared.
I sat beside you, but I wasn't with you.
I felt invaded by your need – a visceral fear invading me
Your colourless-blue eyes expectant with the terror of death
And hope – that I might reach out to you and give you what you needed.
Your reminded me of my father and his brother
Their pale eyes also held that staring look of needy unfulfilment
And somehow slightly mad
But very, very sad.
You repulsed me and I looked the other way
Your death was horrible
You died alone.
I found you on your bed, covered in a caul of sticky mucous you have coughed or sicked up
And as you lay gasping, drowning
And your eyes widened, appealing, desperate
Your hands reached out. . . . .

The pictures and poem deepened Judith's understanding of herself and her work with these particular patients, as well as her work as a whole, and resonated with the experiences of other group members, enabling them to recognize the shared nature of their clinical experience. The focus of this particular group session was the supportive restorative function, but other sessions might focus on other aspects by staff bringing a specific conversation with a patient or someone close to a patient that they had found difficult or interesting. Sharing ideas and practising skills through role play can enable new learning. Trust is a very important aspect of supervision, whether one-to-one or in a group, and can only be built up over time.

Scheduling the opportunity to debrief at the end of each shift, and particularly after a difficult or traumatic situation, is as important as the other things we regularly structure, such as team handovers. Debriefing is a specific opportunity to reflect upon the events of the day with a colleague or group and actively to leave these behind. In addition, it can be helpful to have a specific place on your journey home where you stop thinking about work and begin to think about home and perhaps vice versa. Writing a list of things undone to empty your head of work, and knowing that the list is holding them for you, can also be a useful way of clearing the mind.

Having a counsellor available for staff is a valuable investment in staff support and high-quality holistic care, but the confidentiality and trust involved in this service need to be absolute.

INDIVIDUAL AND ORGANIZATIONAL FRAMEWORKS THAT BOTH CONTAIN AND INFLUENCE PSYCHOSOCIAL PRACTICE

Framework for our individual practice

Boundaries and continuity of care It is often helpful to be clear about the amount of time you have to spend with a person, sharing this gives you control over both time and what is, and is not, explored in the time available. Clarifying the nature of your relationship with the person, and confidentiality, are important: what is shared with whom in what circumstances is important and should be made explicit. You also need to clarify who should be developing an emotionally supportive relationship and why it needs to be kept under scrutiny to ensure that there is continuity of emotional support from a person with an appropriate type and level of skill.

Personal awareness We often find ourselves feeling rather 'braced for action' when in a difficult situation. If we can feel our feet on the ground and breathe more fully, we can act from a more solid and centred space inside ourselves. Then we can meet our patients where they are in an open-hearted way.

Being aware of one's strengths and blocks is central to the creation of a supportive 'emotional cradle'. Developing a sense of witnessing yourself in action and reflecting on how you handle situations uses new insights to help you to build up your skills and enhances your effective use of supervision, reflection, debriefing, supervision and counselling.

Framework for the organization

This should include:

- *the purpose or mission statement*;
- *human resource policies:* for example on staffing and related structures, skill mix, individual performance review, supervision, reflective practice, professional development and education, debriefing and formal and informal support;
- *regular specific opportunities to review people's psychological needs:* monitoring psychological needs is an ongoing process so formal review and discussion related to this can be integrated into the clinical evaluation of care in a way similar to the traditional ongoing review of physical symptoms such as pain on ward rounds and in handovers and documentation;
- *clinical documentation:* it is important for teamworking that psychological documentation uses a shared, agreed structure;
- *audit and transparency in clinical accountability.*

These set the context in which we carry out our roles. A diagrammatic representation of the relationship between psychosocial care and staffing and organizational frameworks can found in Figure 7.1. This illustrates how psychosocial care is 'held' by specialists, culture-carriers, the members of the interprofessional palliative care team and the organizational frameworks at different levels, these levels being interdependent.

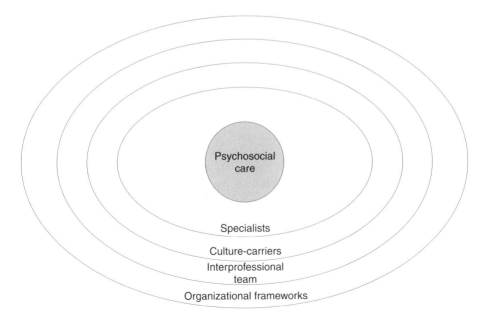

Figure 7.1 The relationship between psychological care and organizational frameworks

CONCLUSION

In conclusion, being present with people facing life-threatening illness is challenging, rewarding and sometimes distressing. In the community of palliative care we are all sharing each other's journey. It is hoped that the skills outlined in this chapter will enable you to share the journeys of patients and those close to them in an effective and meaningful way.

I am part of all that I have met and all experience is an arch where through gleams that untravelled world whose boundary fades forever and forever as we move.

Alfred, Lord Tennyson

REFERENCES

Bukberg, J., Penman, D. and Holland, J. 1984: Depression in hospitalised cancer patients. *Psychosomatic Medicine* **43**, 199–212.

Burnard, P. 1985: *Learning human skills: a guide for nurses.* London: Heinemann.

Butterworth, C.A. and Faugier, J. 1992: *Clinical supervision and mentorship in nursing.* London: Chapman & Hall.

Dean, C. 1987: Psychiatric morbidity following mastectomy: pre-operative predictors and types of illness. *Journal of Psychosomatic Research* **31**, 385–92.

Fainsinger, R.L., Tapper, M. and Bruera, E. 1993: A perspective on the management of delirium in terminally ill patients on a palliative care unit. *Journal of Palliative Care* **8**, 4–8.

Fallowfield, L., Hall, A., McGuire, G. and Baum, M. 1990: Psychological outcomes of different treatment policies in women with early breast cancer outside a clinical trial. *British Medical Journal* **301**, 575–80.

Fisher, M. 1995: Psychological needs and care in the hospice setting. *European Journal of Palliative Care* **2**(3), 115–19.

Fisher, M. 1996: How do members of an interprofessional clinical team adjust to hospice care? *Palliative Medicine* **10**, 319–28.

Foley, K.M. 1985: The treatment of cancer pain. *New England Journal of Medicine* **3**(3), 84–95.

Green, D. and Mor, V. 1983: *A preliminary final report of the national hospice study.* Providence: Brown University.

Heaven, C. and Maguire, P. 1997 Disclosure by hospice patients and their identification by nurses. *Palliative Medicine* **11**, 283–90.

Kaye, P. 1996: *Breaking bad news pocket book.* Northampton: EPL.

Kearney, M. 1996: *Mortally wounded stories of soul pain, death and healing.* Dublin: Marino.

Kübler-Ross, E. 1970: *On death and dying.* London: Tavistock.

McNiff, S. 1994: *Art as therapy: creating a therapy of the imagination.* London: Piatkus.

McKay, A., Davis, M. and Fanning, P. (1983): *Messages.* Oakland, CA: New Harbinger.

Meltzer, H., Gill, B., Pettigrew, M. and Hinds, K. 1995: The prevalence of psychiatric morbidity among adults in private households. In: *OPCS surveys of psychiatric morbidity in Great Britain.* OPCS Report No. 1. London: HMSO.

National Council for Hospices and Specialist Palliative Care Services. 1997: *Feeling better: psychosocial care in specialist palliative care – a discussion paper.* Occasional Paper No. 13, London: NCHSPCS.

Nerken, I. 1993: Grief and the reflective self: toward a clearer model of loss, resolution and growth. *Death Studies* **17**, 1–26.

Nichols, I.C. 1993: *Psychological care in physical care.* London: Chapman & Hall.

Pinder, K., Ramirez, A., Black, M. et al. 1993: Psychiatric disorder in patients with advanced breast cancer: prevalence and associated factors. *European Journal of Cancer* **67**, 341–6.

Power, D., Kelly, S. and Gilseman, J. 1993: Suitable screening tests for cognitive impairment and depression in the terminally ill – a prospective study. *Palliative Medicine* **7**, 213–18.

Proctor, B. 1986: Supervision: a co-operative exercise in accountability. In: Marked, M. and Payne, M. (eds). *Enabling and ensuring: supervision in clinical practice.* London: National Youth Bureau.

Raphael, B. 1980: A psychiatric model for bereavement counselling? In: Shloenberg, B.M. (ed.) *Bereavement counselling: a multidisciplinary handbook.* Connecticut: Greenwood Press.

Rodim, G. and Voshort, K. 1986: Depression in the medically ill – an overview. *American Journal of Psychiatry* **143**, 696–705.

Worden, J.W. 1983: *Grief counselling and grief therapy.* London: Tavistock.

FURTHER READING

Bosnack, R. 1998: *A little course on dreams: a basic handbook of Jungian dream work.* Boston, Shaftsbury: Shambala.

Buckman, R. 1992: *How to break bad news: a guide for health care professionals.* London: Papermac.

Rowan, J. 1983: *The reality game: a guide to humanistic counselling and therapy.* London: Routledge & Kegan Paul.

Shuman, R. 1996: *The psychology of chronic illness.* London: Basic Books.

Tschudin, V. 1982: *Counselling skills for nurses.* London: Bailière Tindall.

Wellings, N. and Wilde-McCormick, E. (eds) 2000: *Transpersonal psychotherapy: theory and practice.* London: Continuum.

chapter 8

SPIRITUAL PAIN

David Stoter

For everything there is a season, and a time for every matter under heaven –
– a time to be born and a time to die,
– a time to weep and a time to laugh,
– a time to mourn and a time to dance,
– a time to keep and a time to lose,
– a time to love and a time to hate,
– a time to keep silence and a time to speak.

Ecclesiastes: Ch. 3., vv. 1–7

THE NATURE OF SPIRITUAL CARE

Spiritual care is one of the most overlooked aspects of palliative care, probably because it is so often ill defined and misunderstood, being for many of us fraught with unanswered questions and difficulties. Because of the many surrounding misconceptions, some professionals tend to 'back off' and 'leave it to the clergy'. Nurses may ignore it apart from recording the patient's stated religion as part of the nursing process record (Faulkner, 1985). Spiritual care is so often seen as religious care for the few who request it and therefore becomes dismissed as a footnote just for the report. Although it is important to recognize and meet the needs of those from all cultures and creeds, seeing spiritual care only as religious care trivializes and diminishes its true nature. This perception may lead to paying lip service to meeting spiritual needs, but in reality giving it a low priority.

It is not only those of us who are involved in the day-to-day aspects of practical care who find this a difficult subject. In research studies considering the care of the dying person there are surprisingly few references clarifying the nature of spiritual care, although our own hospice movement has its roots in Christian foundations (Owen et al., 1989). This omission was recognized during an international conference of experts at Yale University when they faced difficulty in searching for a definition of the nature of spiritual care.

WHAT IS SPIRITUAL CARE?

The uncertainties mentioned above make it important to clarify from the beginning of our explorations the positive aspects of spiritual care. Spiritual care involves valuing individuals for themselves, all having their own values and beliefs with the absolute right to be an individual needing affirmation of who they are and an acceptance of their personal views and attitudes to life. Every person is a spiritual being with a spiritual dimension, although only a few reflect a specific religious dimension.

Spirituality includes the whole range of people's life experiences, their successes and failures, joys and sorrows, strength and weaknesses. It embraces background, culture, work experience, home and social life – everything in fact that makes for the uniqueness of the person, with a unique capacity to respond to life events and situations. If this view is broadened to encompass a partner or family group, it follows that they form a unique couple or family group and that the patient actually exists within that setting, with the thoughts, hopes, fears, beliefs, doubts and expectations all influenced by, and individual to, that group. As in physical care, each factor – and not just a simplistic symptom response – is taken into account so in spiritual care it is important not to look into symptom control alone but to respond to the situation as a whole for that person or family.

This means an acceptance of that individual in totality and an affirmation of people just as they are wherever we find them. It means accepting their range of beliefs, doubts, fears and anxieties as a valid expression of where they are, and affirming them with no preconditions of our own. This is a sound starting point from which to approach spiritual care, which is a gift of love with no preconditions, reflecting as it does the highest forms of human love and, for some, a belief in God's love and acceptance of each of us as we are.

This then is our positive approach and starting point – that everyone has a spiritual dimension and that we need to differentiate between this and a religious dimension; that each individual is unique with personal values and needs, and each responds to a situation and to care in an individual way. This was summed up in a nicely defined statement from the above-mentioned conference at Yale: 'it is the patient who defines the territory (for spiritual care) not the caregiver' (Fiefel, 1986). What is important is to recognize the potential of the spiritual dimension to be a healing force for the whole person, body, mind and spirit. Arriving at a real understanding of the spirituality of the patient is essential if care plans and care-giving are to deliver patient-centred care that genuinely reflects the patient's needs and wishes.

THE SPIRITUAL NEEDS OF THE INDIVIDUAL

Before looking at ways of offering spiritual care appropriate to each individual, it helps to identify what the specific needs are rather than embarking on a programme derived from our own perspective. The starting premise that each individual has a spiritual dimension, with certain values and beliefs that are unique, indicates that it is difficult to give an easy overall definition of spiritual need. We can however, say that it will vary between individuals and that needs manifest themselves in several ways. Sometimes they are openly expressed, at other times felt but not expressed. They also exist relative to other conditions and may as such change at different times (Bradshaw, 1972).

It is therefore important to avoid sweeping value judgements, making assumptions about what people 'need' and thinking that there are set answers to the questions asked. The discussion of spiritual care highlights the general factors that can help in meeting needs, such as recognizing that there is a universal requirement for affirmation and unconditional acceptance, and a need for the opportunity to discover the way forward in a safe and caring environment, acknowledging that everyone is at a different stage on a personal spiritual or life journey.

THE RELIGIOUS ASPECTS OF SPIRITUAL CARE

An important component of spiritual care is religious care, which needs to be related specifically to the individual's preferences and needs. Some knowledge of different denominations and of other religions and their practices is necessary here to bring about an understanding of their complexities. Although it is widely recognized that there are obvious differences when considering other faiths, it is important to note that there are denominational differences not only within the Christian faith, but also within all religions. Even within a particular denomination, Christian or otherwise, there is a wide spectrum of beliefs and attitudes with a diversity of practices. It is important to realise that although some 'immigrants' remain orthodox within the origins of their culture or faith, others absorb aspects of Western living and education, and thereby express more complicated transcultural needs. If religious/cultural care is to be approached with sensitivity, it is therefore important to understand these perspectives and find out what is acceptable and comfortable for the individual patient or family.

In today's multi-racial and multi-cultural society, the range of religious beliefs encountered may present a confusing variety of different approaches and practices; it is thus helpful to have some information available on wards or units for reference, for example a list of denominations and other faiths, outlining their attitudes, practices or specific needs, together with local contacts who can be approached for further information if required. In large hospitals, the chaplain's department will frequently act as a resource base. A practical example (Case study 8.1) may illustrate why these differences must be understood.

CASE STUDY 8.1

The nursing staff in a special care baby unit were highly concerned when they found a small dagger under the sheet of a baby in an incubator. They were considering calling in the social worker to follow up a perceived threat of non-accidental injury until they were reassured that a dagger is one of the five religious symbols with significant meaning for Sikhs and had as such been placed close to the child's body.

Several reference books are available that provide clear descriptive accounts of specific beliefs and practices, giving the carer valuable insights into religious and cultural preferences relating to food, privacy, worship and especially death. An understanding of any of these can make an important contribution to the patient's general well-being and quality of life (McGilloway and Myco, 1985; Neuberger, 1987).

WHO GIVES SPIRITUAL CARE?

We have already seen that some professionals see spiritual care as the responsibility of the clergy or religious people alone, but when viewed in its true dimension, it becomes clear that in involves the whole team rather than any one person. Sometimes, however, one particular person, one with whom they feel comfortable, may emerge or be selected by the patient or family as the key person to facilitate their own support. The contribution of the family should also be recognized, as should the need for back-up support from the rest of the team and any necessary specialist input.

The implications for the care-giver will be considered more fully later, but at this point it should be noted that it is often the nurse, because of the nature of the work involved and the time spent with the patient, who is responsible for the majority of spiritual care. The nurse has a very special relationship with the patient and family, making it possible to give spiritual care of the highest quality, especially if there is a willingness to remain open in the relationship and try not to give predetermined answers. Although the observations made in this chapter are addressed primarily to nurses, the principles considered are applicable to any professional involved with palliative care.

SOME APPROACHES TO SPIRITUAL CARE

Spiritual care poses many questions where few answers are on offer, which may make it seem a threatening aspect of care. It deals with the kinds of question that often appear with the onset of serious illness – questions that need to be explored for each individual in a safe environment starting from where the person is in his or her own belief and experience and allowing the discovery of answers when the time is right: 'Why?', 'Why me?', 'What have I done?', 'What has he or she done to deserve this?', 'What is happening to me?', 'Is there life after death – if so what is it like?', 'Is there a God – if so what is He like?' Other expressions often heard are 'I've done nothing worthwhile with my life', 'Who will remember me when I'm gone?' and 'Why should anyone care about me?' To these questions or statements there are no direct answers or responses that can be handed out like pills or medicine for specific ailments.

An even more complex situation may appear when the patient has a religious origin different from that of the professional carer, or, more difficult still, has no faith at all, views death as oblivion, or has a particular faith when the carer has either none or considerable doubts. A useful starting point is to begin by listening to and receiving the questions and doubts as they are presented, allowing individuals to *be* who they are, as they are. This is the baseline from which to move forward – just to be alongside, in a non-threatening, non-authoritarian relationship that is not demanding or invasive of the patient's personal world of belief. This may present difficulties for some nurses as it is a relationship that requires some departure from the more traditional nursing role of 'delivering care'. It is, however, important to be sensitive to the fact that the patient may not wish to enter into any relationship other than the professional one.

The 'history-taking' approach, using a question and answer method, can have a depersonalizing effect, giving a preconceived, stereotyped, photo-fit picture leading to false assumptions about the kind of care to offer. Such direct questions may be intrusive, a more 'oblique approach' often being more rewarding. For example, instead of using a question like 'Have you any children?', it may be more suitable to make a comment such as 'That's a lovely picture of your family', an approach that may open up a relaxed conversation giving a sense of warmth and trust.

It is natural and desirable to talk about family life, which may well lead on to patients sharing details about themselves, their families, fears, preferences and beliefs. The essential ingredient is for patients to become aware that someone is willing to share their humanity. This should not, however, be used as an opportunity for the professional to work out personal problems in this relationship or to project personal needs onto the patient.

The patient may need to 'test out' the nurse to see whether he or she has really been 'heard'. For many, once they are assured of being heard, the opportunity comes for a release of fears and doubts, the 'felt' anxieties and needs being openly 'expressed' as the patient takes the nurse into the darker areas of experience. Some may need to focus on impending death, its nature and a projection into what it is like to be dead. These are powerful areas of pain and distress that are related to the unknown. Other common fears relate to burial, cremation or being in a coffin, to dying alone, to losing control of oneself or suffering pain and to anxieties about the family. Forms of loss, in terms of dignity or personal identity, loss of role or loss of control over personal destiny, also arouse emotion. All of these are powerful fears, especially for the younger patient, for whom a loss of body image may be particularly important. Some of these anxieties may well also find an echo in the carer.

THE PROFESSIONAL CARER IN THE TEAM

PERSONAL SKILLS NEEDED

It is clear that the nurse or professional carer needs to have good listening skills to enable the patient fully to share these painful areas. Such a relationship can create a very exposed situation for the nurse, particularly when there is an expression of despair, as the patient enters into and shares the darkness. The situation may well be so threatening that the temptation is to stop the process to avoid becoming completely lost, dealing with one or more aspects through a problem-solving model. This feels safer but is less helpful to patients, who are looking for someone to be with them on the journey as far as they feel able to go, to stay close without judgement or ready answers that could trivialize the situation and their need. Professional carers may experience a strong temptation to reinforce their own security by comforting the patient through trite sayings such as 'Don't be frightened' or 'Don't worry, we will look after you.'

This may be a particular area of difficulty for those trying to express comfort in religious terms. It is easier to do something positive to fulfil the nursing role by attempting to bring hope or a relief of pain and distress, at a time when the patient is aware of the situation that has to be faced but wants to express it to someone who can hear and accept the rawness and weakness of pain and darkness. It is helpful to know that others do not have the answers to death and dying, and that professionals have their own fears and uncertainties related to these issues.

The response of the carer is then, not in words but in staying, listening, hearing and being the eyes and ears of the person expressing the pain as he or she enters the darkness. With this accompanying hand and presence in the shared experience, individuals may be enabled to express the depth of their distress. Having been heard and accepted in the deepest place of darkness or despair, they may find that their hopelessness begins to lift as they discover that they feel heard in that most threatening place of all and now know that it is in future safe to share in depth with that person.

This may be followed by a change in perspective as a glimmer of hope develops. An example of a similar kind of experience familiar to most of us is travelling through a long tunnel when the darkness deepens and becomes more oppressive as we approach the centre. After that point, the darkness is always behind, and whenever we look ahead we are looking towards the light, which is, even if only a glimmer at first, getting brighter all the time. The carer needs to accept that this glimmer may be very faint and may indeed remain so.

Part of the process that brings relief to patients is being given permission to express these feelings without being told that they are silly or that there is an easy way out. It is the professional's role not to give hope but to enable patients to discover a meaningful hope for themselves. This may well be the point at which patients know that their despair is understood and accepted but that this insight is something which cannot easily be put into words. It is tempting for the carer to respond by saying, 'I understand how you feel', which is never helpful or true – it is the receiving of the shared experience that brings reassurance where words may trivialize the moment. When patients feel understood, they may quietly say, 'I'm glad you understand.' This listening process is perhaps best summarised in the words of Dr Cicely Saunders – for her, the phrase 'Watch with me' epitomized her approach to spiritual care in hospice work, and she also wrote, 'Watch with me, means above all, just "Be there"' (Saunders, 1965).

SKILLS OF CO-OPERATION IN THE TEAM

The whole process and relationship for the nurse in this experience is rather like being strapped into a roller coaster at a funfair. The harness needs to be fixed at the beginning of the ride, and the passenger must stay harnessed until the end of the journey and not try to get out. Trying to side-step or solve the problem is like attempting to remove the harness and failing to reach the end of the journey. The professional needs to 'fix the harness' and stay in until the end.

This may present practical difficulties in terms of continuity of care and is a problem that needs acknowledgement, hence the importance of teamwork and support. It is important for most people to have one key worker whom they can trust – very few can reveal themselves at this depth to more than one or two people. It is not always advisable or necessary for more than one person to hear the whole life story, which means that trust must develop between members of the team, and more senior staff may need the humility to value the contribution of less experienced ones. No one person can be effective for everyone at all times.

A difficult issue may arise for the team as far as confidentiality is concerned. By definition, the sharing of deep feelings should be recognized as confidential as it is threatening for the patient to feel that his or her personal revelations are common knowledge. There is a fine line to be negotiated between sharing confidences within the team and holding them absolute. Some kind of contract or agreement with the patient and the family may be necessary if information needs to be shared for a very good reason. This is a highly important area for the professional, who needs to be aware of personal limitations and of when to call in the specialist or a more experienced person, at the same time showing a sense of discrimination concerning what can be shared.

There may well be a need for the professional to seek back-up and support in coping with personal insecurities when moving forward in a difficult relationship. It is important for a nurse not to pull out but to know where such support can be found, have ready access to it and know that help is available to identify the problem areas and enable a return to the situation with renewed insight and confidence to see it through, while exploring new territories. It is preferable for a person with specialist skills or more experience to work with the carers, supporting and helping them to carry on rather than taking over the key role, which might have the effect of 'deskilling' that member of staff in future helping relationships. It is sometimes necessary for a chaplain or other professional to be involved in some aspects of the work, which may remain confidential to them. Even in such cases, it is important that the nurse retain a continuing responsibility for spiritual care.

The whole area of adequate preparation and available support for staff working in these areas of palliative care is one of utmost importance as it will ultimately affect the quality of care given. These issues will be discussed more fully later in the chapter. Professionals in this field need to be aware of their personal limitations and of the importance of receiving help in resolving these areas of difficulty and of sharing their own pain, anger, doubt and helplessness.

THE CARING TEAM

THE PATIENT IN THE FAMILY

When considering the provision of spiritual care, it is central to the observations made so far that the patient is not just the recipient of care offered, but rather a full member of the caring team (Owen et al., 1989). The traditional terminology of talking about the delivery of care militates against an approach that involves the patient fully in all discussions about progress and nursing, medical and spiritual care. A now more acceptable approach locates the individual within the setting of the family and environment as a partner or fully involved member of the decision-making team. It is thus an integral part of spiritual care to help the whole family to feel involved and accepted, and to enable them also to question and express fears with both the professional and/or the patient, which will facilitate open communication within the family.

Unresolved anxieties can create barriers and lead to negative communication – it is important that the legacy left for the family is a good one that has not been destroyed by premature disengagement or inappropriately expressed anger. Anger expressed at the appropriate time is unlikely to be remembered with bitterness after the death is over. Feelings openly expressed within the family may be painful at the time but are, if accepted in love and openness, likely to be resolved. On the other hand, if the patient feels alone, separate and unable to express feelings openly with the family or a sympathetic professional, the feelings of isolation that may follow may well be expressed in anger and bitterness.

THE PROFESSIONAL'S ROLE

The professional's role is therefore one of enabling rather than taking over. The patient and family need to remain in control of the relationship, with one or two provisos. First, it is unwise to enter the conspiracy to deceive that is often set up in the early stages of illness when the family is shocked and vulnerable; such a conspiracy may well prevent the ability to relate openly, and disable family communication from the time of diagnosis or prognosis. Second, the patient needs to relate to the nurse in two different ways, feeling confident both that there is professional clinical control present for patient safety, and recognizing that, in the spiritual dimension, the patient has the control.

In addition, the patient and family have the right to establish the parameters of what they are willing to receive and the style and cultural form in which they desire this. They have a right to have their own religious faith or no faith at all, to be individual or unorthodox in approach.

It is important to remember that no one has the right to try to impose upon another their own way of thinking in this situation. It is one thing to attempt to share our faith with others by knocking on people's doors or preaching from a pulpit, but in palliative care we have no right to expect them to listen just because they are captive in bed and reliant on us for care. If we establish good caring relationships, it is highly probable that patients will ask for our opinions and will then want to listen – we can then share because, and for as long as, we are invited to do so. We also have the responsibility to provide care for patients of every race, culture and creed, these principles being an integral part of the international code of nursing ethics.

One area in which the nurse may be helpful and have an educative role is in enabling the family to understand what the patient needs and helping them to see how inappropriate it is to deceive and how this deception reduces the possibility of communication. It may help if they understand that many patients know that there is a strong possibility that death may not be far off, but may not find it easy to express this knowledge in words.

SOME IMPORTANT ISSUES FOR THE PROFESSIONAL

One difficult issue is accepting that some patients remain angry and never appear to come to an acceptance of their situation, even with constant encouragement and support. This may be more apparent in the hospice approach to care, where patients sometimes find that the intensely caring atmosphere inhibits their need to express anger forcefully. Nurses need to beware of the danger of matriarchialism in palliative care – of overprotecting the individual from his or her stronger feelings by a 'cosseting' approach. While acknowledging the enormous contribution of the hospice movement (both past and present), the gentle accepting aspect of its philosophy may present difficulties for some, the patient feeling unable to express the intensity of emotions and personal experience in an uninhibited way. Professional carers need to be aware of and sensitive to the sharp face of the spiritual response and the whole area of pain and the harsh reality of loneliness in suffering, as exemplified in the experience of Jesus in Gethsemane before his crucifixion (*Luke*: Ch. 22, vv. 39–46).

Kindness and gentleness have a very positive input for some patients, indeed for most patients for some of the time, but many need harsh reality to be met with naked realism. It is most unsatisfying to thump a soft pillow when angry or to throw anger at a 'pillow-like' person. Professional carers need to accept the patient's right to die angry, or to die not accepting their illness or death – they have a right to continue to fight or to give up. Carers have no right to dictate how or when patients will die, but they must affirm each patient's right to be themselves.

GUILT FOR THE PROFESSIONAL

Much guilt often surrounds professionals in palliative care, generated by the fact that they cannot give clear answers. This is especially true when it has not been possible to relieve pain or distress, or if there is no demonstrable acceptance of the situation. Because of our human nature, it takes a great deal of maturity to realize that the expression of uncontrolled tears, anger or naked fear is an affirmation of our skills in providing spiritual care rather than the reverse, even though this is a negative and more traditional interpretation. These emotions need to be translated into a model that is acceptable to the patient. In the acceptance of these naked emotions, healing and a sense of peace may well follow. There are some for whom these emotions will remain intense up to the time of death, but that should not be seen as a failure on the part of the professional.

Another difficult area concerns individuals' rights to receive their own religious or cultural care in whatever manner and from whom they wish to receive it, irrespective of how that may appear to the carer. This means that the nurse may at times need to bring in someone – a priest or a representative of another faith or religion – to provide a form of care that is felt to be 'wrong'. (One obvious exception to this is if someone is asking for an action that is against the law of the land.) There is a need for true humility in all carers, to acknowledge that while they know what they think truth is, others may well see things differently and have a right to do so.

Misunderstanding can arise if lay and professional people use the same words with different meanings, resulting in confusion. It is important to avoid the use of jargon, which is not really applicable in the field of spiritual care. Another helpful area of preparation lies in assisting the professional carer to identify and clarify his or her personal beliefs. This will encourage a sensitivity to the patient's uncertainties and explorations, and also increase awareness of any possible prejudices arising from a particular personal perspective or belief.

SUPPORT IN THE PROFESSIONAL ROLE

There are many ways of offering support through existing networks within a particular organization. These may include group settings or one-to-one relationships, in which the feelings of helplessness and questions arising in the palliative care situation may be explored in a non-threatening and non-authoritarian environment. Here, the individual is in turn acknowledged, accepted and given care for his or her own personal pain or doubt. In some places, programmes of self-awareness and self-development are available through educational channels, these being enhanced if they can be accompanied by adequate 'on the spot' back-up and debriefing in the workplace, where real-life experiences occur. Such programmes are valuable in helping individuals to be aware of their own personal humanity and therefore better able to accept the frailties of others and to become less afraid of failure.

Although there may appear to be constant factors within the body of truth, if people look carefully back through their lives, truth is not a static commodity but one that develops and evolves; indeed, most people have a broader and different perception of life and faith from that which they held 10 years ago. While the core of people's understandings of truth may remain essentially unchanged, their perception of truth develops when they make new discoveries on the journey through life. If it does not change, they are not engaging with life in the world around them or growing within their own knowledge, faith or belief.

PREPARATION FOR THE PROFESSIONAL ROLE

In looking at these aspects of spiritual care, it is apparent that they demand a certain level of maturity and experience in situations that may at times feel threatening to the carer. This calls for a degree of adequate preparation and support provision that presents a major area for consideration, one which cannot be fully explored here. It is, however, worth indicating some ways in which carers can be prepared, or equip themselves, for this kind of work. It is helpful to build up as wide a personal knowledge as possible on different religions, cultural and denominational groups, and to understand the thinking of agnostics, atheists and humanists (McGilloway and Myco, 1985). The patient will thus be met on a basis of mutual understanding. A knowledge of local resources and culture is also important so that one can learn to communicate effectively with the patient and family.

The team is an important source of support, engendering an atmosphere of trust and openness that acknowledges the threatening nature of the work and values each member's contribution. It should also be remembered that chaplains are increasingly becoming involved right across the whole spectrum of care and many make a specific contribution to staff support as well as patient and family care.

CONCLUSION

Good spiritual care is never heavy or intrusive but natural, human and warm. Above all else, it is the acceptance by a very human being of another very human being within a safe, affirming and loving environment. Although there are common responses and ingredients within the process of dying and bereavement (Kübler-Ross, 1969; Carr, 1982), and models of the dying person are excellent for understanding the process of dying and grieving, these can be dangerous if they are used in a prescriptive manner to push or steer people along their journey. Each pathway to death and each personal grief is essentially individual and a unique experience for that person, and therefore cannot be standardized in any way (Clench and Neville, 1982). The recognizable stages may not all be present, or they may appear all at the same time or in a different sequence. Therefore, these models, albeit a useful aid to acknowledging the process, cannot be seen as a definitive statement (Sims, 1988). Good spiritual care demands a close empathy – a closeness and ability to touch and hold appropriately, one of the greatest skills being to use and value silence.

Never speak unless you think you can improve upon the silence.

Archbishop Michael Ramsey

REFERENCES

Bradshaw, W.J. 1972: The concept of need. *New Society* **30**, 640–3.

Burnard, P. 1990: Learning to care for the spirit. *Nursing Standard* **4**, 38.

Carr, A.T. 1982: Dying and bereavement. In: Hall, J. (ed.) *Psychology for Nurses*. London: British Psychological Society/Macmillan Press.

Clench, P. and Neville, M. 1982: *Introducing Nursing*. Series 1, **34**, 1475.

Faulkner, A. 1985: *Nursing: A Creative Approach*. Eastbourne: Baillière Tindall.

Fiefel, H. 1986: Foreword. In: *In Quest of the Spiritual Component of Care for the Terminally Ill*. Proceedings of a Colloquium, Yale University.

Kübler-Ross, E. 1969: *On Death and Dying*. New York: Macmillan.

McGilloway, O. and Myco, F. 1985: *Nursing and Spiritual Care*. Lippincott Nursing Series. London: Harper & Row.

Morrison, R. 1989: Spiritual health care and the nurse. *Nursing Standard* **4**, 28.

Neuberger, J. 1987: *Caring for Dying People of Different Faiths*. Lisa Sainsbury Foundation Series. London: Austin Cornish.

Owen, G.M. *et al.* 1989: The dying person. In: *A Study of the Marie Curie Nursing Service*. London: Marie Curie Memorial Foundation.

Saunders, C. 1965: Watch with me. *Nursing Times* **61**, 48.

Sims, S. 1988: Cancer and ageing. *Nursing Times* **84**, 26–8.

FURTHER READING

Stoter, D.J. 1995: *Spiritual Aspects of Health*. London: Mosby.

Stoter, D.J. 1997: *Staff Support in Health Care*. Oxford: Blackwell Science.

chapter 9

THE ISSUES OF SEXUALITY AND INTIMACY IN PALLIATIVE CARE

Elizabeth Grigg

> Sexuality involves the totality of being a person and therefore nurses and patients are only given their full respect as people when nursing care has firm foundations in a truly holistic approach incorporating sexuality as a vital aspect of humanity.
>
> Webb (1985)

Nursing care has since the 1970s tried to focus more on a holistic model of care encompassing the patient's psychosocial, environmental, cultural, biological and physiological components. Prior to this, nursing care followed a largely medical model of cure in which the biology and pathology of illness persisted and took priority. The 'sexual part' of this holistic care has always been problematic and is indeed often ignored by nurses.

In the 1980s the recognition of human immunodeficiency virus (HIV) and acquired immune deficiency syndrome (AIDS) placed sexuality and sexual health care on the political agenda and hence the professional schema (Faugier, 1993). HIV and AIDS highlighted the ignorance and prejudice of many care-givers and the serious deficiencies in their ability to meet the psychosocial and sexuality needs of their patients. HIV and AIDS are now not quite as highly placed on the political programme, which may mean that sexuality and sexual health-care education will be lost within the nursing curriculum, and nurses will lose sight of the vital importance of patients' perceptions of their sexuality and sexual identity when they are ill. Nurses and nurse educators must continue to address the fact that the patients' sexuality continues almost always to be overlooked – whatever their condition. Despite the 'rhetoric of holism' (Boughton, cited in Lawler, 1997) nursing care still concentrates upon the physical rather than the whole.

According to Gilley (1988), and latterly Cort (1998), attention to concerns of sexuality is, and remains, singularly lacking in relation to palliative care, at a time when people often long for intimate closeness with their loved ones. As Webb (1987) argues:

communication and love between different people depends upon the integration of somatic, emotional, intellectual and social components comprising the sexuality of each individual...human beings are sexual in every way all the time; human sexuality is an integral factor in the uniqueness of every person.

(Stuart and Sundeen, cited in Webb, 1987)

People thus remain sexual beings until they die.

If nurses are knowledgeable about sexuality *in its totality* and have learned to accept their own and other people's feelings and beliefs about sexuality, they will be more comfortable in dealing with both professional situations possessing a sexual connotation, such as washing patients of the opposite sex, and broader issues of sexuality, for example working with patients undergoing an abortion (Webb, 1985). According to Webb, such nurses will also be able to integrate the concept of sexuality into their nursing care. In the process of assessing, planning, implementing and evaluating care, they will be perceptive to signs that draw attention to people's concerns in relation to sexuality and use nursing judgements on the kinds of approach needed.

Nursing has its own techniques and skills, which are evident in its area of expertise – the sensitivity that most nurses show to the experiences of their patients. Lawler (1991) suggests that this is 'how' rather than 'what' things are done. This makes nursing more of a social entity than merely a science, an art or a mixture of the two. Expert nursing practice results not only from knowledge, but also from the experiences of the social world of nursing (Benner, 1984).

AN HISTORICAL AND SOCIETAL PERSPECTIVE OF SEXUALITY

The concept and definition of sexuality is complex, experts differing in their perceptions of and explanations on it. Henslin and Sagarin (1978), Pocs (1989), Sardi (1992) and more recently Parker and Gagnon (1995) have stated that people of a variety of different civilizations in different historical periods have engaged in a variety of different modes of sexual expression and behaviour. Despite this cultural and historical diversity, one important principle should be borne in mind: that sexual awareness, attitudes and behaviours are learned within the sociocultural context that defines the appropriate sexuality for that society's members.

Changes in the social environment, such as the 'liberation of women from the home' (Pocs, 1989) have strengthened the concept of people as sexual beings and posed a challenge to the 'anti-sex ethic' that has traditionally served to orient Western society. Such society is now witnessing a gradual convalescence from a disease that Brecher (1988, cited in Sardi, 1992) called 'Victorianism', which reinforced the moral teaching of Christianity and was characterized by the belief that all sexualities were wicked and loathsome, and would lead to disaster. Sexual repression would, on the other hand, lead people into being frugal and hard working.

In pre-Christian times, however, sexuality was open and accepted as being part of the normal expression of a culture. According to Sardi (1992), for example, G. Rattray Taylor's work *Sex in History* showed that nudity was, in pre-Christian Ireland, no cause for shame. In contrast, women in Victorian England covered their bodies from the neck to below the ankle with layers of clothes; Richard Lewinsohn's research *A History of Sexual Customs* (cited in Sardi, 1992), indicated that their bodies were neither seen nor spoken about. Women were in fact often so prudish that they would not let themselves be examined by physicians, instead indicating on dummies especially set up for the purpose the spots where they felt pain.

Social change is not easily accomplished. Sociologists generally acknowledge that changes in the social environment are accompanied by the presence of interest groups that offer competing versions of what 'is' or 'should be' appropriate social behaviour (Denisoff and Wahrman, 1979). The contemporary sociocultural changes surrounding sexuality are highly illustrative of such social dynamics (Henslin and Sagarin, 1978; Parker and Gagnon, 1995).

In relation to nursing care, Salvage (1987) states that the different meanings given to sexuality, in terms of both a global and a personal perspective, are endless. She highlights the fact that each individual nurse and patient may have a very different perception of what sexuality means to them and to each other. This makes it difficult for nurses to define the meanings that their patients give to actual or perceived alterations in their sexual persona as a result of diagnosis, illness or treatment.

Moreover, given the nature of sexuality and sexual behaviour in Western culture, it is not surprising that by far the most problematic areas of nursing are those associated with sexuality (Lawler,1991). Sexuality comes with a great deal of cultural 'baggage' so that when nurses are confronted with patients, cultural meanings that attend being either a nurse or a patient and the context of care all require management. According to Lawler (1991), much of that management concerns meanings attached to: 'The *definition* that patients and nurses place upon the relationship between the physical body and sexual expression' (original emphasis).

Research over the past two decades has led to the conclusion that nurses do not have the necessary theoretical knowledge to be able to teach, counsel or otherwise care for their patients in this area; nor are they sufficiently aware of and comfortable with their own sexuality to be able to act non-judgementally. Sexual behaviour and sexual health care were once never mentioned in nurse training. When they did begin to appear on the curriculum, what was taught was restricted to anatomy, physiology and altered body function – biological aspects only. Although this information is obviously important and necessary, so too is the opportunity to explore personal feelings and attitudes, and their relevance to providing complete care for others.

Webb (1987) suggests that the rigid and conservative attitudes that many nurses have to a definition of sexuality are likely to influence both the quality and the quantity of their relationships with patients and amongst themselves.

THE DEFINITION OF SEXUALITY, SELF-CONCEPT AND BODY IMAGE

'Human beings are sexual in every way, all of the time...[sexuality] is an integral part of the uniqueness of every person' (Poorman, cited in Stuart and Sundeen, 1991). Sexuality and self-concept (or self-esteem) are essentially interlinked, self-concept being the perception that individuals have of their personal and physical self. The personal self is related to beliefs, ethics, morals, spirituality and ideals, whereas the physical self is related to body image, body sensations and feelings. Body image can be seen as 'body reality', 'body ideal' and 'body presentation' (Crouch, 1999); an altered body image, through surgery or illness, may drastically impact upon a person's self-concept. Even a diagnosis can immediately affect self-concept and threaten body image.

Andrew and Andrew (1991) defines sexuality as including body image, sexual activity and self-esteem. The definition of sexuality is many sided, but acknowledging its multiplicity and fluidity will enhance an understanding of the relevance of sexuality to nursing, both to nurses themselves and to the care that they give their patients and clients. Webb (1987) states that the term 'sexuality' 'can mean as many different things to as many different people, and a single understanding cannot be reached'. She not only argues that it reflects the norms and beliefs of a society, but also describes sexuality as 'the capacity of the individual to link emotional needs with physical intimacy'. Similarly, Hogan (cited in Webb, 1985) defines sexuality as follows: 'considering that sexuality is more than the sex act, it is all that we are as men and women, it encompasses the most intimate feelings and deepest longings of the heart to find meaningful relationships'.

Lion (cited in Webb, 1985) expands upon this definition and explains sexuality as:

> being much more than the biological side of sex acts, it is the all encompassing emotional aspects of human relationships. It involves the totality of being human and includes all those aspects of the human being that relate to being boy or girl, man or woman, and is an entity subject to lifelong dynamic change. Sexuality reflects a person's character as well as their genital nature.

According to Webb (1987), this perspective emphasizes the changing nature and expression of sexuality throughout the life cycle.

Sexuality has historically been conceptualized as a biological construct in which social processes play a secondary part. Nurses need to understand the definition of sexuality *in its totality* if they are to provide holistic care (Lawler, 1991). Thomas (1989), and – a decade later – Cort (1998) contend that, despite the literature on the subject of sexuality, the 'real' matter of sexuality is still not even mentioned in nurse training. The rich social meanings that accompany sexuality remain ignored.

SEXUALITY EDUCATION FOR NURSES

Research by Lewis and Bor (1994) revealed that 65 per cent of the nurse respondents questioned never addressed sexuality with patients or had indeed ever had any 'sexuality training' *per se*. Bell (1989) refers to three objectives in educating nurses with regard to sexual health – attitude, knowledge and skills – all of which involve an examination of the sexual self, an awareness of one's own sexuality and an awareness of the possible diversity of other people's sexuality. This, Bell argues, will create tolerance and acceptance, and enhance attitudes. She presupposes that a knowledge of sexual issues, such as the effects of illness on body image, the consequences of ethnic and religious beliefs relating to sexuality and a knowledge of sexual functioning, response and anatomy, will create a more positive attitude. This should help nurses to become more comfortable and competent when interacting with their patients.

Bell (1989), Thomas (1989) and Savage (1990a) stress that skill in both verbal and non-verbal communication is vital in facilitating the interaction between the patient and nurse in the area of sexuality:

> Nurses need support and encouragement to cope with the presence of sexuality in their work and to incorporate sexual health care into their nursing practice. But at the same time the difficult nature of sexuality has to be acknowledged and the expectations we have of nurses must be realistic.
>
> (Savage, 1989)

ADDRESSING SEXUALITY WITHIN NURSING CARE

Nurses will not truly be meeting the needs of their patients if the issues of sexuality in care are not addressed. Moreover, if palliative care is to be practised sincerely it must adhere to holism and thereby include sexuality. Thomas (1989) claims that, despite the number of definitions of sexuality that 'encompass the totality of being', it continues to be misunderstood as solely a biological sex act, which makes it difficult for nurses not only to consider their patient's sexual needs, but also actually to help them to express these needs.

According to Lawler's (1991) research, the complex 'social construction of the sexualised body' makes it impossible for some nurses even to mention body parts, especially those in the genital area. Savage (1987) and Lawler (1991) propose that one reason why many nurses have difficulty here is because sexuality has shaped the structure of nursing itself. Society dictates that men and women behave differently, and nowhere has the gender role been acted out more faithfully than in nursing. Male and female nurses are stereotyped, men because they cross their gender role and women because they do not. Because they have taken on the role of personifying womanhood, female nurses are most commonly portrayed as 'golden-hearted sex objects' (Savage, 1989), whereas male nurses are emasculated by taking on work involving caring and gentleness – supposedly only women's qualities.

Webb (1985), Savage (1987, 1989) and Lawler (1991) suggest that sexual stereotyping, which has been reinforced by the media's portrayal of female nurses as 'pornographic sex-symbols' (Savage, 1987), helps to shape the relationship between nurses and their patients. They stress that sexuality is integral to the nurse–patient relationship because of the very nature of nursing and the physical and emotional intimacy it involves. The nurse has however, to make it clear that these acts are non-sexual. How nurses cope depends on their attitudes towards their own sexuality and the knowledge they have about what sexuality really is.

According to research by Waterhouse and Metcalfe (1991), the majority of patients would like nurses to initiate addressing issues of sexuality with them. It may be that the influence of medical treatment is directly affecting their biological sexual functioning or that they have a poor self-concept because of the perception of a changed body image as a result of illness, so that they no longer feel sexual or attractive. Whatever their concerns, these should be identified and discussed. Bor and Watts (1993) argue that some patients are willing to answer the most intimate questions about their sexual behaviour as long as they are not judged or ridiculed.

This ignoring of the sexual side of patients may be attributed to nurses being too embarrassed to address such needs, but it might also be because nurses fail to recognize or acknowledge that they exist. This lack of communication on matters of sexuality ends up in a conspiracy of silence (Savage, 1989), nurses using evasive tactics when dealing with this area (Lawler, 1991).

Current nurse training does not even address the fact that nurses may feel uncomfortable when they provide care. Thompson (1990) for example, refers to the need for privacy for adolescent patients on oncology units in order for them to develop their sexual and social relationships, but Savage (1990a) argues that nurses feel uneasy about allowing their patients privacy. She continues that it would be simple for nurses to create partial privacy simply by pulling the curtains around the bed, allowing even those who are seriously ill physical closeness with their partners or friends, but many nurses are reluctant to do this. According to Savage, the suggestion of private rooms being provided for patients if they need sexual intimacy causes even more unease among nurses than does the use of screens.

Thompson (1990) believes that the interest, attitudes and skills of health professionals determine the quality of sexual health care received by young cancer patients who have educated themselves. When initiating an intimate discussion with patients, the PLISSIT model (cited in Waterhouse, 1996) is useful:

P = permission
LI = limited information
SS = specific suggestions
IT = intensive therapy

Giving 'permission' or establishing comfort, trust and openness with a patient is the first and most vital step in any relationship to promote the addressing of sexual concerns. It is hard even for some nurses to create this step, maybe because of a lack of privacy or, more commonly, feeling inadequately trained.

The step of 'limited information' should also be manageable for nurses. This is simply the ability to discuss with patients the possible effects of treatment or disease upon their sexual functioning. After establishing trust and safety, it should be possible to discuss more intimate matters with patients and therefore provide partial information and empowerment.

The next steps may necessitate a specialist input so nurses must be able to judge when it is appropriate to 'refer on' without feeling inadequate; they should also remember that even just listening to patients' fears may help them with unburdening and provide them with relief. Providing a silent, but responsive, presence can help people to organize their thoughts and come to terms with issues of self-concept (Dumas, 1996).

The role of reflection in and upon practice can also help to provide a framework within which nurses can analyse their thoughts and feelings towards a patient's sexuality in an instructive way. A simple adaptation of Carper's (1978) model of reflection (Johns, 1995) could, for example, be applied to look at an incident that has cause discomfort related to the area of sexuality (Box 9.1). However, as Savage (1990b) asserts, if sexuality is to be more centrally incorporated into nursing care, the support available for nurses must be improved.

BOX 9.1 A MODEL OF REFLECTION (ADAPTED FROM CARPER, 1978)

A description of the experience:	What contributed?
	What were the key processes?
Reflection upon the experience:	What was I trying to achieve
	Why did I respond thus?
	What were the consequences?
	How must the patient have felt?
	How did/do I feel?
	How do I know this?
Influencing factors:	What made me act thus?
	What knowledge informed me?

COULD I HAVE DONE THINGS DIFFERENTLY?

How does this connect with previous experiences?
Could I handle this better in a similar situation?
What would then be the consequences for the patient, others, myself?
How do I now feel about the experience?
Will it ultimately help me in the future?
Has the experiences expanded my knowledge?

SEXUALITY AND PALLIATIVE CARE FOR THOSE WITH CANCER: EXEMPLARS FROM PRACTICE

The key elements of sexual health as defined by the World Health Organization are relevant and helpful as they recognize that sexuality is related to sexual activity in health, disability or illness. These key elements are:

1. A capacity to enjoy and control sexual and reproductive behaviour with a social and personal ethic.
2. Freedom from fear, shame, guilt, false beliefs and other psychological factors inhibiting sexual relationships.
3. Freedom from organic disorders, diseases and deficiencies that interfere with sexual and reproductive functions.

(Weller, 1993)

Nurses must continually remember that chronic disease and disabling illness can have a serious effect upon a person's sexuality, sexual expression and identity, and thus upon their sexual health. This may be because of agents influencing physiological functioning, it may be the consequence of psychological or social factors. Whatever the reason, the nurse's ability to be aware of the concerns of a patient or their loved ones can have a profound impact on the quality of care given.

Palliative care is caring about the whole person and their world – physical, psychological, social and spiritual – and all these components must encompass sexual elements in order to be absolutely and unconditionally holistic. However, as Bor and Watts (1993) argue:

Conversations about death, dying, relationships and sexual matters are among the most challenging and difficult that nurses and other health care providers have with their patients. Cultural taboos, the fear of upsetting patients and underdeveloped counselling and interpersonal skills may present obstacles to more open an effective communication.

Many nurses in fact find it easier to initiate a conversation about death than about sex.

Although there is an increase in the literature pertaining to sexuality, there is still very little that addresses palliative care and sexuality or intimacy (Carr, 1996). The sexuality side of palliative care is still not routinely addressed; when it is mentioned, it is tackled with little confidence (Cort, 1998). As stated above, however, the majority of patients want nurses to address issues of sexuality with them, and some patients are willing to answer intimate questions about their sexual behaviour provided they are not judged or ridiculed.

Body image is immediately threatened when people are given a diagnosis of 'cancer'. They may fear that the effect of their illness will prevent them coping in their current role as a particular family member, an employee and so on. Treatment and illness will also affect their body image, perhaps because of shortness of breath and coughing from cancer of the lung, scarring as a result of surgery or hair loss from chemotherapy.

Thompson (1990) considers issues such as body image and self-concept in relation to adolescents with cancer, discussing the potential effects of cancer treatment that may influence sexual adequacy in adolescents. She argues that adolescents are more sensitive about their bodies than adults: 'Any deformity or imperfection, obvious or hidden, can be so unacceptable to the adolescent that disgust and shame result. Acceptance of personal sexuality also presents problems'.

Adults can, however, be as sensitive about their bodies as younger people. As 62-year-old Rita Mackenzie (1984) stated during her illness:

> Not being able to rely on my own body made me feel sexually insecure, and I withdrew from my relationship because of this... I'm really worried that men will stop looking at me now. I'm scared that I've suddenly got no sex appeal. I don't feel any less but it worries me that people will start treating me as though I am sexless.

Thompson (1990) provides a useful table of the potential effects of cancer treatment on adolescents that could be equally applied to adults (Table 9.1). The person with advanced cancer has probably gone through the traumas of one or many of these consequences of treatment. The processes underlying a highly developed cancer will result in further significant physiological changes to the body, which may have a profound effect upon sexual image and sexual feelings.

Weight loss, or weight gain caused by oedema, can cause deep depression for some people. It is vital that nurses are sensitive to this and are able to provide the appropriate care. If changed body shape is concerning the patient, all that may be necessary is the provision of garments that feel as if they fit. New clothes may go a long way towards providing an improved body image and increased self-concept. Many patients will feel valued and nurtured if they are given embellishments to their outfits – especially by loved ones.

Table 9.1 Potential effects of cancer treatment that may influence sexual adequacy

Surgery	Radiotherapy	Chemotherapy
Testicular biopsy	Testicular radiotherapy	Hair loss
Fear of mutilation	*Skin changes*	Sterility
	Sterility	Weight gain/loss
		Skin changes
All surgery	Spinal radiotherapy	Nausea
Residual scarring	*May result in asymmetry*	Vomiting
Amputation of		Use of steroids
affected limb/body part		Facial hair
Leads to poor body image		Vaginitis
		Weight gain/loss

Hair loss can have a profound effect upon some people's body image and therefore self-concept or esteem. I have heard patients state that, once hair loss is evident, they cannot be private about 'having cancer…my hair loss was almost a statement to the public that I was ill and therefore on chemotherapy…I could no longer hide and knew that people were looking at my dreadfully changed body and thinning hair'. Crouch (1999) suggests that 'body reality', as in hair loss caused by chemotherapy, occurs when people know what they look like, 'body ideal' is how they want their body to be, and 'body presentation' is how they present their body to others or how others see them.

The body and sexuality are intimately interrelated (Lawler, 1991). According to Lawler's research, nurses who have the least difficulty in addressing *total* body care are those with a relaxed and open attitude towards the body and touch. The British are culturally 'non-touching', and some nurses have to overcome their own sociocultural background and adjust to a particular professional subculture and its established methods, which permit handling other people's bodies. Lawler (1991) continues:

> They must also confront the symbolism of certain parts of the body, in particular, parts which have sexual significance, and they must find ways to manage social interaction during those times when they break taken-for-granted rules about the body.

Recent research on mastectomy, body image and therapeutic massage identified how body-centred intervention had an extensive positive impact on a small cohort of women who had great difficulty coming to terms with their body image, sexuality and self-worth after losing a breast (Breden, 1999). The study showed that these women responded to massage in two ways. First, the intimacy of the touching made them 'open up' and disclose their beliefs about losing a breast. It helped them to talk and to express their deep and suppressed feelings with their carers. One woman said that she had concealed her anger at losing a breast because she was afraid that it would make her appear ungrateful towards the doctors who had 'cured her cancer'.

Second, touching made them feel 'touchable', acceptable, feminine and worthwhile. Therapeutic touch can have a very soothing influence (Case study 9.1).

Similarly, people who have an Kaposi's sarcoma arising from HIV infection may respond to the lesion being touched, and even more so to it being camouflaged: some patients may experience great comfort from help with hiding blemishes. Male as well as female patients should be offered specialized make-up to cover flaws that may, to them, be horrendous.

According to Lawler (1991), female nurses have more difficulty addressing the sexuality of male patients than vice versa, but it is just as important for men to feel pampered and loved, so nurses must be able to:

> Negotiate not only normal social boundaries when they touch patients, but, because the body is heavily inscribed with meaning – much of it sexual – nurses' work is socially fragile, and they must learn ways to make their work manageable.

CASE STUDY 9.1

I remember one beautiful elderly lady of about 70 years who was admitted for terminal care. During her dying, she struggled to bathe every day and to apply make up, perfume and powder, insisting that she have her hair 'done' once a week. She seemed very peaceful when she felt that she looked beautiful. The nurses were aware of her needs, and when she could no longer continue with this care herself, they were comfortable with doing it for her. This was an important part of her total care as she was happy when her hair was washed, when she was wearing make-up and when she knew she smelt 'nice'. She needed this gentle touching and pampering of her body; she needed to be able to express her sexuality. Towards the end of her illness, all she needed was help to do so. This seemed to matter to her as much as being without pain.

How they cope depends upon expert nursing practice resulting from not only knowledge and empathy, but also the experiences of the social world of nursing.

According to Lawler, there is a point in the male patient's illness when sensuality is not an issue that is considered by female nurses. If a patient is very ill, experiences of a sexual nature are overtaken by the seriousness of the patient's condition. It thus appears easier for nurses to manage body care for men when they are dying because the care that they give cannot be perceived as sexual.

Some men do not, however, want care from women. Homosexual men, for example, often request that intimate care be given to them only by male nurses. They may fear they are being judged or ridiculed by heterosexual staff because of their sexual orientation. As Hancock (1991) states:

> Anything which has sexual overtones stimulates an unholy trinity of inhibition, hypocrisy and prejudices, all of which can and do have a detrimental effect on . . . care . . . this combined with ignorance produces a seemingly impenetrable barrier.

It is possible that this is what some nurses subscribe to. In 1991, for example, Dennis was requested to run some compulsory HIV/AIDS awareness sessions for all of the staff within his particular health authority, nurses forming the largest single occupational group. Dennis's observations drew attention to some participants, including nurses, being overtly prejudiced towards HIV and AIDS patients because they were perceived as being 'different' or 'not like us', and 'they shouldn't do such things', that is 'take drugs' or 'have relationships with partners of the same sex' (Dennis, 1991). Dennis's courses, however, did nothing to change the negative attitudes of some of the participants – these negative attitudes have worrying implications for good patient care. As the Royal College of Nursing (cited in Sim, 1992) states: 'Discrimination against particular individuals for whatever reason, should never be tolerated . . . the adoption of a professional attitude requires that all those who need nursing care should receive it without discrimination'.

I worked for a year as a nurse tutor on a palliative care ward for AIDS patients, many of whom were diagnosed with cancer. The atmosphere on the ward was warm and loving: there were red hearts hanging over some of the beds, and flowers and plants everywhere. The nurses, mostly male, were very tactile with their patients and with one another. The patients, also mostly male, seemed content. Most of them had partners or loved ones with them for most of the time, sitting or leaning on their beds, holding hands or stroking each other. Sometimes the curtains were drawn around a bed. If this was the case, the nurses would never assume access and always asked before going in. Savage (1990a) suggests that once patients have rights over a personal space, nurses hesitate and think twice before disturbing someone whom has sought seclusion. There was also a bedroom available with a double bed for patients who wished to sleep with their partners.

The care given to the patients, by both the nurses and the partners, was conducted almost with reverence. Death seemed to be accepted as a natural progression. Some patients requested that a celebration be arranged after they had died, parties often being held on the ward for staff, friends, other patients and their loved ones. These parties were an expression of the intimacy between everybody involved in the care of people with AIDS in this loving environment.

The nurses cared as much for the loved ones of the patients as they did for the patients themselves. Partners and relatives were encouraged to provide intimate care if that was what was wanted, which helped them to feel as if they were 'doing something' at a time when there is a strong belief that, for someone dying, 'there is nothing else anyone can do'. Lawler (1991) describes the time of dying as a time when patients are totally dependent on others for body care. Nurses suggest that they are 'doing nothing' for the patient during this time, but, as Lawler argues, this is possibly the most difficult time for carers in terms of emotional and practical implications.

Some patients do not, however, wish to be dependent upon their partner or relatives for intimate care. They may, for whatever reason, feel uncomfortable if body care is provided by those closest to them, and nurses need to be responsive to this too (Case study 9.2).

Gilley (1988) provides an example of intimacy that is in complete contrast to the one cited in Case study 9.2:

> There was a couple in their seventies...Mrs E became very ill with metastic carconoma. Mr E nursed her, supported by the district nursing team...There was an intimacy in the flat. The curtains were usually closed even by day, the warm lights on in the bedroom, the nursing dressings and paraphernalia kept hidden. The outside world seemed far away. Help was accepted from doctors and nurses who were then dispatched kindly on their way, but the real business continued within those four walls. I was called in the early hours one cold night. She was near to dying and had been incontinent in their shared bed. Exhausted, he asked me to help change the sheets. As we sorted linen, I shared with him the likelihood that she would die during the night. He knew. 'We've slept together for 50 years. I want one last night with her.' Together we made up the bed with fresh sheets. It was impossible not to think of a bridal bed being prepared. I helped him clean and tidy her. She died in the night.

CASE STUDY 9.2

Bob wished to be perceived by his wife as strong and totally independent, even though his illness gradually made him totally dependent upon the care of others. He was nursed at home, the district nurses initially carrying out all his care. When he deteriorated and needed almost constant care, his wife began to intervene. This caused him great distress and he asked to be admitted to hospital, eventually dying peacefully there. It appeared that Bob wished his wife to remember him as an independent figure who was strong enough not to rely upon her for the sort of care a mother gives to a child. He once said that he wanted her 'to remember me as a man, not as a baby'. Bob never spoke to her about the care he was receiving, and even during the time she stayed at the hospital when he was dying, she always left his bedside while the nurses provided intimate care. She appeared to love him so much that even though he was at times probably unaware of her presence, she understood and accepted why he would not have wished her to witness his vulnerability. She was also never made to feel guilty by the other carers for not joining in with his intimate care.

Kitzinger (1983) describes the sexual relationship of a couple after the woman has undergone a hysterectomy for cancer. She believes that often the man will start to think more about love-making from the woman's perspective, and a more sensitive understanding of her needs evolves: 'Appalled by the idea that she has had surgery, he slows down, gives more body stimulation and is more gentle'.

Some couples need this type of intimacy even though their loved one is very ill. To some, continuing to have intercourse is a symbol of virility and vital to their self-esteem. It may be important for them to have an orgasm with intercourse in order to prove to themselves and to their partner that they are still worthwhile sexual beings. To others, sexual intercourse may be a way of giving and receiving comfort and closeness, and it can be very distressing for loved ones to be denied the opportunity for it. When intercourse becomes too difficult to manage, couples can still pleasure each other by touching and caressing. Nurses should be able to reassure patients that sexual intimacy can be expressed in this way.

A few hospices provide rooms with double beds so that people can have the freedom to lie together for comfort. Some people want to die in their partner's arms, others wish for isolation, so nurses and care-givers must be aware of and respect the diversity of intimate expression. They should accept, empathize with and respond to all such differing sexual needs during a time when total care is of paramount importance:

> In the same way that a good sexual relationship is the private pleasure of a couple, so must the relationship in terminal care be respected as unique to that couple and a part of their intimacy.
>
> Gilley (1988)

CONCLUSION

Sexuality, disease, loss and death are some of the most vulnerable aspects of our lives, often arousing strong feelings and challenging deeply held values. Nurses, as part of society, reflect the same tolerance (or intolerance) to things that have 'sexual' connotations as others in society do.

If nurses are provided with knowledge on sexuality and are facilitated in becoming more comfortable with their own sexuality and accepting of other people's feelings and beliefs about sexuality, they will be more likely to implement good care in this area for their patients (Bell, 1989; Thomas, 1989; Savage, 1990b). Knowledge alone is, however, not sufficient to enhance nursing care and lessen apprehension concerning unresolved sexual anxieties (Dennis, 1991; Robbins et al., 1992) – 'sexuality' care needs support for its implementation. Expert nursing practice results not only from knowledge and empathy, but also from the experiences of the social world of nursing.

It is the responsibility of nurse educators to assist learners with holistic and humanistic practice. By providing a safe learning environment, educators specializing in sexuality education should be able to facilitate learners in developing the skills and solutions they will need in implementing sexuality care for patients. In the clinical setting, it should be the responsibility of peers and/or supervisors to offer further support. Observing practice can reinforce changes that have taken place in the classroom, but this reinforcement does not always take place, so what is learned in the classroom is not always backed up by observation at the bedside (Birchenall, 1991).

As stated by the Department of Health and the English National Board for Nursing, Midwifery and Health Visiting (Faugier, 1993), the outcomes of sexuality education will be adequate only if all professionals (clinical and educational) have access to it. Clinical specialists must be comfortable with sexuality issues so that they are able to act as role models for learners, but learners also have to be equipped to critically examine and reflect upon their practice. Sexuality is continual so sexuality education should be an ongoing process.

Webb (1987) argues that the biological, psychological, social, philosophical and social policy aspects of sexuality in its widest definition need to form part of the curriculum for all nurses, as does work on communication skills, including those of assessment, teaching and counselling. Sexuality is one area in which nurse educators must pay full attention as part of the process of accountability for the quality of care that nurses give and patients receive.

As well as personal attitudes, knowledge and skills affecting sexual assessment, so too does the philosophy and culture of the clinical environment and the ward documentation relating to 'sexual policy'. Privacy must be implemented and encouraged so that all patients, whatever their condition, are allowed to access it with comfort and ease, discussing, dealing with and enhancing their intimacy and love for both their loved ones and themselves.

REFERENCES

Andrew, C. and Andrew, H. 1991: Sexuality and the dying patient. *Journal of District Nursing* (Nov), 8–10.

Bell, J. 1989: Promoting fulfilment. *Nursing Times* 85(6), 35–37.

Benner, P. 1984: *From Novice to Expert.* Menlow Park, CA: Addison-Wesley.

Birchenall, P.D. 1991: Preparing nurse teachers for their future role. *Nurse Education Today* 11, 100–3.

Bor, R. and Watts, M. 1993: Talking to patients about sexual matters. *British Journal of Nursing* 2(13), 657–60.

Breden, M. 1999: Mastectomy, body image and therapeutic massage: a qualitative study of women's experience. *Journal of Advanced Nursing* 29, 1113–20.

Carper, B. 1978: Fundamental patterns of knowing in nursing. In Johns, C. 1995: Framing learning through reflection within Carper's fundamental ways of knowing in nursing. *Journal of Advanced Nursing* 22, 226–34.

Carr, G. 1996: Themes relating to sexuality that emerged from a discourse analysis of the *Nursing Times* during 1980–1990. *Journal of Advanced Nursing* 24, 196–212.

Cort, E. 1998: Nurses' attitudes to sexuality in caring for cancer patients. *Nursing Times* 94(42), 54–6.

Crouch, S. 1999: Sexual health, sexuality and nurses' role in sexual health. *British Journal of Nursing* 8(2), 601–6.

Dennis, H. 1991: Getting the message. *Nursing Standard* 5(17), 55–6.

Dennisoff, R.S. and Wahrmam, R. 1975: *An introduction to sociology.* New York: Macmillan.

Dumas, M.A.S. 1996: What's it like to belong to a cancer club? *American Journal of Nursing* 96(4), 40–2.

Faugier, J. 1993: *Sexual health education: breaking down the barriers. A report of the National Conference for Health and Social Care Professionals.* London: ENB/D.H.

Gilley, J. 1988: Intimacy and terminal care. *Journal of the Royal College of General Practitioners* 38, 121–2.

Hancock, C. 1991: The challenge for nurses. *Nursing Standard* 5(17), 50.

Henslin, J.M. and Sagarin, E. 1978: *The sociology of sex.* New York: Schocken.

Johns, C. 1995: Framing learning through reflection within Carper's fundamental ways of knowing in nursing. Journal of Advanced Nursing 22, 226–34.

Kitzinger, S. 1983: *Women's experience of sex?* Sydney: Penguin Books.

Lawler, J. 1991: *Behind the screens.* Melbourne: Churchill Livingstone.

Lawler, J. (ed.) 1997: *The body in nursing.* Melbourne: Churchill Livingstone.

Lewis, S. and Bor, R. 1994: Nurse's knowledge of and attitudes towards sexuality and the relationship of these with nursing practice. *Journal of Advanced Nursing* 20, 251–9.

Mackenzie, R. 1984: *Menopause.* Auckland: Reed Books.

Parker, R.G. and Gagnon, J.H. 1995: *Conceiving sexuality.* New York: Routledge.

Pocs, O. (ed.) 1989: *Human sexuality 88/89.* Illinois: Illinois State University.

Robbins, I. Cooper, A. and Bender, M.P. 1992: The relationship between knowledge, attitudes and degree of contact with AIDS and HIV. *Journal of Advanced Nursing* 17, 198–203.

Salvage, J. 1990: *The politics of nursing.* London: Butterworth-Heinemann.

'Sardi' 1992: *Erotic love.* London: Dorset Press.

Savage, J. 1987: *Nurses, gender and sexuality.* London: Heinemann Nursing.

Savage, J. 1989: 'An uninvited guest'. *Nursing Times* **85**(5), 25–8.

Savage, J. 1990a: Sexuality privacy and nursing care. *Nursing Standard* **4**(40), 37–9.

Savage, J. 1990b: Sexuality and nursing care: setting the scene. *Nursing Standard* **4**(37), 24–5.

Sim, J. 1992: AIDS, nursing and occupational risk: an ethical analysis. *Journal of Advanced Nursing* **17**, 569–75.

Stuart, G. and Sundeen, S. (eds) *Principles and practice of psychiatric nursing*, 4th edn. St. Lowis: C.V. Mosby

Thomas, B. 1989: Asexual patients. *Nursing Times* **86**(1), 49–51.

Thomas, B. 1990: 'The human side'. *Nursing Times* **86**(28), 28–30.

Thompson, J. 1990: Sexuality: the adolescent and cancer. *Nursing Standard* **4**(37), 26–49.

Waterhouse, J. 1996: Nursing practice related to sexuality. *NT Research* **6**, 412–18.

Waterhouse, J. and Metcalfe, M. 1991: Attitudes toward nurses discussing sexual concerns with patients. *Journal of Advanced Nursing* **16**, 1048–54.

Webb, C. 1985: *Sexuality, nursing and health*. London: John Wiley.

Webb, C. 1987: Nurses' knowledge and attitudes about sexuality in health care – a review of the literature. *Nurse Education Today* **7**, 75–87.

Weller, B.F. 1993: *Education for sexual health and sexuality. Report of York and Guildford workshops*. London: DoH/ENB.

FURTHER READING

Glover, J. 1985: *Human sexuality in nursing care*. London: Croom Helm.

chapter 10

SUPPORTIVE (COMPLEMENTARY) THERAPIES IN PALLIATIVE CARE

Jane Brewer and Jenny Penson

There are more things in Heaven and Earth, Horatio, than are dreamt of in your philosophy.

Shakespeare (*Hamlet*)

Palliative care and complementary therapies are two movements that have grown almost in parallel. Both are committed to a holistic approach and recognize that the mind, body and spirit are all connected and that we are each connected to each other. They see health as being about wholeness and balance, the experience of being at peace with one's internal and external worlds. Palliative care has the expressed aim of enhancing quality of life, and complementary therapies help to capture something positive about the human spirit's ability to confront difficult issues and painful emotions, and to grow in strength and wisdom.

The nursing profession has responded enthusiastically to the increasing interest in complementary therapies by integrating them into orthodox health-care settings as part of holistic nursing practice. Those working in palliative care and oncology have led the way, an increasing number of therapies being offered and research studies undertaken.

The focus of this chapter will be on what Wells and Tschudin (1994) term 'supportive therapies', indicating that they are approaches that may be incorporated into nursing care. It is not however, intended that these should be seen as what Sayre-Adams and Wright (1995) refer to as 'just another technique'. The authors suggest that they form a philosophy of care with attitudes and skills that are in tune with those of palliative care. They have therefore chosen to highlight therapies that are most likely to be available to patients and offer suggestions for enhancing nursing practice.

EVIDENCE

In her report on complementary therapies in cancer care for Macmillan Cancer Relief, Kohn (1999) found that complementary therapy provision was enthusiastically received by patients, especially for emotional and psychological support. The therapies that were most widely used by cancer patients were the touch therapies and psychological interventions (visualization, meditation and relaxation).

North Devon Hospice offers acupuncture, aromatherapy, art therapy, counselling, healing, hypnotherapy, massage, nutritional medicine, reflexology, relaxation with guided imagery, and therapeutic touch free of charge to hospice patients and their main carers. Research on the patient and carer experience of the complementary therapy programme demonstrated that complementary therapies were well integrated into orthodox palliative care – it was in fact difficult to separate them out. The personal qualities of the therapists were deemed to be a crucial factor, pointing to the importance of the therapeutic relationship. Another advantage of complementary therapies identified by North Devon Hospice patients was that they helped to change the hospice image because people were coming to get better rather to die (Hill, 1997).

Research at Rossendale Hospice showed an increased experience of well-being for all therapies, the greatest improvement being demonstrated with hypnotherapy, psychotherapy and neurolinguistic programming. A marked improvement was shown for reflexology, reiki, and reflexology and reiki combined, the increase for aromatherapy being less marked. An improvement was however, observed for all therapies after four sessions. The greatest reduction of anxiety was found using hypnotherapy. Reflexology combined with reiki demonstrated the greatest benefit for sleep disturbance.

The superior results in their hypno-chemo programme are not surprising as patients were referred for the specific psychological treatment of anxiety, depression and the side-effects of chemotherapy. The approach utilizes traditional cognitive-behaviour therapy coupled with the complementary approaches of hypnotherapy and neurolinguistic programming. The approach is designed to reprogramme the mind into more adaptive responses: this is a true self-help programme harnessing fighting spirit. Staff offer self-help as appropriate, naturally taking the stage of disease and personal preference into account. Some patients are highly motivated to pursue this option, whereas others, weary from medical treatment and psychological struggling, need the gentle complementary therapies of reiki, reflexology and aromatherapy to relax them and raise their energy level.

Both hospice complementary therapy programmes have been financed by the National Lotteries Board.

The National Health Service reforms of April 1999 present challenges to complementary therapies in wanting purchase-based evidence of value. Many healthcare Trusts are now putting together policies on the use of complementary therapies in their areas and documenting the training courses their staff have undertaken in order to practise. One of the first was formulated by Bath District Health Authority (Armstrong and Waldron, 1991). The Drugs and Therapeutics Committee is often involved in setting these standards for practice, but whatever the procedures and policies laid down for use by any staff in any clinical area, the trained nurse is always accountable for his or her own practice.

RESEARCH

Research into the effects of complementary therapies in general is notoriously difficult because of the complexity of the holistic approach. A measurement of the effectiveness of complementary approaches is lacking, and claims of success rest on evidence that is largely anecdotal. Leibrich (1990), however, in her critical evaluation of research methodologies for complementary therapies, pointed out that there is nothing inherently unscientific about anecdotal evidence, when published by a world authority, which can yield valuable scientific information without the use of a randomized controlled trial – the world's first heart transplant being one example. Yet it is often argued that quantitative data are not useful. There is some agreement that the approaches used in complementary therapies do not lend themselves to the rigid criteria of scientific research. Wells and Tschudin (1994) believed that complementary therapies did not necessarily need validating by science and medicine: if a patient felt better, that was his or her justification for supportive therapies. Indeed, the Calman-Hine Report (Department of Health and Welsh Office, 1995) sees complementary therapies as an essential component of best practice in cancer care.

One spur to the process of legitimizing complementary therapies is the existence of the department of complementary medicine at the University of Exeter. In 1993, Edzart Ernst became the first professor in the UK to hold a Chair in complementary medicine. Ernst (1995) takes the view that we need more rigorous research in order to answer even the most fundamental questions about the effectiveness, safety and cost of complementary therapies, although he recognizes that there are options that can be shown to ease suffering in complementary care. He believes that the key issue is competence and points to the need for proper training and sufficient experience as where this does not exist, serious adverse effects are virtually unavoidable (Ernst, 1997).

An attempt to address this issue was made by the Bristol Cancer Help Centre, founded in 1979 by Penny Brohn, who had herself suffered from cancer. The centre is used by those who want an alternative approach as well as by those who want to use orthodox treatment at the same time. It took the courageous step of submitting its methods to scientific research, the resulting study (Bagenal et al., 1990) causing a furore when the findings indicated that a group of patients with breast cancer who attended the centre did not live as long as a control group. There now seems however, to be general agreement that the design of the study was flawed and its findings inaccurate. It would seem invidious, as Mantle (1999) suggests, to reject any of the therapies as a treatment, based on old and often poorly designed research. Practitioners should keep an open mind and assess the evidential strength of the research, as described by Muir Gray (1997).

Despite recognizing the need for documentary evidence, Brewer (1989) believes the success of complementary methods to be both tangible and immediate. Subtle changes in body language, breathing rhythm, facial lines and sleep patterns all point to success:

> With a very depressed lady who wanted to die, I noticed with wonder that, as I talked her through a guided healing visualization, the lines of sorrow and sadness quickly faded and a flow of contentment and peace spread across the lady's face and person.

Brewer (1999) further suggests that graphology can help therapists to identify a person's response to therapy.

PERCEIVED BENEFITS

The literature abounds with patients' comments on their personal experiences of complementary therapies in palliative care. The following two experiences could, in the authors' experience, sum up the feelings of many recipients:

- To be treated as a person and fears and concerns are noted.
- Treatments are all gentle.
- Bach flower remedies were demonstrated and I still use Rescue Remedy in times of strain.
- Many treatments are natural, inciting the body's own defences to re-establish homeostasis.
- Improvement in the quality of life.

Thwaite (1996)

> Marion's massages were one of the only things that I actively looked forward to. Something nice that happened in the daily round of unpleasantness. She was particularly good at massaging my head and feet, and I would always drift off into a rare and refreshing sleep when she had finished....My survival is due to the administering of high doses of cytotoxic drugs, and the skill of the surgeon's knife. However, I was able to accept what was happening to me, more ready to deal with the treatment and was in a better frame of mind to heal myself because Marion came and gave me something to look forward to and sent me off into a good sleep.

Izon (1996)

MISUNDERSTANDINGS

Kassab and Stevenson (1996) clarify common misunderstandings about complementary therapies for patients with cancer.

Massage spreads cancer
There is no evidence to suggest that massage spreads cancer around the body. Direct pressure is obviously not advised over an area where there is an active tissue

tumour, for example a lump in the breast, or over any associated lymph nodes, but gentle forms of massage to other areas in the body are unlikely to break off tumour cells. The stimulation offered to the circulation and lymphatic systems of the body via massage is thought to be no more than that obtained from daily exercise.

Reflexology stimulates the excretory channels of the body and therefore the early elimination of chemotherapeutic drugs, leading to a reduction of their effect in the body

An increase in urination and of body discharges has been observed so patients often fear that the therapeutic effects of their drugs will be reduced by this enhanced elimination. Chemotherapeutic drugs have, however, a definitive half-life, so their effect is not affected by the gentle stimulation derived from reflexology. Reflexology may even limit damage caused to the normal body cells by its strengthening effect on the body as a whole, reducing intolerance to chemotherapy and possibly limiting neutropenia.

Some therapeutic essential oils are carcinogenic

The essential oils used in clinical aromatherapy are not oils considered to be carcinogenic or toxic. Possible carcinogenic oils found in camphor oil, tarragon oil, sassafras oil and methyluegent are not usually found in the range commonly used by aromatherapists, and indeed improved training courses and well-informed texts have assisted in the improvement of safety (Vickers, 1996).

Kassab and Stevenson (1996) believe that misunderstandings are often the root of fear, and there is no exception in the case of complementary cancer therapies. For patients to be deprived of the complementary approaches because of fear or misinformation may mean that their needs are not addressed.

NURSING

Nurses who wish to practise complementary therapies as part of their professional role need to have undertaken a recognized course or period of study for the practice of the therapy; they then can be covered by the United Kingdom Central Council for Nurses, Midwives and Health Visitors (UKCC) *Code of Professional Conduct*, clause 4. Knape (1998) outlined the UKCC position on complementary therapies as being about meeting clients' needs and offering the best possible standard of care while being free of risk to clients. It is stated that the trained nurse must 'acknowledge any limitations in her knowledge and competence and decline any duties or responsibilities unless able to perform them in a safe and skilled manner' (UKCC, 1992). The problem here is that there is still little agreement on what may be considered to be a 'recognized' course. We have found that the period of study undertaken by nurses in order to prepare them to practise aromatherapy, for example, varied between one weekend and 3 years.

One way forward is for nurses to work closely with complementary therapists to plan and deliver courses in complementary therapies in nursing. The

English National Board for Nursing, Midwifery and Health Visiting (ENB) course A49 provides an holistic pathway as one route to obtaining the BSc Hons/ENB Higher Award (Manchester University and Tenda, the European Nursing Development Agency), which has the added bonus of the nurse becoming either a nurse aromatherapist or a nurse reflexologist. The Sacred Space Foundation is validated by the ENB to provide (in association with St Martin's College) post-basic courses in therapeutic touch. What is needed now is a standardization of the competencies required and a validation of all the training courses by one professional body.

The Royal College of Nursing (RCN) holds a complementary therapies in nursing forum, which has over 2000 members. Its insurance covers nurses who practise complementary therapies providing they can demonstrate that they have the knowledge and skills to do so safely. It has, among other projects, produced some helpful information on what to look for when choosing a course. It would seem good advice to seek a course that involves hands-on practice and requires case study work as part of its assessment strategy. The RCN also recommends that the patient's consent should be obtained before using any therapy.

Nurses are well aware that much can be communicated to patients while they are involved in nursing procedures of many kinds. Attempting to meet the needs of someone who is incapacitated by illness is a demanding task, one that requires a willingness to share, to some extent, in the patient's experience. The development of self-awareness and ways in which lateral or divergent thinking can be encouraged leads to an openness in taking more creative risks, secure in the knowledge that there are a variety of possible strategies to help a patient.

It can only be when patients feel secure enough in their relationship with the nurse that they will be able to ask difficult questions or share their deepest doubts and fears. Penson (2000) explored the nature of hope and how nurses might foster and support hope as a key aspect of care. What she refers to as the climate of care includes therapeutic aspects such as the layout of the room, colours, art, music, smells and touch, these being enhanced by the attitudes, actions and presence of the health professional. Campbell (1987) describes this kind of nurse–patient relationship as 'graceful care', which he sees as 'not being about anxious people trying to earn love, but about sensitive people who release us from bonds of our own making in spontaneous and often surprising ways'. It would seem that complementary therapies have the potential to facilitate hope and comfort.

Well-developed interpersonal skills are always needed when putting them into practice. Brewer and Cadman (2000) highlight the essential ingredient of emotional intelligence in influencing patient outcome and providing clinical excellence. The authors also acknowledge the transformative power of spiritual intelligence in creating a better situation.

Brewer (1989) recognizes that there is an intimate connection between the quality of care a nurse gives and his or her self-confidence. She believes that high-quality nursing and self-confidence go hand in hand, and that using complementary therapy where appropriate can aid both. Most nurses, she points out, have felt helpless and trapped over serious deficits in the comfort of patients who feel anxious, frightened, in pain or depressed. Just having the experience of a couple of eclectic approaches (extracting the relaxation response, for example) not only provides a higher chance of doing something positive for patients, but also gives nurses more confidence in themselves.

TOUCH

Nurses know that touch is an effective way of communicating warmth and acceptance to patients who are faced with cancer. Touch therapies can help to induce relaxation, aid sleep, enhance feelings of well-being and convey warmth and caring. They can also be used to complement the observations made during nursing assessments. The element of touch is important in palliative care because, in the authors' experience, many patients find that people are afraid to touch them – probably one of the greatest gifts that complementary therapies have to offer is an acceptance of the person and his or her body.

MASSAGE

Massage provides physical contact in what is, for many people, a very acceptable way. When massage techniques are used for patients with cancer, the nurse must be careful to use only gentle touch and to avoid any areas where cancer is known to be present. The hands and feet provide places where massage is likely to be safe, and stroking of the forehead and face may be especially relaxing. When doing this, only a very little oil, cream or even powder (unless the skin is dry) needs to be used.

AROMATHERAPY

The complementary therapy that has grown in use most in recent years, and has been enthusiastically adopted by nurses, is massage using oils extracted from plants, which are usually referred to as 'essential oils' and are the pure, concentrated essences of plants, flowers, trees, fruits and herbs. They are considered to act not only on the body, by stimulating physiological processes, but also on the emotions and the mind. Although aromatherapy is usually applied through massaging the oils into the skin, they can also be used in the bath or in water used for washing. They can in addition be inhaled by being disseminated into the air via a fan or a diffuser, or by being heated in a burner, usually by floating a few drops on water that is heated by a candle. Knowledge and care are needed when using oils because it is often not realized that these substances can be highly potent.

The safety of the nursing staff as well as the patient needs to be considered, a particular point being that various oils should not be used during pregnancy. If oils are disseminated into the air in a hospital ward or department, thought needs to be given to the safety of everyone who may inhale them. Some attention also has to be given to whether the smell is attractive to those other people who may come into contact with it.

Patients with cancer may have their sense of smell altered by the disease or its treatment, for example chemotherapy. They should therefore, always be asked first to smell the oil to be used in order to decide whether or not the therapist's choice is attractive to them. Essential oils are always diluted by mixing them in a carrier oil, and they can be diluted still further (*for example, two drops of essential oil in 10 ml of a carrier oil such as almond oil*) if the person is particularly sensitive to them.

Passant (1990) demonstrated that the need for conventional sedatives for elderly people in hospital was reduced when the patients received aromatherapy. She found that using oils in baths and putting a drop on the patient's pillow often induced a peaceful night's sleep.

REFLEXOLOGY

Reflexology, also known as reflex zone therapy, is a form of massage that concentrates on the feet. Each part, or zone, of the foot represents a part of the rest of the body. Therefore, when massaging the feet, differences in tone, colour, temperature and sensitivity to touch may be found, which reflect imbalances in other parts of the body. This can be used to diagnose problems and to help to eliminate them (Case study 10.1). Reflexology scores have been demonstrated to show a substantial improvement in depressive symptoms helped by the touch involved, which is an important component of palliative care (Peters et al., 1996).

CASE STUDY 10.1

A student nurse in the community encountered a man with bone cancer in severe pain, who was angry at everybody and everything, most of all at the thought of dying. The student asked whether she could try modified reflexology and relaxing music (modified meaning extrapolating the relaxation response of reflexology and thus ensuring safety). The man agreed, and the nurse's intervention helped. Not only was his pain alleviated, but his wife was also shown the technique, using it in his final days, which helped them to grow closer together.

RELAXATION

Relaxation is a bridge between orthodox and complementary therapies with a wide use in many health-care settings. Relaxation is about releasing tension from the physical body and is a desirable precursor to meditation and visualization because these work better if the body is less tense.

We are all familiar with the concept of relaxation. The word is often used loosely, to suggest times when one is socializing or not at work, but true relaxation of the body and the mind is much more than this. Watching television or dozing in a chair is not sufficient to reduce tension that has accumulated and will continue unconsciously.

Techniques for relaxation can be quickly learnt via groups or classes or by listening to tapes or reading guides. There are many different methods of relaxation. Some people find that the progressive type, with its focus on clenching and then letting go of each muscle group, and on the control of the breath, suits them best. This is the one with which many women are familiar because it is taught in antenatal classes (Benson, 1988).

This is an area in which it is particularly important to practise what is being preached, and nurses can benefit from learning the skill of relaxation and how to incorporate this into their lifestyle.

GUIDED IMAGERY

Guided imagery makes use of the imagination in order to focus the mind and induce relaxation through pleasant thoughts, a form of planned daydreaming perhaps. Words create a picture for the mind of some pleasant scene, those involved visualizing themselves travelling to a place that is special to them and that they can revisit at any time in the future. All the senses are called on to make the mind-picture come alive, with descriptions of perhaps the feel of the sun on one's face, the sound of the breeze in the trees, the taste of the salty air. If a tape is used, it may contain music or the sounds of, for example, the sea or birdsong.

Van Fleet (2000) concluded that the use of relaxation training and imagery offers potential benefits to patients to reduce side-effects and enhance well-being and a sense of control. Nurses can learn to employ basic strategies to help patients manage their symptoms and enhance their quality of life. The most effective strategies engage patients according to their beliefs, values, preferences and needs. Careful assessment must precede intervention.

VISUALIZATION

Visualization techniques applied to the fight against cancer are associated with the work of Carl and Stephanie Simonton in the 1970s. The underlying hypothesis is that physical processes in the body are affected by what the imagination creates and that, with training, an individual can learn to develop his or her powers of imagination and use them to combat the cancer. People with cancer who are interested in this approach are helped to visualize their cancer and their immune system as if in a battle; the actual images used should be chosen by them. Brohn (1987) makes the important point that the cancer must be represented by something that is weaker than the image chosen for the immune system. The main picture is to be that of a strong, powerful force that is battling against a weak and feeble opponent. An important end to the visualization is one of seeing oneself healthy and active in the future. It is usually suggested that the image should be used for a short period once or twice a day, and is combined with relaxation techniques.

Visualization can give back feelings of control to the person with cancer; it is a positive approach that can counteract the negativity surrounding the disease itself. It seems feasible that nurses could learn to assist people who would like to try this approach, although they need to be aware that, for some people, the regular focusing of the mind on having cancer could be detrimental.

MEDITATION

Although meditation may be thought of as a form of religious exercise, it can also be viewed as another form of relaxation or visualization technique, depending on the beliefs of the individual using it. Its aim is to quieten the mind and body. This can be achieved by learning to concentrate, perhaps upon an object such as a candle or on a word that is special to the individual, their own mantra. Thinking about their breathing may be another way into this peaceful state. Then they learn to let go of the busyness of the day and the incessant chatter of their mind, letting thoughts come and go until they reach a state of inner quiet, a silent space. Like other skills, this takes time to learn. Books, tapes and classes are available to help, and scripts to guide meditation can be found in the books by Bond (1986), Brewer (1998), Rushworth (1994) and Zahourek (1985).

THERAPEUTIC TOUCH

'Therapeutic touch' is a term that may be confused with 'massage techniques'; here, it refers to a specific form of touch first used by Krieger (1986). She is a professor of nursing in the USA who was much influenced by the work of, among others, Rogers (1980), her model of nursing containing the concept of 'unitary man', whom she saw as being an open energy system in continual interaction with the energy fields of others. In other words, we do not end at our skin but at the boundary of the energy field that surrounds us and is constantly changing. We may imagine that, when we feel good, our energy field is expanded and we feel open to others, whereas when we feel ill, our energy field contracts and we feel closed in.

In order to carry out this technique, the nurse places her hands a few centimetres away from the body and runs them over the patient so that she has 'felt' all the surfaces. With practice, she can learn to detect subtle differences in the sensations she receives and to interpret them. She can learn to smooth them out, thereby helping to enhance feelings of relaxation. A study by Giasson and Bouchard (1998) supported the hypothesis that three non-contact therapeutic touch treatments increase the sensation of well-being in those with terminal cancer. Therapeutic touch is the most researched therapy used by nurses.

HEALING

Healers believe that they can become channels through which the healing force, which can perhaps be described as energy, power, heat or light, can be transferred to the patient. This can be done via the laying on of hands or by simply being with the person or even attending to them from a distance.

Healers believe that the source of the healing lies outside themselves but may describe this in different ways, some seeing it as coming from God, others from some other form of Universal Consciousness. Most healers do not make claims to cure people but see their work as helping people towards equilibrium and wholeness. In this process, a healing of mind and spirit can take place, and this may sometimes be accompanied by physical improvement (Case study 10.2).

CASE STUDY 10.2

Sally, a patient in her late 20s, spoke of her experience of healing as a complement to orthodox chemotherapy treatment. She had no idea what to expect from healing but soon realized that asking for help was the first step on the road to recovery. She was feeling angry with her body for letting her down, and very confused about her inner feelings. *When the healing started, she began to calm down and realized that this was her time to receive...she began to connect with her inner feelings, acknowledging her emotions. She became aware of hotspots in certain areas of the body, where she imagined the healing energy being intensified and received. Coloured images, usually of strong sunlight with rays pouring in through an open door, were seen. After approximately four sessions, Sally began to feel huge surges of energy, a high, following the healing.* Her healer made sure she was grounded before she left, and Sally learnt to direct and use the energy herself when needed. Happily, some months later, she was told that she was cured (Penson, 1998).

Healing can be very therapeutic for people even when they are dying. It is important to protect patients from unrealistic expectations and to emphasize that healing concerns wholeness, balance and a sense of well-being.

It may not always be appreciated that most healers undergo training courses and register with a professional body, such as the National Federation of Spiritual Healers, thus protecting the public. Their code of conduct was drawn up in consultation with the British Medical Association, the General Medical Council and the RCN.

MUSIC

An analysis of the music therapy literature by O'Callaghan (1996) yields numerous reports to support the role of music in the alleviation of pain in palliative care.

Brewer (1998) explores the benefits of music therapy as she relates her therapeutic interaction with Pat, a 50-year-old woman recently diagnosed with carcinoma of the bronchus with bone secondaries. Fear and pain were portrayed in her face. The following steps were used in preparation for her musical experience:

- gentle relaxation in the form of modified reflexology (extracting the relaxation response);
- active listening, via personal stereo headphones, to the sounds of nature, water and the continual Ohm vibration;
- therapeutic suggestion, implemented by saying to Pat, 'allow the soothing music to wash over and through the body and a more relaxed and comfortable feeling will occur'.

The music chosen flowed evenly and was soothing, gently lulling Pat into sleep. Her face softened as her body visibly relaxed: 'Music can do in minutes what weeks of meditation in practice strives towards' (Rose, 1988). Pat later commented on the value of the chosen music in alleviating her discomfort and providing a calm space. A simple music listening session combined with therapeutic touch and suggestion thus seemed to make a difference to her treatment.

There are many reasons why music often seems effective in alleviating emotional conflict; it brings order to our experience and is rhythmic, melodic and harmonic. It is suggested that music may be introduced as a supportive therapy combined with other therapeutic strategies. Music and colour may gently soothe depressed individuals and awaken feelings of restoration. It has been successfully combined with relaxation for individuals with insomnia. 'Tranquil rest' by Jane Brewer uses soothing music that gently calms the mind and body into tranquillity. This was confirmed by observations of patients who had softened facial lines of tension, relaxed bodies and enhanced sleep. Anecdotal evidence demonstrated that 'Music for healing', by Stephen Rhodes, was effective for soothing children and anxious individuals. Again, careful preparation leads to success.

HYPNOTHERAPY

Hypnosis is a natural state of an altered awareness and can occur naturally and spontaneously when our mind wanders, our attention focuses inwards and we become, while still alert and awake, not 'there' but rather where our daydream has taken us. In a therapeutic trance state, this is an opportune time to give individuals helpful and positive suggestions.

Zahourek (1985) offers stunning insights into clinical hypnosis and therapeutic suggestion in nursing, with clear guidelines on making a difference to dying patients and those who fear death. Clinical hypnosis and therapeutic suggestion in nursing help nurses to conceptualize what they have intuitively been doing for years. In the Rossendale Hospice study, hypnotherapy was found to be the most effective in reducing anxiety (Taylor et al., 2000).

NURSING PRACTICE

Rushworth (1994) draws on a wide range of disciplines using hypnotherapy, neurolinguistic programming, meditation and relaxation to help patients to live with the implications of their condition. She gives an example of a 'change the picture and change the pain' technique with a patient suffering from pain from bony metastases despite receiving diamorphine via a syringe driver. The importance of focusing on the positive and achieving an altered state of awareness is highlighted:

> 'I have been asked to come and see you to find a way to make you more comfortable.' (The pre-supposition is that there is a way; this is where the congruence begins, and the brain starts to recognise a possible exit from the situation.) 'What colour is your pain?' The patient, looking perplexed, said, 'Red, it's definitely red!'
>
> Then she was asked what size and texture it was; she replied that it was about the size of two hands and was spiky. Rushworth's next question was, 'And what colour will it be when it has gone?' (Pre-suppositioning the positive suggestion that it would go.) 'What colour is totally comfortable?' The patient decided on pale blue; the size and texture was to be of a cotton wool ball. Then, resting my hand very lightly on her hip to focus her attention on the area, she was invited to change it from red to blue! She couldn't imagine it, so it was suggested to begin by changing it to purple because that was half way. 'Tell me when you've done it' (another pre-supposition). After half a minute she said, 'I've done that!'
>
> Now you've got the hang of it! Now change it all the way to pale blue and tell me when you've done it! 30 seconds later she opened her eyes and exclaimed, 'It's gone!' She was told she now knew what to do. She had a good night's sleep and continued to improve physically and emotionally, mobilising cheerfully.
>
> Rushworth (1994)

The technique described has a definite hypnotic element in that the patient is being asked to enter an altered state of awareness by 'going inside' and making a picture of the pain. Once patients have given you their representation of 'pain' and 'comfort', it follows that if they can change the picture, they will be able to change the pain, gaining some measure of control over it. The 'colour, texture and size' method described can be used to change sensations other than pain, such as feelings of tightness, tingling or a churning stomach.

A patient suffering from severe nausea was asked to imagine that his stomach was the surface of a lake during a storm. The desired image was to be that of the storm having passed and the lake surface being as smooth and calm as a millpond. If a little discomfort remains, the nurse can say, 'Now shrink it as small as you can...then put it outside on the window sill.' It is important to act as if you expect it to work, eliminating tentative words such as 'try', 'hope' or 'might' from your vocabulary.

The most commonly used hypnotic methods for symptom management in palliative care are relaxation, suggestion and ego-strengthening. When relaxed, a general ego-strengthening suggestion is:

As each day and every day passes, you will find yourself getting less and less depressed, discouraged or nervous. As each and every day passes, you will find yourself getting more and more cheerful and happy, more calm and relaxed. You will be more confident and accepting of yourself than previously.

An example of a specific ego-strengthening coping strategy is:

'You will find these [coping strategies] to be more and more effective'...'It will automatically occur to you to think of [specific coping strategy] whenever you notice [specific problem] beginning to happen.'

Liossi and Mystakidon (1996) argue that quality of life and comfort before death can be considerably improved by hypnosis and that it should be seen as an integral part of care. The view of hypnosis as a means for individuals to transform themselves from within both physically and mentally, through their own potential, is consistent with the accepted philosophy and practice of palliative care.

Kraft (1990) found a combination of psychotherapy and hypnotherapy to be beneficial in the alleviation of anxiety in patients suffering from widespread cancer and in the treatment of problems such as chemotherapy phobia, intractable pain, dyspnoea, insomnia and itching. Hypnosis provides the patient with a tool by which he or she can exert a measure of control over the effects of cancer. This feeling of personal control reduces the sense of helplessness that many patients experience, heightening a person's ability to concentrate and live for the moment.

'CALMNESS, RELAXATION AND CONFIDENCE' TECHNIQUE

The calmness, relaxation and confidence technique has been successfully used by the author as an ego-strengthening technique (Brewer, 1998, 1999). It uses a positive approach, meditation, visualization and hypnotherapy combined with deep relaxation. Deep relaxation is first induced, positive suggestions then being introduced, for example:

As each and every day goes by, and you become more calm and more relaxed, so you become more competent and more confident about your ability to become peaceful, happy and successful in whatever you choose.

In this technique, the participant uses the imagination to release tension by visualizing it drifting and floating away, for example:

> In a few minutes' time, I will be saying the word 'now', and I will be remaining quiet; I would like you if possible to think about any tension that you have left and if possible to put a shape and colour to it; just let it float away like a cloud.

To reinforce the feeling of relaxation and introduce a deeper state of altered awareness, the participant is asked to focus on the word 'Calm' and keep repeating it without giving it a meaning, like the sound of a distant bell. This is to negate intellectualizing over the meaning of the word and to allow a meditative state to occur in which there is an increase in the number of alpha brain waves, denoting a state of relaxed alertness, this ideally leading to theta brain waves, as advocated by Silva and Miele (1978) This corresponds to Benson's (1988) method of relaxation, in which, in stage 1, one word is used as a focus. The number of sessions can vary but the essence of this technique is the inculcation of a habit.

CONCLUSION

The benefits of incorporating complementary therapies into palliative care have highlighted an improvement in quality of life and empowerment. All the techniques involved require knowledge and understanding on the part of the nurse so they are completely safe for the patient and others who may be involved. There are, however, as we have seen, important issues that have to be addressed. These include appropriate and validated training programmes, the setting of standards for safe practice and the need for qualitative research studies to provide a sound knowledge base for nursing practice.

Nurses have a professional responsibility to respond to the wishes of the patient and act as his or her advocate. By supporting the use of complementary therapies as part of conventional nursing care, people with cancer can be offered the best of both worlds by receiving care that is truly holistic.

The poem 'In the mind' (King, 1990) exemplifies what the authors believe is the aim of complementary therapies in palliative care.

IN THE MIND

Come, massage my mind,
I'll lay quite still for you now,
And gently caress, with your fingers so fine,
The hardness to melt, as if I'd had wine,
Then let me just rest, in simple recline,
Your fingers just dip in the essence of peace,
And gently, just gently, whisper so sweet
Now stay near me close, your presence is balm,
Just unwind me a little until I am calm.
Oh why do I let all the pressures of life,
Come rob me of daisies and dandelions bright?

Yes, now I am drifting on clouds soft and white.
Above all my troubles of feeling so tight.
Suggest with your skill, caress with your tongue,
Just like a mother cat would purr to her young.
Now paint me a picture to hang in my mind,
More precious than all that money could find.
Use the fragrance of colour, and use with great care,
For the picture you paint, will be forever there
In the hall of my mind,
And I'll treasure it always, for the peace that I find.

REFERENCES

Armstrong, F. and Waldron, R. 1991: A complementary strategy. *Nursing Times* 87, 34–5.

Bagenal, F., Easton, D.M. and Harris, E. 1990: Survival of patients with breast cancer attending the Bristol Cancer Help Centre. *Lancet* 336, 606–10.

Barnett, K. 1972: A survey of the current utilisation of touch by health team personnel with hospitalised patients. *International Journal of Nursing Studies* 3, 195–209.

Bell, L. and Sikora, K. 1996: Complementary therapies and cancer care. *Complementary Therapies in Nursing and Midwifery* 2, 57–8.

Benson, H. 1988: *Your maximum mind*. Wellingborough: Aquarius.

Bond, M. 1986: *Stress and self awareness: a guide for nurses*. London: Heinemann.

Brewer, J. 1989: Alternative approach – profile. *Nursing Standard* 3(50), 46.

Brewer, J. 1998: Healing sounds. *Complementary Therapies in Nursing and Midwifery* 4, 7–12.

Brewer, J. 1999: Graphology. *Complementary Therapies in Nursing and Midwifery* 5, 6–14.

Brewer, J. 1998 and Cadman, C. 2000: Emotional intelligence enhancing student effectiveness and patient outcomes. *Nurse Educator* 25(6), 264–6.

British Medical Association 1993: *Complementary medicine: new approaches to good practice*. Oxford: Oxford University Press.

Brohn, P. 1987: *The Bristol programme*. London: Century-Hutchinson.

Burke, C. and Sikora, K. 1993: Complementary and conventional cancer care: the integration of two cultures. *Clinical Oncology* 5, 220–70.

Campbell, A. 1987: *Moderated love: a theology of professional care*. London: SPCK.

Clover, A. and Kassab, S. 1998: Complementary medicine for patients with cancer. *European Journal of Palliative Care* 5(3).

Department of Health and Welsh Office 1995 *A policy framework for commissioning cancer services: a report by the expert advisory group on cancer*. The Calman–Hine Report. London: DoH.

Ernst, E. 1995: Complementary cancer treatment: hope or hazard. *Clinical Oncology* 7(4), 259–63.

Ernst, E. 1997: Evidence-based complementary therapies. *Complementary Therapies in Nursing and Midwifery* 3, 42–5.

Fleet, S. van 2000: Relaxation and imagery for symptom management: improving patients' assessments and individualising treatment. *ONF* 27(3), 501–9.

Giasson, M. and Bouchard, L. 1998: Effects of therapeutic touch on the wellbeing of persons with terminal cancer. *Journal of Holistic Nursing* 16(3), 383–98.

Hartland, J. 1984: *Medical and dental hypnosis and its clinical applications*. London: Baillière Tindall.

Hill, R. 1997: Report on Complementary Therapies at North Devon Hospice. Unpublished study, University of Exeter.

Hodgkinson, L. 1994: Therapy with complements. *Independent*, May 19.

Izon, D. 1996: A patient's perspective. *Complementary Therapies in Nursing and Midwifery* **2**, 66–77.

Kassab, S. and Stevenson, C. 1996: Education – common misunderstandings about complementary therapies for patients with cancer. *Complementary Therapies in Nursing and Midwifery* **2**, 62–5.

King, F. In the mind. *Health Herald*, No. 9, 14.

Knape, J. 1998: Complementary therapy and the registered nurse, midwife and health visitor. *Complementary Therapies in Nursing and Midwifery* **4**(5).

Kohn, M. 1999: *Complementary Therapies in Cancer Care*. London: Macmillan Cancer Relief.

Kraft, T. 1990: Use of hypnotherapy in anxiety management in the terminally ill: a preliminary study. *British Journal of Experimental and Clinical Hypnosis* **7**(1), 27–33.

Krieger, D. 1986: *The therapeutic touch: how to use your hands to help or heal*. New York: Prentice-Hall.

Liossi, C. and Mystakidon, K. 1996: Clinical hypnosis in palliative care. *European Journal of Palliative Care* **3**(2).

Mantle, F. 1999: Complementary therapies: is there an evidence base? Nursing Times Clinical Monographs No. 1.

Muir Gray, J. 1997: *Evidence-based healthcare. How to make policy and management decisions*. Edinburgh: Churchill Livingstone.

O'Callaghan, C.C. 1996: Complementary therapies in terminal care: pain, music creativity and music therapy in palliative care. *American Journal of Hospice and Palliative Care* **13**(2), 43–9.

Passant, H. 1990: The holistic approach in the ward. *Nursing Times* **86**, 24–6.

Penson, J. 1998: Complementary therapies: making a difference in palliative care. *Complementary Therapies in Nursing and Midwifery* **4**, 71–81.

Penson, J. 2000: A hope is not a promise – fostering hope within palliative care. *International Journal of Palliative Nursing* **6**(2), 94–8.

Rogers, M. 1970: *An introduction to the theoretical basis of nursing*. Philadelphia: F.A. Davies.

Rose, C. 1988: *Accelerated learning*. Great Missenden: Accelerated Learning Systems.

Rushworth, C. 1994: *Practical techniques in palliative care and curative treatment. Making a difference in cancer care*. London: Human Horizon Series/Souvenir Press.

Sayre-Adams, J. and Wright, S. 1995: *The theory and practice of therapeutic touch*. Edinburgh: Churchill Livingstone.

Sayre-Adams, J. and Wright, S. 1995: Change in consciousness. *Nursing Times* **91**(41).

Shamash, J. 1997: Complementing the NHS. *Nursing Standard* **12**(6).

Silva, J. and Miele, P. 1978: *How to balance your mind with the Silva mind control method*. London: Grafton.

Spiegel, M.D. and Moore, R. 1997: Imagery and hypnosis in the treatment of cancer patients. *Oncology* **11**(8).

Taylor, E.E., Hills, H.M., Hoyle-Wood, J., Rimmer, P.A., Pepper, H.D. and Sweeney, A.V. 2000: Holistic resources: complementary therapies in palliative care – evaluation of service provision. *Holistic Health* **64**, 14–18.

Thwaite, J. 1996: Complementary therapies 1996. A patient's choice. *Complementary Therapies in Nursing and Midwifery* **2**, 65–70.

United Kingdom Central Council for Nursing, Midwifery and Health Visiting 1992: *Code of professional conduct*. London: UKCC.

Vickers, A. 1996: *Massage and aromatherapy. A guide for health professionals*. London: Chapman & Hall.

Wells, R. and Tschudin, V. (eds) 1994: *Wells' supportive therapies in healthcare*. London: Baillière Tindall.

Zahourek, P.R. 1985: *Clinical hypnosis and therapeutic suggestion in nursing*. London: Grune & Stratton.

FURTHER READING

Balkam, J. 1994: *Aromatherapy. A practical guide to essential oils and aromassage*. Blitz Editions.

Brown-Saltzman, K. 1997: Replenishing the spirit by meditative prayer and guided imagery. *Seminars in Oncology Nursing* **13**(4), 255–9.

Davis, P. 1991: *Subtle aromatherapy*. Saffron Walden: C.W. Daniel.

Featherstone, C. and Forsyth, L. 1997: *Medical marriage: the new partnership between orthodox and complementary medicine*. Findhorn: Findhorn Press.

Gimbel-Theo, X. 1997: *Healing with colour*. London: Gain Books.

Pietroni, P. 1993: Complementary medicine – its place in the care of dying people. In: Dickensen, D. and Johnson, M. (eds) *Death, dying and bereavement*. Buckingham: Open University.

Siegel, B. 1989: *Love, medicine and miracles*. New York: Harper & Row.

Simonton, C. Matthews-Simonton, S. and Creighton, L. 1978: *Getting well again: a step by step self-help guide for patients and their families*. London: Bantam Books.

Snyder, R.J. 1997: Therapeutic touch and the terminally ill. Healing power through the hands – Knieger/Kunz method. *American Journal of Hospice and Palliative Care* (Mar/Apr).

Wilkinson, S.D.C. 1999: Quality Study. *Cancer Research for BBC News/Health/ Complementary Cancer Care Books*.

Wright, S.G. and Sayre-Adams, J. 2000: *Sacred space: right relationship and spirituality in healthcare*. London: Churchill Livingstone.

Zohar, D. and Marshall, I. 2000: *Spiritual intelligence. The ultimate intelligence*. London: Bloomsbury Publishing.

USEFUL ADDRESSES

Bristol Cancer Help Centre (BCHC)
Cornwallis Grove
Clifton
Bristol BS8 4PG

Cancer Alternative Information Bureau (CAIB)
PO Box 285
405 Kings Road
London SW10 OBB

Department of Complementary Medicine, University of Exeter
25 Victoria Park Road
Exeter
Devon EX4 4NT

Sacred Space Foundation
Ravenscroft
Renwick
Cumbria CA10 1JL

chapter 11

NUTRITIONAL CARE

Charlette Gallagher-Allred

Let food be thy medicine.
Corpus Hippocraticum

THE MEANING AND VALUE OF FOOD AND NUTRITION

Food and drink are among life's greatest pleasures, and our perception of food and drink varies throughout life. When we are healthy and our appetite is good, food and drink are enjoyed and often taken for granted. When we are ill and our appetite may be poor, food and drink can be a source of conflict and take on a greater importance. Food carries biological, emotional and sociological meanings as well as religious, cultural and ethnic values. In my many years of work with cancer patients who receive palliative care, I have learned that when I am able to share the meaning that food and drink have in my life, I am more able to appreciate the meaning that they have in the lives of others.

It is important for health-care providers to understand the psychological aspects of cancer. A diagnosis of cancer elicits powerful emotions, including fear and grief. It can have a shattering effect on patients' self-image, particularly with those who have undergone any type of disfiguring surgery. A common feeling among cancer patients is a loss of control of life's events and an anxiety over the perceived incompleteness of their lives. Many patients experience guilt associated with their past or present lifestyle, and many focus on failed or strained relationships and a failure to accomplish their goals. There are also dreadful fears surrounding cancer, such as fear of abandonment, fear of pain, fear of the dying process, fear of physical and mental disability, and fear of dependency upon others.

The emotions that burden cancer patients often manifest themselves as eating disorders. Sometimes there is overeating, but more often these emotions dampen the appetite. Furthermore, many tumours produce chemical substances that promote anorexia. The dying process itself can diminish a patient's appetite as well as alter nutritional needs in the following ways:

- The anatomical, physiological and metabolic changes that occur because of various diseases can decrease gastrointestinal absorption and increase nutrient requirements, as frequently occurs in patients with acquired immune deficiency syndrome (AIDS), who often develop severe diarrhoea and malabsorption.
- The dying process itself slows many body functions, including gastric emptying, which results in increased satiety, decreased hunger and frequent food intolerances.
- Medical interventions such as chemotherapy alter metabolic processes and frequently result in an increased nutrient requirement. Even palliative medications, such as narcotics, alter nutrient needs when side-effects such as nausea, vomiting and constipation occur.

GOALS OF NUTRITIONAL CARE

Although patients with cancer often feel a loss of control, nutrition is one aspect of their care over which they feel they have some influence. Giving patients the feeling that they can help with their own well-being through what they eat and drink is important, and a proactive approach to nutrition care early in the diagnosis of cancer is usually desired by patients.

Although anorexia and weight loss are commonly associated with cancer, improved appetite and weight gain have been observed in patients with prostate and breast cancer. Patients with cancer may also be overweight prior to the diagnosis of cancer. In addition, many patients gain weight as a result of lymph-oedema or steroids, these being taken either as part of the chemotherapy programme or as appetite stimulants.

The responsibility of health-care providers to patients early in the diagnosis of cancer is to encourage a varied food intake, weight maintenance for the overweight patient, and weight maintenance or increased weight if possible for those who are underweight. Encouraging a good intake of fruits, vegetables and wholegrain breads and cereals, along with dairy products, meat, fish, poultry and fats as needed to meet calorie requirements, is appropriate so that patients can regain control.

The families of cancer patients frequently feel impotent so they can be brought into the care of their loved one by being included in nutrition counselling sessions. Family members can reinforce nutritional principles and encourage eating, but they should be cautioned not to be too overbearing as there is a fine line between nagging, which is counterproductive, and encouragement.

The goals of nutritional care for patients with cancer whose choice is for palliative care are as individual as the patients themselves. Goals may also vary as the patient's illness progresses. The nutritional goals for patients whose life expectancy is several months or longer may, for example, be to provide tube feeding to prolong both the length and the quality of life. Nutritional support via percutaneous endoscopic gastrostomy tube feeding can achieve this goal for a patient with amyotrophic lateral sclerosis who has dysphagia and is at risk of suboptimal caloric and fluid intake, worsening of muscle atrophy, weakness and fatigue. Similarly, tube feeding is appropriate for patients undergoing aggressive cancer therapy or for a patient following a stroke when rehabilitation is the primary goal.

On the other hand, the nutritional goal for a palliative care patient with cancer whose life expectancy is short may be to use food and drink as desired by the patient to maximize enjoyment and minimize pain. When eating and mealtimes can accomplish either of these goals, they should be used to advantage. If eating is not an enjoyable experience, however, its practice should not be overemphasized. It is at this time that health-care providers can be strong patient advocates and family allies by reassuring both that loving care can be demonstrated in ways other than feeding.

THE HEALTH-CARE PROVIDER'S ROLE IN ACHIEVING NUTRITIONAL GOALS

> The role of the nurse…is first, to come to terms with personal, psychological, and moral and ethical issues surrounding nutrition and hydration on an individual level; and second, to enter into a partnership with the patient and family and guide them through the storm of emotions and questions using a framework based on principles of ethics, crisis intervention, and effective communication.
>
> Mauer Baak (1993)

Mauer Baak's admonition to nurses applies to all members of the palliative care team. Following such self-understanding, the nurse, dietitian and others will perform several functions in order to achieve the goals in the provision of nutritional care, including the following:

- assessing the patient's physical and psychological condition for the role that curative and palliative treatments, food and mealtimes have in causing symptoms; ascertaining whether dietary modifications can alleviate these symptoms and improve well-being;
- identifying the patient's and family's nutritional concerns and dietary questions;
- establishing goals of treatment and integrating dietary interventions as appropriate into the overall plan of care;
- counselling the patient and family on specific and practical dietary modifications that can enhance well-being;
- periodically re-evaluating nutritional goals and intervention, and implementing changes when appropriate.

ASSESSING THE PATIENT'S CONDITION

Assessment is the first component of the provision of nutritional care, a plan of care being only as good as the completeness and accuracy of the data collected and the assessment of the patient's condition and family's situation.

Box 11.1 outlines an assessment instrument including important nutrition-related questions that the nurse might ask the patient and family during initial and ongoing visits. Answers to these questions will give clues to the nutritional status and eating behaviour of the patient. In addition, they might alert the nurse to the need for the services of a dietitian or nutritionist. The involvement of a dietitian or nutritionist is generally necessary when conditions or issues such as those shown in Table 11.1 are present.

BOX 11.1 NUTRITION ASSESSMENT INSTRUMENT

1 Does the patient experience any of the following problems?
   - nausea and/or vomiting
     If so, is this associated with:
       - the taste of specific foods
       - the sight or smell of particular foods
       - the temperature of foods?
   - diarrhoea
   - constipation or gastrointestinal obstruction
   - mouth sores
   - difficulty swallowing
   - dry mouth
   - poor appetite
     If so, is this caused by:
       - pain or other symptoms
       - depression or anxiety
       - early satiety, fatigue or weakness?
   - pressure sores

2 Does the patient take any vitamin, mineral or other food supplements?

3 Does the patient have a gastrointestinal or intravenous feeding tube in place?

4 Are the patient or family expressing significant remorse about weight change?
   - If the patient has lost a lot of weight, does the weight change make the patient more dependent on others?
   - Does the patient or family want to try to reverse the weight loss with enteral or parenteral nutritional support?
   - If the patient has gained weight, is the weight change acceptable to the patient?

5 Do the family exhibit any of the following?
   - an inappropriate use of food as a crutch for emotional problems
   - a belief that disease is caused by what the patient did or did not eat
   - fear that if the patient does not eat, he or she will feel hunger pains
   - fear that if the patient becomes dehydrated, he or she will soon die
   - a belief in unorthodox nutritional therapies such as vitamin C, laetrile, macrobiotic diets or enzyme supplements

---

Table 11.1 Suggested reasons for referral to a dietitian or nutritionist

Examples

Physiological intake issues
- Presence of tube feeding or total parenteral nutrition
- Patient has concerns about weight loss
- Patient has concerns about weight gain
- Difficulty with oral intake because of mouth sores, dysphagia or poor dentition
- Concerns with the continued loss of appetite
- Inadequate fluid intake
- Patient or family would like additional nutritional suggestions

Clinical issues
- Presence of wounds
- Uncontrolled diabetes
- End-stage renal disease
- End-stage liver disease (with or without encephalopathy)
- Symptoms not controlled by medication, such as nausea, vomiting, diarrhoea, constipation, dyspepsia or fluid accumulation
- Intestinal obstruction when oral intake is not contraindicated
- Chronic bleeding with weakness
- Patient taking alternative nutritional therapies such as herbs or supplements

Psychological/social issues
- Conflicts regarding the use of food and drink
- Patient or care-giver difficulty in giving up past dietary restrictions
- Issues concerning initiating, withholding or withdrawing nutritional support
- Patient or care-giver needing clarification on dehydration issues
- Financial difficulties affecting intake
- Living conditions affecting intake

IDENTIFYING PATIENT AND FAMILY CONCERNS

Box 11.1 above also includes questions on specific nutritional issues and dietary concerns that patients and families may wish to pose. The health-care team need to be attentive to off-hand concerns that expose hidden fears, such as:

- 'If I don't drink anything, will dehydration be painful?'
- 'If I give up alcohol, will my liver tumour shrink?'
- 'I'd like to eat, but I'm afraid I'll choke and be unable to breathe if I eat too much.'
- 'If I had eaten "right", would I have avoided cancer?'

INTEGRATING NUTRITION INTO THE PLAN OF CARE

After the information from the nutritional assessment tool has been collected and assessed, and the patient and family concerns identified, a nutrition problem list can be drawn up. Nutritional goals that are consistent with other medical and nursing goals should then be established. Following the delineation of appropriate palliative nutritional therapies, the problems, goals and therapies are written into the plan of care.

The patient and family's ethnic, cultural and religious background must be taken into consideration when identifying goals and suggesting appropriate treatment. Despite the well-known adage that it is hazardous to apply stereotypes to individual patients, peoples of various backgrounds do have different views and do respond differently to food, symptoms, pain, health-care delivery systems and dying. The views and responses of others are often greatly different from our own. To be helpful to patients and their families, health-care providers must not only recognize that individual differences exist, but also be supportive of these differences.

COUNSELLING ON APPROPRIATE DIETARY MODIFICATIONS

The patient is generally highly motivated at the beginning of therapeutic cancer intervention. Therefore, after minimizing the patient's and family's guilt related to the cancer, health-care professionals should focus their attention on the current diet – whether the patient is eating properly and what changes may be appropriately made. The value of proper nutrition in promoting overall good health and physical well-being should be emphasized but not overpromised: teach the patient that diet cannot cure cancer and that, regardless of diet, cancer can recur. Nutrition quackery is tempting to patients at this point, the health-care professional's responsibility here being to provide facts without being judgemental and to advise the patient if the contemplated therapy is potentially injurious to health. As with any counselling, however, the patient makes the final decision, and his or her decision should be respected even if health-care professionals disagree with it.

During the time of cancer therapy, the patient and family need to focus their dietary concerns on meeting the patient's immediate needs for calories, protein, vitamins, minerals and fluid. Patients sometimes have trouble understanding why the concentrated-calorie diet that may be high in fat, protein and carbohydrate is different from a prevention diet that they may consider to be low in fat and high in fruits, vegetables and whole grains.

During active cancer therapy, nutrition is often one of the only areas over which the patient feels control, the patient's ability to manipulate their intake to consume sufficient calories bringing a great sense of accomplishment. Courage and determination to survive are often reflected in a patient's efforts to eat well despite his or her symptoms. If patients know that they are not eating well and are losing weight, they may wish to discuss aggressive nutrition interventions with health-care professionals. Health-care team members need to demonstrate an awareness that patients may be afraid to verbalize their wish to discuss tube feeding or parenteral feeding by offering in advance a discussion of these issues should they become important to the patient and family at any time.

When the cancer therapy has been completed, the emotions of the patient and family may range from severe depression to unbridled (but cautious) joy, depending on the outcome of the treatment. Relief will be to some extent felt by all. When the therapy is complete, nutrition to promote the return of physical strength is important. Weight goals need to be set, possibly with a margin of safety for future therapy. The merits of diet in secondary prevention need to be considered if the patient and family desire, but these need to be tempered to avoid reimposing guilt or promising a cure or a prevention of recurrence.

Patients and their families often go through a period of fear of abandonment at this time, but a cessation of treatment should not mean a cessation of care. Most patients and families appreciate being told their options in straightforward but empathetic terms.

Counselling the dying patient should address issues such as:

- how the disease process and the process of dying affect the patient's desire for food;
- how changes in a patient's appetite and ability to eat cause changes in food intake, bodily appearance and bodily function;
- specific dietary measures for symptom control;
- relief measures that will be available as the patient's condition deteriorates;
- the availability of community nutrition and food resources;
- how to reach the nurse and dietitian when questions arise and assistance is needed.

RE-EVALUATING GOALS AND INTERVENTION

Self-evaluation, an evaluation of the established plan of care, and an evaluation of the patient's and family's ability to achieve the desired goals are standard procedure during and after visits by members of the health-care team: it is only with such evaluation that progress can be noted and the care plan be modified as necessary. When the goals have not been achieved, blame should not be imposed on patients, families or health-care team members. Instead, realistic revisions to the plan should be made.

Two dietary situations that nurses and dietitians frequently encounter are those of the patient who cannot and will not eat and the patient who can and wants to eat but needs assistance in knowing what to eat and how to maximize the quality of mealtimes.

HELPING THE PATIENT WHO CANNOT AND WILL NOT EAT

Anorexia and cachexia are common phenomena that occur in cancer patients who are receiving palliative care. Tumours cause early satiety (especially seen with those of the lung, stomach and pancreas), specific food aversions (with almost all tumours, particularly to protein-containing foods such as beef and pork), nausea and vomiting (especially with liver cancer or metastases to the liver, and as a result of narcotics and other therapies) and a decreased interest in foodstuffs (particularly with an external tumour compression or partial obstruction of any part of the gastrointestinal tract). Although weight loss in the cancer patient is a worrisome sign, treatment unfortunately does not necessarily improve the patient's well-being or survival.

Anorexia and cachexia are not always a problem to the patient and family, although when they are, they are generally more problematic for the family than the patient. Cachexia may be a concern because patients and families do not understand what causes it or how it occurs. They should be told that, contrary to the popular misconception, cancer does not cause a loss of body weight by eating away body parts like a worm eats a leaf. Hearing this can help to alleviate the fear that something ugly is happening inside the body.

When working with an anxious family and a patient who cannot or will not eat, attempts should be made to diminish the effects of the no-win situation. Treatment is best directed at ameliorating social consequences such as the embarrassment of the patient at his or her gaunt appearance and physical complications. Teaching the family about the effects of the disease and the dying process is also important. The family's anxieties can be diminished and the patient freed from the pressure to eat when attention is shifted from maintaining the patient's nutritional status to enhancing patient comfort through providing small, appetizing meals. It is sometimes most appropriate to offer the patient no food unless he or she requests it. Although this change in approach may at first be difficult, it often brings considerable relief to both patient and family in the long run. Helpful phrases in discouraging the 'he must eat or he will die' syndrome include:

- 'The disease controls his appetite; pushing him to eat won't change the course of the disease.'
- 'He's sick and will be sick even if he eats.'
- 'Pushing him to eat may only make him feel uncomfortable.'
- 'Let him sit with you and eat what he wants.'
- 'Try not to worry that he eats poorly; it doesn't seem to bother him.'

DEHYDRATION

Patients and families often assume that dehydration is an uncomfortable state; on the contrary, when dehydration occurs close to the time of death, it appears to become a natural anaesthesia by decreasing the patient's perception of suffering, perhaps by reducing the level of consciousness or increasing the production of endorphins and dynorphin. The concomitant dry mouth effect associated with dehydration can be relieved by ice chips, lubricants and other simple measures (Table 11.2, and Box 11.2 below).

If the patient's life expectancy is being measured in weeks or days, dehydration, as a natural course of events, may be preferred over aggressive nutritional support through tube feeding and/or total parenteral nutrition (TPN) if such feeding causes discomfort. By forgoing aggressive therapy, the patient may benefit from the following:

- decreased gastrointestinal and venous distension;
- decreased nausea, vomiting and potential for aspiration;
- decreased diarrhoea;
- decreased pulmonary secretion, resulting in less coughing, less fear of choking and drowning, and fewer rattling secretions;
- decreased urinary flow and need to void.

Table 11.2 Suggestions for improving oral intake

- Feed the patient when he or she is hungry, changing mealtimes if needed. Note the patient's best meals and make these the largest
- Serve a small serving of the patient's favourite foods on a small plate
- Gently encourage, but do not nag, the patient to eat; remove uneaten food without undue comment
- Cold foods are generally preferred to hot ones. Reassure the parents of a dying child that they do not have to serve a hot, nutritious daily meal for the child; encourage them not to feel guilty if the child wants nothing or wants only a fast-food hamburger or fries
- Set an attractive table and plate, using a plate garnish or table flower if enjoyed by the patient. In an institutional setting, serve the patient's food on trays set with embroidered tray cloths and pretty china or stoneware rather than using traditional paper underliners and dishes. If feasible, allow the patient's personal china and utensils from home to be used
- Make mealtimes sociable (when desired by the patient) and enjoyable, vary the place of eating, and remove bedpans from the room
- Children can be encouraged to drink by playing games; it is fun for a child to drink fluids in an unusual way, such as through a syringe or from a small medicine cup, or by eating juice bars or ice lollies. Remove toys from the bed, turn off the television and bring in friends for a meal. Children will enjoy a packed lunch on occasions, and they like eating foods that have been cut into interesting shapes or look like their favourite characters
- Suggest that the patient rests before eating as most children and adults feel more like eating when they are relaxed
- Encourage high-calorie foods day or night, including eggnog, milkshake, custard, pudding, peanut butter, cream soups, cheese, fizzy drinks, pie, sherbet and cheesecake. In an institutional setting, consider serving foods from a hot trolley instead of or in addition to allowing patients to choose their meals in advance. Consider soup and soft sandwiches for midday meals. Try to supply as much variety in food selection as possible, including regional favourites
- Provide lipped dishes for those patients who have arm and hand weakness; use rubber grips on ordinary cutlery for those with a weak grip
- In an institutional setting, have a dining room with a home-like atmosphere available, where patients and families can eat together if they wish. Allow the family to eat with the patient in the patient's room if desired. Have staff available to feed patients who are unable to feed themselves, and do not hurry patients to eat
- Liberalize the diet as much as possible; diabetic or low-sodium diets are rarely essential, but if they are, consider simple low-sugar foods and a lack of regular salt packets instead of more restricted diets

---

Adapted from Gallagher-Allred (1989), with the permission of Aspen Publishers.

BOX 11.2 DIETARY THERAPY FOR COMMON SYMPTOMS IN PALLIATIVE CARE

(Note that not all of the identified treatments may be appropriate for all diseases or conditions)

Belching

- Allow the patient to make the final choice of foods to eat and avoid, but consider testing the patient's tolerance to gas-producing foods such as beer, carbonated beverages, alcohol, dairy products if lactose intolerant, nuts, beans, onions, peas, corn, cucumbers, radishes, cabbage, broccoli, Brussel sprouts, spinach, cauliflower, high-fat foods, yeast and mushrooms
- Encourage the patient to eat solids at mealtimes and drink liquids between meals instead of with solid foods
- Advise the patient to avoid eating quickly and reclining immediately after eating; encourage the patient to relax before, during and after meals
- Advise the patient to avoid overeating, to avoid sucking through a straw, to avoid chewing gum and to keep the mouth closed when chewing and swallowing

Constipation

- Encourage the patient to eat foods high in fibre (bran, whole grains, fruits such as pineapple, prunes and raisins, vegetables, nuts and legumes) if an adequate fluid intake can be maintained. Avoid high-fibre foods if dehydration, severe constipation or obstruction is anticipated
- Increase the fluid intake as tolerated. Encourage fruit juices, prune juice and cider; 30–60 ml of a mixture of 2 cups of apple sauce, 2 cups of unprocessed bran and 1 cup of 100 per cent prune juice can be drunk with the evening meal if the patient likes it and may reduce laxative use
- Discontinue calcium and iron supplementation if used. Limit cheese, rich desserts and other foods if constipating

Diarrhoea

- Let the patient make the final choice of foods to eat and avoid, but suggest omitting the following foods if they cause diarrhoea: milk, ice cream, wholegrain breads and cereals, nuts, beans, peas, greens, fruits with seeds and skins, fresh pineapple, raisins, cider, prune juice, raw vegetables, gas-forming vegetables, alcohol and caffeine-containing beverages
- Encourage the patient to eat bananas, apple sauce, peeled apple, tapioca, rice, peanut butter, refined grains, crackers, pasta, cream of wheat, oatmeal and cooked vegetables
- Encourage the patient to avoid liquids with their meals but instead to drink an hour afterwards
- Encourage the patient to relax before, during and after a meal
- Enteral and/or parenteral nutritional support in the AIDS patient may be appropriate if the patient has a lengthy life expectancy and the cause of the diarrhoea is known and treatable. If tube feeding or an oral diet is appropriate, this should be high in calories and protein and low in fibre, lactose and fat
- If dehydration is a problem, encourage high-potassium foods

Hypercalcaemia

- Allow hypercalcaemic patients to eat foods high in calcium, such as dairy products, if desired, but encourage them to avoid calcium and vitamin D supplementation. The restriction of high-calcium foods is rarely helpful
- Encourage the patient to drink lots of fluid, particularly carbonated beverages containing phosphoric acid if the patient enjoys them

BOX 11.2 (*Continued*)

Mental disorders

- Encourage the patient to avoid alcohol and caffeine-containing foods, such as coffee, tea and chocolate, if they contribute to anxiety, sleep deprivation or depression
- If the patient is drowsy or apathetic, suggest that the family may need to feed the patient. Encourage them to prepare the patient's favourite foods, usually in soft form to be served with a spoon or in bite sizes so that the patient might be able to self-feed. Help the family to protect the patient and others by shutting off or removing knobs from stoves, removing matches and locking doors to cabinets or closets that contain poisons, alcohol or medications. Put away electrical appliances such as mixers, food processors, can openers and waffle ononirons, and unplug microwave ovens
- If the patient is agitated or confused, caution the family on the dangers of hand-feeding the patient. Suggest feeding with a spoon and not allowing the patient to handle feeding utensils, plates, glass, etc. Encourage the family to tell the patient what time of day it is, what meal is being served and what foods are there. Remind the patient that the foods served are his or her favourites. Make mealtimes enjoyable by reminiscing about pleasant events in the patient's life. Consider the pros and cons of waking the patient if asleep at mealtimes
- If the patient is stuporous or comatose, counsel the family that semi-starvation and dehydration are not painful to the patient. Explore with them the pros and cons of enteral and parenteral nutritional support if they request information

Mouth problems

- If the patient says that foods taste bitter, encourage poultry, fish, dairy products, eggs, milk and cheese; bitter-tasting foods usually include red meat, sour juices, coffee, tea, tomatoes and chocolate. Suggest cooking foods in glass or porcelain instead of metal containers, and avoid serving foods on metal dishes or with metallic utensils. Encourage sweet fruit drinks, carbonated beverages, ice lollies and seasonings, herbs and spices to enhance the flavour
- If the patient says that foods taste 'old', try adding sugar; sour and salty flavours often taste 'old'
- If the patient says that foods taste too sweet, suggest drinking sour juices and cooking with lemon juice, vinegar, spices, herbs and mint; add pickles to appropriate foods
- If the patient says that foods have no taste, suggest marinating appropriate foods, serving highly seasoned foods, adding sugar and eating meals at room temperature
- If the patient has difficulty swallowing, suggest small, frequent meals of soft food (puréed if needed), advise against foods that might irritate the mouth and oesophagus, such as acidic juices or fruits, spicy foods, very hot or cold foods, alcohol and carbonated beverages
- If the patient has mouth sores, suggest blended and cold foods; gravies, cream soups, eggnog, milkshakes, cream pies, cheesecake, mousses, macaroni cheese, soufflés and casseroles are well liked. Suggest that the patient avoid alcohol, acidic fruit juices and vegetable juices, and spicy, rough, hot and highly salted foods. Antifungal preparations are available if necessary
- If the patient has a dry mouth, suggest frequent sips of water, de-fatted bouillon, juice, ice chips, ice lollies, ice cream, fruitades or slushy frozen baby foods mixed with fruit juice. Sucking on hard sweets and chewing sugar-free gum may stimulate the flow of saliva, as may dry alcoholic beverages. Solid foods should be moist, puréed as needed, with sauces and gravies, and not too tart, too hot or too cold if mouth sores are present. Synthetic salivary substitutes (some prefer citrus added, some prefer them refrigerated) are often helpful

---

BOX 11.2 (*Continued*)

Nausea and vomiting

- Encourage the patient to avoid eating if nauseated or if nausea is anticipated
- Suggest small meals of cool, non-odorous foods such as dry biscuits, cream crackers, soft toast, dry cereals, lean and white meats, milk, yoghurt, pudding and cheese. Many patients find it helpful to avoid fatty, greasy or fried foods. Avoid also mixing hot and cold foods at the same meal, high-bulk meals and nausea-precipitating foods such as overly sweet foods, alcohol, spicy foods and tobacco with meals
- Encourage the patient to eat slowly and avoid overeating. Relaxing before and after meals, and avoiding physical activity and lying flat for 2 hours after eating, may also help
- Suggest that the patient does not prepare his or her own food

Gastrointestinal obstruction

- If an oral intake is not contraindicated, encourage the patient to eat small meals that are low in fibre, low in residue and blended or strained. Many patients will prefer to eat their favourite foods, enjoy large meals and then vomit frequently. A gastric tube, open to straight or intermittent drain, may alleviate the need for regular vomiting
- With 'squashed stomach syndrome', encourage the patient to eat small, frequent meals, avoiding nausea-producing foods, odorous foods, gas-producing foods and high-fat or fried foods. Limit the fluid with meals, taking drinks an hour before and after meals

---

Adapted from Gallagher-Allred (1989), with the permission of Aspen Publishers.

When life expectancy is longer, fluid intake should be encouraged, implementing creative ways to increase intake such as varying the flavour and temperature of water and providing liquid nutritional supplements, juices, bouillon and other liquids. Inadequate fluid intake contributes to constipation, a common problem that detracts from quality of life.

There is also a role for low-volume parenteral hydration to increase comfort for patients who manifest symptoms of opioid toxicity (such as agitated delirium, myoclonus and seizures), accompanied as appropriate by switching the opioid and using less-sedating treatments. Hypodermoclysis for rehydration (usually around 1000 ml per day) is inexpensive, has few complications and can be administered at home (Bruera et al., 1995).

HELPING THE PATIENT WHO CAN AND WANTS TO EAT

For those who want to eat and who can be helped to eat better, the importance of improving their appetite and enabling them to eat as normally as possible cannot be overestimated. Medications such as corticosteroids, megestrol acetate, tricyclic antidepressants, dronabinol, and alcohol as an aperitif, can be administered to heighten appetite and mood. Improving a poor self-image by preferred clothing, a hairdresser's appointment or a visit to the dentist can also improve a patient's appetite.

If the anorexia has a correctable cause and the patient has a predicted life expectancy of several months, these causes should be treated aggressively if desired by the patient. Similarly, treatment should be aggressive if the patient's anorexia appears to be an isolated symptom and the suspected consequence is malnutrition that could compromise both the quality and the quantity of the patient's remaining days. Suggestions for improving the oral intake of adults and children through use of food have been summarised in Table 11.2 above.

Commercial medical nutritional supplements are warranted for adult patients and children who need a high calorie intake in a small volume. Medical nutritional supplements are often appreciated by weak patients and their families because the patient can drink the highly fortified liquid products with minimal effort and the family members feel that they are providing 'something special'.

If enteral tube feeding, either in addition to oral intake or as the sole source of nutrition, is desired by the patient, liquid commercial nutritional products can be administered via a small-bore, flexible catheter that is, in most patients, passed directly into the stomach through the abdominal wall, or through the nose into the stomach or upper small intestine. The formulas to be administered should generally be isotonic solutions. Depending on the patient's ability to tolerate the solution, feeding should be started with a continuous drip at full strength if an isotonic solution is being used, or at half strength with a hypertonic one. An appropriate starting rate is usually 50 ml per hour (up to a final rate of 100–125 ml per hour); alternatively, the concentration can be increased (half to three-quarter to full strength) over several days, depending on patient tolerance and nutritional goals. Many patients and families prefer intermittent tube feeding to a continuous drip feed because it seems more like a meal than does drip delivery via a pump.

For most patients, a continuous drip administration of 100–125 ml per hour of full-strength (1 kcal/ml) solution is in theory the maximum amount needed if weight maintenance (2400–3000 kcal per day) is the goal. In practice, however, only 1000–1800 kcal per day (a continuous drip for 10–15 hours) is generally needed to achieve satiety and comfort, greater amounts frequently causing complications that include fluid overload, cramps, diarrhoea, reflux and aspiration.

A case can be made for the limited use of TPN in palliative care. When patients are in the early stages of their disease, they are often able to lead a full and active life. TPN may, however, be appropriate if patients are unable to ingest enough calories orally or via enteral tube feeding to sustain their activity level, as the result of a poorly or non-functioning gastrointestinal tract. Inoperable bowel obstruction and short bowel syndrome are two examples of such situations.

TPN is, on the other hand, generally not well tolerated by terminally ill patients, and rarely does parenteral feeding reduce the distress of anorexia and cachexia when the terminal stage is reached. Instead, TPN often subjects the patient to new problems that are more distressing, and to prolonged suffering that would not have been faced had parenteral feeding been avoided. If TPN is desired, it is generally best started in the hospital setting before the patient returns home or to a long-term care facility. Administration in the home or long-term care setting should be closely monitored by a specially trained care team.

It has been the experience of this author that palliative care patients with advanced cancer rarely find any advantage in aggressive nutritional support via tube or parenteral feeding. Instead, allowing patients to eat and drink as they desire, and not pushing them to do so if they do not desire or are unable to do this, is a viable alternative. A tube previously placed for enteral feeding, or an intravenous line for TPN, may not, however, need to be discontinued unless the patient wishes, but even though the feeding tube may be in place, there is no moral reason for using it for feeding.

DIETARY THERAPY FOR COMMON NUTRITIONAL PROBLEMS

Although the process of dying often brings many less-than-desirable side-effects, it is wrong to view it as a 'disease' hungry for medical 'remedies'. The health-care team can, however, give the patient and family many helpful dietary suggestions for symptom control so that they can maximize comfort during the dying patient's remaining days.

Box 11.2 provides suggestions for appropriate dietary therapy for common symptoms in palliative care. Because the majority of palliative care patients are diagnosed with incurable cancer, the suggestions are primarily based on responses from cancer patients. The reader must remember that not all of the treatments identified may be appropriate for all diseases or conditions.

FOOD SERVICE SUGGESTIONS

Food service in an in-patient palliative care setting must reflect the philosophy of maximizing patient comfort and enhancing quality of life (Drew Kidd and Lane 1993), with menu development reflecting the ethnic, cultural and regional food preferences of the population. Regardless of the meal pattern selected (e.g. three or four meals, lighter meals, heavier meals, etc.), there must be flexibility for reheating menu items and preparing quick meals when patients desire. Allowing patients to select menus as close to serving time as possible may help to allay anorexia. Small portions attractively garnished and plated in a dining atmosphere conducive to patient and family socialization also contribute to better meal acceptance. Family members' assistance with feeding further enhances the dining experience.

In the palliative care setting, some patients and families may express a desire for additional fibre, others for low-fat foods, still others for meals that reflect personal nutritional beliefs, and specific dietary modifications such as low-sodium, low-fat and diabetic requirements may be needed. In most cases, however, these restrictions are liberalized to allow the patient maximum pleasure, variety and choice. Fluctuations in patients' mental alertness, level of responsiveness, dental status and swallowing difficulty may indicate the need for modifications of consistency to provide soft, mechanical soft, puréed or blended foods. Simple, easy-to-prepare foods served in smaller portions are more acceptable to patients than complicated, labour-intensive recipes. Comfort and familiar foods are also better enjoyed and tolerated. Some examples of universally selected comfort foods are macaroni cheese, grilled cheese sandwiches, peanut butter or jam sandwiches, toast, crackers, soups, fresh fruits and soft salads.

In-patient palliative care facilities often provide a family kitchen, including personal china, flatware and glassware cupboards, refrigerated storage and a reheating system to handle foods brought from home. A family kitchen allows meal flexibility and supports the family and friends in their caring efforts. Public health rules for labelling and dating food items, and safe storage time limits, should be enforced: the importance of food sanitation and safety cannot be overemphasized in a setting in which many patients are immunocompromised.

By serving nutritious, attractively prepared food to heighten visual and physical pleasure, the palliative care facility's food service staff have the opportunity to enrich patients' lives at a time when the smallest pleasure is truly treasured.

ETHICAL AND LEGAL CONSIDERATIONS IN NUTRITIONAL SUPPORT

The ethical and legal considerations involved in the nutritional support of palliative care patients are increasingly being debated, in part because of recent technological advances in nutritional support that enable professionals to keep people alive for longer than meaningful life sometimes can be maintained. Tackling the dilemma of 'to feed or not to feed?' requires, as with other methods of medical treatment, that those involved in palliative care ask the underlying questions 'What good will it do for the patient?' and 'Do the benefits of nutrition support outweigh the burdens?'

To answer these questions, it is important first to establish the clinical facts of each patient's situation and effectively communicate these to the patient and family. The benefits and burdens that the patient may experience from the provision or withholding/withdrawal of nutritional support should also be delineated for both patient and family. The benefits and burdens identified in Table 11.3 can help health-care professionals when discussing this issue with patients and their families. The patient's and family's educated perspectives, based on their personal value systems should then be the cornerstone of the decision-making process.

The process of providing artificial nutrition and hydration to avert cachexia and dehydration is so onerous for some patients that the benefits are inconsequential or meaningless. To others, not to intervene is unacceptable and tanta-

Table 11.3 Potential benefits and burdens of artificial nutrition and hydration

Benefits
- Added calories and other nutrients may prolong life and give the patient and family more time to:
  - allow denial to serve as a natural coping mechanism that protects one from the fear that death is nearing
  - provide emotional support by reducing the fear of abandonment
  - get their psychosocial and material affairs in order
  - allow for a significant family event to occur
  - improve patient and family interrelationships
  - add confidence that 'everything is being done' to prolong life as long as possible
- Prevent perceived suffering from a fear that death from dehydration and/or starvation is a painful way to die
- Increase the ability to recover from the effects of other medical therapies
- Improve the patient's overall sense of well-being and self-esteem
- Improve nutritional status to decrease the risk of infection, pressure ulcers and aspiration pneumonia
- Nutrition is obligatory if it alleviates discomfort from hunger, cachexia, malnutrition and/or dehydration
- Fulfil the moral belief that all persons should be fed
- Fulfil the moral belief that artificial nutrition and hydration are basic humane care and society's responsibility to 'be thy brother's keeper'

Burdens
- Pain and physical suffering from:
  - tube or line insertion and usage
  - uncomfortable distension, nausea, vomiting, diarrhoea, possible aspiration and pneumonia, and excess stomal leakage and wound dehiscence with tube feeding
  - fluid overload, ascites, peripheral oedema, pulmonary oedema, thrombosis and possible lung puncture and sepsis with total parenteral nutrition
  - possible restriction of activities by tethering the patient to an infusion apparatus
  - increased need for catheterization in those too weak to void large volumes
  - increased nasogastric and/or pulmonary secretions, which may require suctioning
  - increased pharyngeal secretions with increased fluid intake, resulting in a death rattle
- Psychological distress, including the possible indignity of being kept alive beyond the time life is meaningful, and the sadness of imposing hardships on family and friends
- Spiritual and moral conflict
- Financial hardship

mount to murder. The choice lies in doing what is in the patient's best interests after the goals to be accomplished have been considered and the expected benefits and burdens have been analysed by the patient, the patient's family and competent health-care professionals. There are a multiplicity of reasons why patients and their families may choose or oppose initiating or withholding/

withdrawing artificial nutrition and hydration, as there are many reasons underlying the preferences of health-care professionals.

Case law rarely provides definitive answers to the question of whether or not to feed, but three relevant opinions are often expressed, which appear to transcend national boundaries:

1 Withholding and withdrawing nutritional support have the same ethical significance.
2 Artificial nutrition and hydration are considered to be medical therapy and can be refused by competent patients and, in certain circumstances, the surrogates of incompetent patients.
3 Patient autonomy is a guiding ethical principle.

It is necessary to emphasize that, in circumstances in which the patient dies when artificial nutrition and hydration is withdrawn, the cause of death is the underlying disease or condition rather than the withdrawal of the nutritional support. In the past, prior to the availability of nutrition and hydration support technology, patients would have died of their disease. Advances in nutrition and hydration support technology have not changed this so the absence of such support is not the specific cause of death. It is highly important to emphasize this concept to patients and their families. Families already carry a sufficiently heavy load without adding to it the burden of guilt caused by the decision to withdraw nutrition and hydration.

As mentioned above, 'withholding' and 'withdrawing' artificial nutrition and hydration are considered to have the same ethical significance even though the removal of artificial nutrition and hydration may be psychologically and emotionally much more difficult. This should not, however, lead to withholding this therapy in an attempt to avoid a difficult decision regarding the future withdrawal of support.

CONCLUSION

Nutrition and hydration issues are common when caring for patients with cancer. The health-care team will experience a great deal of satisfaction in individualizing and implementing an appropriate nutritional care plan for the patient and family. Nutrition and hydration have a rightful place in the palliative care team's arsenal of therapies to enhance the quality of a patient's living as well as dying.

REFERENCES

Bruera, E., Franco, J.J., Maltoni, M. et al. 1995: Changing pattern of agitated impaired mental status in patients with advanced cancer: association with cognitive monitoring, hydration, and opiod rotation. *Journal of Pain and Symptom Management* 10, 287–91.
Gallagher-Allred, C.R. 1989: *Nutritional care of the terminally ill.* Gaithersburg, MD: Aspen.

Kidd, K. Drew and Lane, M.P. 1993: Maximising food service in an inpatient hospice setting. *Hospice Journal* **9**(2/3), 85–106.

Mauer Baak, C.M. 1993: Nursing's role in the nutritional care of the terminally ill: weathering the storm. *Hospice Journal* **9**(2/3), 1–13.

FURTHER READING

Fainsinger, R.L. and Bruera, E. 1995: The management of dehydration in terminally ill patients. *Journal of Palliative Care* **10**, 55–9.

Hunt, T. 1996: Nutritional needs. In: Fisher, R. and McDaid, *Palliative day care*. London: Edward Arnold.

Hunt, T. 1992: Nutrition in palliative care. *Journal of Communitive Nursing* **6**, 10–14.

White, K.S. and Hall, J.C. 1999: Ethical dilemmas in artificial nutrition and hydration: decision-making. *Nursing Case Management* **4**, 152–7.

HELPING THE BEREAVED AND HELPING OURSELVES

Jenny Penson

> The loss of a loved person is one of the most intensely painful experiences any human being can suffer, and not only is it painful to experience, but also painful to witness, if only because we're so impotent to help.

These words of Bowlby's (1980) speak to me as both a human being and a nurse because if we do not know how to help, the natural tendency is to avoid the situation. And if we do avoid it, we are likely to feel guilty. The aim of this chapter is therefore to raise awareness and encourage confidence so that we can be helpful to people who are facing the challenge of bereavement. Its focus will be on the therapeutic relationship and the ways in which nurses can handle the effects of the losses they regularly encounter at work.

The experience of being bereaved is as old as life, and death, itself. We are arguably the only species that has an awareness of its own vulnerability and certain death. Although we all know that we will one day die, we tend not to live in the present but in the future, always looking ahead to the next day, the next week, the next year. The palliative care movement has done much to bring issues of death and dying into the open. The provision of some kind of bereavement support is always made, although the ways in which it is offered vary widely.

BEREAVEMENT

Bereavement means being robbed of something valued. This appears to be a helpful definition because the word 'rob' indicates that the person has been wrongfully taken away, that they should not have died. There is therefore, a sense of injustice that often calls up strong and overwhelming emotions. It refers to the situation of anyone who has lost a person to whom they were strongly attached.

Bereavement affects everyone but does so unequally. Some people develop physical or mental illness or even die, whereas others appear to take it in their stride. There are some major factors that appear to influence the individual response to bereavement. First, all relationships carry with them a degree of *ambivalence*, but where there has been an insecure attachment to the deceased or a relationship in which one person has been overly dependent and the other very dominant, there may be particular problems in adjustment. Second, the *nature* of the loss includes factors concerning the kind of relationship with the deceased and whether the death was anticipated or unexpected. A death that has occurred by violence, suicide or catastrophe will usually necessitate skilled help.

LOSS

The key concept in bereavement is *loss*. We have all experienced losses in our lives, including the expected losses that are inherent in any transition from one stage of life to another, and losses that are part of any change, even when it is one that brings many gains as well, for example marriage or the birth of a wanted child. A useful analogy is that losing someone loved can be likened to the amputation of a limb because it feels as it part of yourself has gone and can never be replaced.

There are losses that are in some way *hidden* or even invisible in that others may not be aware that the loss, for example miscarriage or abortion has happened. It could be the death of a more distant family member such as a grandparent or aunt, or that of a special friend. Families from a first marriage may not feature in the everyday life of the families from a second one so a bereavement may not be acknowledged or support be forthcoming.

In our work as nurses, we are familiar with the *physical* losses that are part of many disease processes, and sometimes of treatment. Cancer provides a pertinent example often involving changes in body image caused by weight loss as well as by surgery, chemotherapy or radiation.

As nurses, we may have deliberately concealed a death out of misdirected kindness, perhaps not telling other patients on a ward that someone has died or colluding in not telling a child that his parent is going to die in a misguided wish to protect him. Parkes (1998) refers to these as *disenfranchised* losses.

For many, major loss leads to *multiple bereavement-related* losses. A loss of role, status, financial security, practical support and intimacy may frequently be experienced at the same time. The loss of an imagined future and the loss of assumptions and dreams, as Bowman (1997) suggests, need to be grieved over before new dreams can be created and pursued.

GRIEF

Grief describes the emotional response to loss. It is made up of a strong and sometimes overwhelming variety of emotions, including shock, anger, guilt, despair, sadness, restlessness and anxiety, which can render the bereaved person vulnerable to illness and even death, although the evidence for this is inconclusive. Grief is experienced physically with sensations such as shortness of breath, palpitations, indigestion, headaches, muscle tension and fatigue. Contrary to what one might at first suppose, the end of a troubled relationship may cause some bereaved people great difficulties in grieving, with still more anger, resentment and guilt.

ANTICIPATORY GRIEVING

This starts from the moment the relative knows that the patient is not going to recover. It is often considered to be helpful to adjustment, contrasting with an unexpected death when there has been no opportunity to say goodbye, to resolve family issues or to ask or receive forgiveness (Callanan and Kelley, 1992). Evidence linking an advance warning of death with positive bereavement outcomes is, however, inconclusive.

Costello (1999) found that anticipatory grief had a cumulative rather than a specific influence on bereavement. Another view is that the anticipation of the death intensifies attachment to the dying person rather than leading to detachment (Parkes and Weiss, 1995). In an endeavour to be realistic and not to give false hope, the focus of care may be on a peaceful death rather than on making the most of the time that is left (Penson, 2000). Grieving in advance may lead to treating the person as if he or she has already died. For some, grieving can only begin after the person has died.

PERSPECTIVES

There are many perspectives on the experience of bereavement. Modern theorists tend to define bereavement in terms of stages that have to be passed through in order to reach resolution (Bowlby, 1980; Parkes, 1996, 1998;). Kübler-Ross (1970) looked at bereavement in terms of stages experienced by the dying patient leading to what she termed 'a good death'. Stage theories offer useful signposts on the bereavement journey, although they have been criticized for implying that grieving is a passive process, whereas Worden (1992) sees it as 'grief work'.

Another view is that bereavement is a major source of stress (Holmes and Rahe, 1967; Lazarus and Folkman, 1984). Ricketts (1995) points out that there will be a wide variability in the pattern of bereavement and in his cognitive-behavioural model of grief, identifies specific coping skills that may be enhanced through interventions.

Sanders' (1989) holistic model of bereavement goes beyond stages of adaptation to include a spiritual perspective on grief, with transformation as a goal. A more recent holistic approach focuses on healing and renewal through interventions that include complementary therapies (Miller and McGown, 1997). Mathers (1976) suggests that there are humanistic goals that may be achieved from the experience of being bereaved:

> The pain of bereavement is the price we have to pay for loving: so that, though it is costly, it is not too dear, since the experience of losing what you have loved, and grieving over it, is a challenge, to learn more about yourself, to become more mature, more healthy and more truly human.

This view is endorsed by Solari-Twadell et al. (1995), who see the process of rejoining life as being about surrender and that this requires faith, and 'such faith is not a matter of doubtless certainty but a matter of daring courage'. These approaches move the bereaved from a reliance on external support to the development of inner strength and self-awareness.

The consensus seems to be that the expression of grief, in whatever form, is essential in order to adjust to bereavement and that there is an accepted pattern of grieving. Any deviations from this expected sequence may therefore be viewed as abnormal, complicated or even pathological.

COMPLICATED GRIEF

The aim of assessment is to identify those who may be at risk of getting stuck at some point or not being able to adjust to their loss so that monitoring and support in some form can be offered to those who are more at risk. Good liaison between all those involved will ensure that this is put into practice.

Factors that need to be taken into account include personal information, such as age and state of health, other close relationships, how and where the death took place, whether or not the bereaved person was present at the time of death, and social factors such as financial status and community support. It is generally agreed that *sudden* death is the biggest single risk factor in bereavement. Here, there has been no opportunity to anticipate the loss in any way, and there will be a strong sense of shock, especially if there were disagreements, conflicts or unresolved issues just prior to the death.

The *timeliness*, or otherwise, of the loss is linked to the nature of the relationship. It is considered that the death of an elderly person is easier to grieve than that of a young one. Therefore, the *death of a child* is the hardest loss to grieve, this holding true even when the 'child' is an older person being grieved over by an elderly parent.

Social isolation is a common factor, especially in the elderly. Although a few people seem to have deep inner resources and little need for contact, most of us need to be in relationship with others in order to thrive. *Psychological fragility* may make the bereaved person more likely to be at risk. A previous history of mental illness, particularly depression, an inability to cope with a previous life crisis or an unresolved loss from the past will impact on the present bereavement.

In *the dysfunctional family*, there may be physical and/or emotional dependence on the person who died, severe conflict or an extreme family crisis that will render the individual more vulnerable in bereavement. Contrary to what one might at first expect, *an unhappy relationship* with the deceased may also lead to difficulties in adjustment as there is likely to be more anger and guilt involved, and fewer good memories to heal the past.

Understanding a 'normal' pattern of bereavement will enable the helper to know when the process seems to be prolonged, or even excessively shortened, which may be described as being delayed, postponed or blocked (Parkes, 1996). Risk assessment tools can help to identify who might most benefit from intervention. The majority of such tools are derived from the Bereavement Risk Index of Parkes and Weiss (1995).

THE THERAPEUTIC RELATIONSHIP

It is not difficult to offer help; it is often our own feelings of inadequacy or embarrassment that prevent us offering opportunities to listen and give support. The quality of the communication that takes place between nurses and relatives – the caring triangle – impacts on the patient and, arguably, on the adjustment to bereavement. The deceptively simple skill of listening can be very powerful. Many of us may feel that we are rarely listened to in everyday life. As Shakespeare wrote in *Macbeth*, 'Give sorrow words: the grief that does not speak whispers the oe'r-rought heart, and bids it break.' Feeling that we have been fully heard can of itself be therapeutic. We can learn to convey a relaxed and unhurried approach and to resist interrupting in the assumption that we already know what relatives are going to say. The key skill is that of centering ourselves so that we are fully present in the moment.

The hypothesis exists that the care given to the bereaved person before the death takes place can be helpful to his or her adjustment later. In supporting relatives before death, the nurse is often aware that the relatives' prime concern is the quality of the care given to the patient. This is what Hopper (2000) refers to as efficient care, arguing that it is through the quality of their nursing care that nurses address the spirit of their patients. Death is a profound event, not least because each of us is aware that this journey will one day also be ours to travel. It can therefore never be for us something that happens 'out there': it affects us deep within.

The therapeutic relationship is fostered by respect for the patient and family and by the valuing of their unique contribution. A climate of trust needs to be created in which information is forthcoming and encouragement given for the relatives to give to the patient in whatever ways they are able. Support and clear explanations of what is happening needs to be offered. Relatives may need to be gently reminded that, when they look back on this time, there may be things they wish they had said, or other family and friends who might have wanted to do so. The photograph album can be a good focus for sharing memories. Opportunities can be used to review together the achievements, frustrations and satisfactions of lives shared and to express forgiveness and gratitude. These are some of the final gifts identified by Callanan and Kelley (1992).

Questions that might help to encourage communication include: What is the worst thing for you at the moment? When are the low points? How do you handle the difficult times? What do you find helps? How do you see things working out in the future? Encouragement can be very helpful but needs to be balanced by a sensitivity to the times when people are not coping and may need permission to be vulnerable.

Opening up communication between patients and relatives can lead to patients expressing their wishes concerning their will and funeral and burial arrangements. This can help the bereaved relative by easing uncertainty and confusion, and may help to avoid later disagreements between family members.

STRESS

When bereavement is viewed in terms of a major stressor, the growing body of knowledge of psychoneuroimmunology indicates that a persistently high level of cortisol diminishes the effectiveness of the immune system (Pert, 1998) and can arguably lead to physical illness. This is more likely to happen when relatives are left with memories of helplessness, so involvement and support in the patient's care may be helpful.

Techniques for managing stress may be appropriate. Physical exercise such as the gentle art of yoga, swimming, walking, jogging, keep fit, weight training and other sports help to engender a relaxed body and an elevated mood. Tension and anxiety can be relieved by complementary therapies such as relaxation and guided imagery (Jones, 1999), or relaxation with biofeedback (Arnette, 1996). Engaging the unconscious mind by the use of affirmations, metaphors and guided visualizations can help the healing process of grief (Salka, 1997).

Keeping a diary can provide a means of expressing feelings and a way of charting and reviewing progress. Making plans for managing the commonly low points of Saturdays, Sundays, and Bank Holidays and Christmas time, as well as anniversaries known only to the bereaved themselves, can be empowering.

RESOURCES

In acting as a resource to the bereaved family, the helper needs to be aware of the many ways in which support may be offered and what is available in their locality. There are likely to be local branches of national organizations such as Cruse (for widows and widowers) or Age Concern (supporting elderly people). Local churches may have volunteers who offer home visits. Local amenities such as sports and leisure centres provide opportunities to meet others and improve health and fitness, adult Education centres offering a wide range of classes for leisure and learning. Complementary therapists have in common a holistic approach and can be a very valuable source of help and support. The Citizens Advice Bureau, Health Education department and local library provide information that may be helpful, and the Samaritans offer a valuable confidential telephone service for those in distress.

Follow-up services are offered by hospices and Macmillan and other palliative care centres, often including befriending schemes for bereaved people, for example home visits by supervised volunteers. They may also facilitate therapeutic groups for bereaved individuals. If there seem to be gaps in the services available in a particular locality, it may be possible to act as a facilitator to bring a group of bereaved people together for a period, with the aim of others taking it forward later if they wish.

THE WAY FORWARD

In order to help the bereaved person to reach out in this way, what is needed is someone who will sit quietly and listen, and who will not succumb to the temptation to suppress emotional expression. Rejoining life will have painful elements because it will always be different: it involves reconstructing one's existence, developing new strengths and investing energy into new ways of being. C.S. Lewis (1961) described such a turning point in his own bereavement when he wrote about a gradual feeling of hope and the possibility of moving forward in new directions. For some, the crisis of loss will also be seen as relating to the opportunity for personal growth.

Helping people near the end of life touches us personally, reminding us of our own mortality and losses, and can make us feel vulnerable and afraid. In our professional roles, we become attached to certain patients and their families. As we have seen, where there has been an attachment, there will be loss when separation occurs (Bowlby, 1980). It will sometimes be hard for us to let patients and/or their family members go.

THE COST OF CARE

This can be likened to Parkes notion of the cost of commitment (Parkes, 1996). In a relationship in which there is an emotional response of commitment, there will be grief and feelings of loss when it ends. As soon as we involve our heart in the work we do, we are committed to the patients for whom we care, and there will inevitably be feelings of loss when they die. To avoid this, some nurses develop strategies such as distancing. Any dissonance between what we genuinely feel and what we actually display to the world can also lead to stress, but a lack of commitment makes work merely a job and unfulfilling.

This 'emotional labour', as Gray and Smith (2000) describe it, is inherent in the nature of nursing. Nurses form an invisible bond of support with the patient, and the caring relationship becomes suffused with complex emotions. There are risks to us when limits are not recognized, boundaries not set and support not available on a regular basis.

As Parkes (1999) points out, although grief in staff is natural, the idea that it is also a sign of weakness still persists. Nurses care for others but are reluctant to care for themselves. Nor should it be assumed that nurses have all the psychological skills to cope with death and dying. Death is always a profound event; like birth, it never loses its power or its mystery.

The losses that nurses encounter regularly in their work are often hidden losses because others may not define the death of a patient as a loss to be mourned. Members of the nurse's family may take this for granted and expect the nurse to cope. In addition, the nurse may be overwhelmed by several losses happening at once. Grief may become cumulative when multiple losses allow no time to mourn the patients who have died and when no acknowledgement is made of the loss.

EMOTIONAL PAIN

It is painful to witness another's distress, whether this is manifested as physical, emotional or spiritual pain. When we perceive a patient's experience as suffering, feelings of helplessness can lead to avoidance, this being exacerbated when there appears to be no reason for it because 'man is not destroyed by suffering, he is destroyed by suffering without meaning' (Frankl, 1987).

ANXIETY

Feelings of apprehension may be brought to the fore by a loss that appears similar to that which we most fear ourselves. Cassell (1991) points out that we can empathize only with those whom we perceive as being like us and reminds us that, even then, this may be more limited than we might like to think. Social factors such as the same culture, class, age, sex, attitudes, dress, ways of responding and coping styles will affect our responses and ability to empathize.

FAILURE

Caring for people near the end of life is challenging, and the relationship between patient, family and nurse can become very close and intense in a short space of time. Boundaries may be pushed back and limits not set. The close relationship that is often thus created may carry unrealistic expectations and involve complicated family dynamics, which can lead to feelings of powerlessness and failure.

OVER IDENTIFICATION

This is more likely to happen if those we care for represent our feared losses, for example when nursing a dying child if we are a parent. When we perceive the death as particularly unfair, such as the death of someone newly married, or the sudden death of someone who appeared to be responding well to treatment, we feel the grief of unfulfilled hopes.

NOT SHOWING EMOTION

Many nurses have been socialized into the idea that it is weak or unprofessional to show that they care; they may fear that expressing their feelings could make them feel worse. As Goleman (1999) suggests, the more accurately we can monitor our emotional upsets, the more quickly we can recover from distress.

Emotional clarity is required to enable us to manage difficult times, and acknowledging our needs is the key.

STRESS AND SUPPORT AT WORK

Organizations need to put in place systems to recognize and manage stress, valuing staff by acknowledging difficult times and offering support, as the cost of unrelieved stress is potentially high, leading to illness and burnout (Owen, 2000). Supporting teams through stress is a dynamic process that needs regular appraisal and review.

If nurses are to be empowered to cope with their feelings of grief, these feelings need to be acknowledged, first by the nurses experiencing them and then by their peers. However, as Wakefield (2000) points out, this type of support is rarely available, and many nurses are expected to cope and continue to administer nursing interventions as if nothing has happened. Indeed, the self-concept of being a coper fulfils others' expectations of the nursing role and makes it difficult for nurses to express their feelings even when they lose a family member.

Farrell (1992) asserts that it is essential for the emotional needs of caring professionals to be met by a support system. An assumed demand is however, not the same as a realized one. Hughes and Vaughan (1989) found that a support group for nurses was little used and that the offer of pastoral care from personal tutors was not taken up.

Networks of support needs to be individualized as nurses are as diverse as any other group and may therefore find that different approaches suit them. A knowledge of change theory can help the organization to provide ways of supporting the individual that are likely to be accepted. Clinical or team meetings provide an opportunity for feelings to be shared as well as care discussed. These can improve morale, but not everyone feels confident enough to use them. It is important to learn to talk about what has been done well and when we feel we have got it right as well as when we think we have not.

Davies and Oberle (1992) developed the supportive care model to articulate the job components of the palliative nursing role. The final dimension of this model focuses on nurses themselves. Preserving our own integrity encompasses reviewing our experiences, valuing ourselves, feeling good about our work and dealing with personal stress.

It may also be assumed that debriefing for staff when someone dies is always well received. However, Munro (2000) reminds us that people have different ways of coping and that for some it is not helpful to have debriefing forced upon them. One way of coping is not thinking about what has happened. All individuals need to adopt their own preferred ways rather than having such debriefing forced upon them.

Sometimes we do not know where to find support or how to benefit from it. The longer we do not express how we feel, the more difficult it will become to do this. We need to find a safe place to share our feelings.

SELF-CARE

Barber (1994) suggests that 'Professional carers have a duty to care for themselves. If they cannot receive care themselves they have no business forcing care on others.' He goes on to say that:

> when nurses who do not care for themselves try to emit care, they all too often give out 'dead lifeless care'. Care such as this is damaging and is more akin to duty. Though dutiful caring rarely kills anyone, it is at core insensitive and robs the therapeutic relationship of love.

This is echoed by Lewis (1999), who found that a bereavement support programme for oncology nurses led to much less stress, better peace of mind and hopes of increased work longevity. It also created more experienced, superior and compassionate care for the patients and their families. The two are intrinsically linked.

When facing loss on a regular basis, nurses need to develop skills to care for themselves; they cannot give from an empty place. When they do not take care of their own needs, they burn out. Nurses thus need to:

- *recognize* the symptoms of unresolved grief, including a lack of energy and enthusiasm, fatigue, a low tolerance level of stressors, emotions lying near the surface and an inability to relax;
- *anticipate* by planning how to handle these situations: make the most of the positive aspects, and say and do all that can be done, so that there will be few regrets when looking back;
- *let go* of some of the hurt and grief; feel the feelings. Deal with hurt or guilt now so that it is not allowed to collect and be carried over to the next situation. Sort things out, talk it through while it still hangs loose, before it has a chance to harden. Then let it go;
- *say goodbye* as marking endings enables the nurse to move forward. Formalizing this is part of the process of letting go; sometimes it might even be necessary to attend the funeral;
- *reflect* on what happened and the feelings attached to that so that the nurse can make sense of them, find meaning and learn. By understanding ones own feelings, one may better understand others;
- *seek and receive* support, this being a necessary strength required for destressing in demanding situations. It is about learning to receive as well as to give;
- *manage stress.* Stress appraisal, coping skills and the presence of psychological, social and material resources are interrelated and associated with health following stressful experiences (Lazarus and Folkman, 1984);
- *adjust* to the stress of change. Remember that everything passes, and keep life in balance;

- *attend to their own health* holistically through a healthy lifestyle. Receiving complementary therapies is another way of caring for ourselves;
- *care for colleagues* to enable them to feel valued. This can engender good practice and, arguably, lead to an improvement in the health of the total organization.

SKILLS

The skills needed are those of learning to trust others, a willingness to receive the time, attention and care from another and sharing uncomfortable feelings and experiences. It is suggested that being able to receive support as well as give it is an indicator of considerable personal maturity (Nichols and Jenkinson, 1992). Giving support is about learning to be free of the need to:

- be responsible for others and their problems
- put on a performance
- be in control of events
- give advice
- be right
- talk in order to fill a silence.

This freedom from constraints, which are often imagined rather than real, will enable the helper to be more relaxed, open and focused, and thus more helpful. This helps to convey an acceptance of others as people. The experience of being fully listened to can be very therapeutic.

These are all healing behaviours that can, of themselves, transform others' experiences, enabling them to find their own answers and to let go of their painful past.

TIME OF DEATH

Acknowledging that the death has taken place is important for nurses as well as for the other patients in the same ward. All individuals are of course unique and special to those who love them, and each death should be marked in some way. However busy the environment, there needs to be a short space to do this. It is important to address issues at the time and not let them fester.

So stop and take a quiet moment, no matter how brief. Meet in the ward office or back at the health centre. Remember the best things about this person. Tell someone all about it, your story. Show emotion if you need to but do not lose control. The offer of a short prayer is very comforting for relatives, and many nurses find that this helps them too. Create a space between work and home for decompression, a short space in which to let go of the working day before taking on home commitments.

CONCLUSION

The development of self-awareness, giving and receiving support, and education in interpersonal skills are key to adjusting and using the experiences that nursing practice provides for us. As Parkes et al. (1996) point out:

> with proper training and support we shall find that repeated grief, far from undermining our humanity and our care, enable us to cope more confidently and more sensitively with each succeeding loss.

Healing of the spirit takes time and courage, and if we can facilitate this in any way, it is our privilege to do so. There is mutuality in the therapeutic relationship, so in our encounters with bereaved people there is much that we can receive as well as much that we are able to give.

REFERENCES

Arnette, J.K. 1996: Physiological effects of chronic grief: a biofeedback treatment approach. *Death Studies* 20(1), 59–72.

Barber, P. 1994: *Who cares for the carers?* London: Distance Learning Centre, South Bank University.

Bowlby, J. 1980: *Attachment and loss*, Vol. 1. Harmondsworth: Penguin.

Bowman, T. 1997: Loss of dreams: a special kind of grief. *International Journal of Palliative Nursing* 3(2), 76–80.

Callanan, M. and Kelley, P. 1992: *Final gifts: understanding and helping the dying.* London: Hodder & Stoughton.

Cassell, E.J. 1991: *The nature of suffering and the goals of medicine.* Oxford: Oxford University Press.

Costello, J. 1999: Anticipatory grief: coping with the impending death of a partner. *International Journal of Palliative Nursing* 5(5), 223–31.

Davies, B. and Oberle, K. 1992: Dimensions of the supportive role of the nurse in palliative care. *Oncology Nurse Forum* 17, 87–94.

Farrell, M. 1992: A process of mutual support. *Professional Nurse* 8(1), 10–14.

Frankl, V. 1987: *Man's search for meaning.* London: Hodder & Stoughton.

Goleman, D. 1999: *Working with emotional intelligence.* London: Bloomsbury.

Gray, B. and Smith, P. 2000: An emotive subject: nurses' feelings. *Nursing Times* 96(27), 29–31.

Holmes, T.H. and Rahe, R.H. 1967: The social adjustment rating scale. *Journal of Psychosomatic Research* 11, 213–18.

Hopper, A. 2000: Meeting the spiritual needs of patients through holistic practice. *European Journal of Palliative Care* 7(2) 60–2.

Hughes, J. and Vaughan, J. 1989: Counselling for carers, real or imaginary? *Nursing Standard* 32(3), 20–1.

Jones, A. 1999: The use of guided imagery as a mourning intervention. *International Journal of Palliative Nursing* 5(4), 196–201.

Kübler-Ross, E. 1970: *On death and dying.* London: Tavistock.

Lazarus, R. and Folkman, S. 1984: Stress appraisal and coping. New York: Springer.

Lewis, A.E. 1999: Reducing burnout: development of an oncology staff bereavement programme. *Oncology Nursing Forum* **26**(6), 1065–9.

Lewis, C.S. 1991: *A grief observed*. London: Faber & Faber.

Mathers, J. 1976: A healthy society? In Sutherland, I. (ed.) *Health education: perspectives and choices*. London: Allen & Unwin.

Miller, B. and McGown, A. 1997: Bereavement: theoretical perspectives and adaptation: Canberra, Australia. *American Journal of Hospice and Palliative Care* **14**(4), 157–77.

Munro, R. 2000: Post-trauma counselling may do nurses 'more harm than good'. *Nursing Times* **96**(2), 10.

Nichols, K. and Jenkinson, J. 1992: *Leading a support group*. London: Chapman & Hall.

Owen, R. 2000: Relieving stress in palliative care staff. *Palliative Care Today* **9**(1), 4–5.

Parkes, C.M. 1996: *Bereavement: studies of grief in adult life*, 3rd edn. London: Penguin, Routledge.

Parkes, C.M. 1998: Bereavement in adult life. *British Medical Journal* **316**, 856–9.

Parkes, C.M. 1999: Coping with loss: consequences and implications for care. *International Journal of Palliative Nursing* **5**(5), 250–4.

Parkes, C.M. and Weiss, R. 1995: *Recovery from bereavement*, 2nd edn. New Jersey: Jason Aronson.

Parkes, C.M., Relf, M. and Couldrick, A. 1996: *Counselling in terminal care and bereavement*. London: BPS Books.

Penson, J. 2000: A hope is not a promise: fostering hope within palliative care. *International Journal of Palliative Nursing* **6**(2), 94–8.

Pert, C. 1998: *Molecules of emotion: why you feel the way you feel*. London: Simon & Schuster.

Ricketts, T. 1995: Grief: a cognitive-behavioural perspective. *British Journal of Nursing* **4**(17), 992–7.

Salka, S. 1997: Enlisting the unconscious mind as an ally in grief therapy. *Hospice Journal* **12**(3), 17–31.

Sanders, C.M. 1989: *Grief: the mourning after – dealing with adult bereavement*. New York: John Wiley.

Solari-Twadell, P.A., Schmidt Bunkers, S., Wang, C. and Snyder, D. 1995: The pinwheel model of bereavement. *Image* **27**(4), 323–6.

Wakefield, A. 2000: Nurses' responses to death and dying: a need for relentless self-care. *International Journal of Palliative Nursing* **6**(5), 245–50.

Worden, W.J. 1992: *Grief counselling and grief therapy* 2nd edn. London: Tavistock.

FURTHER READING

Ironside, V. 1996: *'You'll get over it': the rage of bereavement*. Harmondsworth: Penguin.

Parkes, C.M. 1998: Bereavement. In: Doyle, D., Hanks, G. and MacDonald, N. (eds) *Oxford textbook of palliative medicine*, 2nd edn. Oxford: Oxford Medical Publications.

Penson, J. 2000: Bereavement. In Cooper, J. (ed.) *Stepping into palliative care*. Abingdon: Radcliffe Medical Press.

Riches, G. and Dawson, P. 2000: *An intimate loneliness: supporting bereaved parents and siblings*. Buckingham: Open University Press.

USEFUL ADDRESSES

Bereavement Care (International journal for those helping bereaved people)
Cruse Bereavement Care
126 Sheen Road,
Richmond
Surrey TW9 1UR
Tel: 020 8940 4818

Bereavement Research Forum
The Linda Machin Rooms
The Dudson Centre
Hope Street
Hanley
Stoke-on-Trent ST1 5DD
Tel: 01782 683155
(A multi-professional group for networking)

National Association of Bereavement Services
20 Norton Folgate
London E1 6DB
Tel: 020 7247 1080
(Support for those providing bereavement services)

National Association for Staff Support (NASS)
9 Caradon Close
Woking
Surrey GU21 3DU
(Support for staff within the health-care services)

Sacred Space Foundation
Ravenscroft
Renwick
Cumbria CA10 1JL
Tel: 01768 898874
(Support and retreats for nurses)

Part 3

PALLIATIVE NURSING: A UNIQUE CONTRIBUTION

chapter 13

PALLIATIVE NURSING

Kerry Macnish

Suffering is an ineradicable part of life, even as fate and death. Without suffering and death human life cannot be complete.

Frankl (1987)

This chapter offers a reflection on the role of the palliative nurse caring for adult patients and their family or carers. It is written in a bid to assist and support nurses' understanding in this exacting and demanding role, one that can also bring great joy and satisfaction.

Death and dying are clearly not new events. At the turn of the twenty-first century, caring for the dying was essentially commonplace within nursing (Nebauer et al., 1996), although palliative nursing as a distinct speciality had emerged only within the past few decades. This chapter begins by looking at some recent and relevant developments within palliative care, particularly in the UK, in order to assist our current understanding of the definitions, concepts and roles that influence palliative nursing.

Palliative nursing is explored using chosen, available benchmark studies and narrative literature, but it must be said that there is a distinct paucity of research on the role of the palliative nurse, particularly in the UK. Therefore, a model produced in Canada by Davies and Oberle (1990) is chosen to illustrate the role as it arguably encapsulates much of the clinical work of the palliative nurse. The model provides the significant focal point for further exploration within the chapter. We will consider mainly the clinical component of the role as this occupies most of the palliative nurse's time (Davies and Oberle, 1990). Educational and research issues for the palliative nurse are also briefly explored. In addition, I have occasionally used illustrations from my own experiences as a practising palliative nurse specialist in palliative care.

There has been rapid expansion and change over the past three decades in hospice and palliative care services. These changes are, both medically and socially, characterized by fluctuations in expectations, responses, economics and priorities, occuring in a society uncomfortable with, yet still surrounded by, loss (National Council for Hospices and Specialist Palliative Care Services [NCHSPCS], 1996a). A tremendous variation has occurred in the range, size and funding of hospice organizations, as well as in the delivery of palliative care within local communities (Clarke, 1993a). Palliative care services cover provision in both community and in-patient settings and may be part of the National Health Service (NHS) or voluntary sector, multi-professional or uni-professional (NCHSPCS, 1995a).

Emerging from locally identified needs, Clarke (1993b) suggests that palliative care has therefore proliferated in a largely unco-ordinated way. If this is true, accounting for individual idiosyncrasies and local practices of palliative nursing may be beyond the remit of this chapter. It is thus important to acknowledge early on that palliative nursing occurs in a wide variety of different general settings, with or without the involvement of specialist palliative care. However, although this chapter will make reference to the main settings in which palliative nursing exists, it focuses particularly on the nurse working within the specialist area of palliative care. It could nevertheless be argued that the following exam-ination of this role could be transferable to nurses working in other contexts. Palliative care is common to all specialities (Graves and Nash, 1992), and most nurses will, at some point in their career or their personal life, be exposed to the realities of loss, grief and death. Each experience, each loss, presents us with the opportunity to learn and grow as unique practitioners.

This chapter exposes just some people's knowledge, personal theory or lived experience of the nature of nursing people who are dying. It is not a blueprint for palliative nursing, but it is hoped that it will stimulate thoughts and ideas that are recognizable within actual practice and assist judgements and inter-ventions that promote ongoing reflections, good practice and research.

PALLIATIVE NURSING – A HISTORICAL PERSPECTIVE

Various authors have documented the historical growth of hospices and the development of palliative care (Clarke, 1993b, 2000; Doyle et al., 1995; Saunders, 1995; Johnston, 1999), but it would be fair to say that the attention on nursing the dying in the UK arose from the inevitable influence of hospices.

St Joseph's Hospice opened in London in 1905, the first so-called 'modern' hospice – St Christopher's Hospice – being established in London in 1967, six decades later (Saunders, 1995). Advances in scientific medicine during the 1960s influenced the social perspectives of death as, in a system designed around cure and rehabilitation, death was viewed as distasteful or even a failure (Clarke, 2000). As such, terminally ill patients were not receiving the quality of care they needed (NCHSPCS, 1996a). Thus, when Dame Cicely Saunders, a trained nurse, social worker and doctor, opened the first in-patient unit at St Christopher's, it was created outside mainstream medicine in a bid to prevent what she later termed 'unrelieved death' (Saunders, 1995).

On the other side of the Atlantic, the pioneering doctor Elizabeth Kübler-Ross published her seminal work *On Death and Dying* in 1969. Her perspective of death as being an opportunity to find hope and resolution established what Clarke (2000) refers to as a 'new discourse' on terminal care. Care that fostered dignity for the dying and promoted an exploration of the meaning of death became prevalent. Kübler-Ross (1970) developed a theory on the five stages of dying based on the coping styles of her patients. This became renowned and remains popular (Levine, 1988), although it has received some criticism (Buckman, 1995; Copp, 1999), including setting the precedence of a biomedical perspective, which contends that there are normal and abnormal grief reactions (Mulhall, 1996). Appraising Kübler-Ross' theory, Buckman (1995) suggests that the emotional responses of the dying patient should be viewed as a mosaic, or palette, of emotions unique to each individual. He adds common emotional responses such as fear, guilt, hope, despair and the use of humour to the model and suggests a new three-stage model in which progress can be made not by changing the nature of emotions, but by the resolution of resolvable elements of expressed emotions (Buckman, 1995).

From the outset, hospice care emphasized high professional standards in clinical care as well as in research, evaluation, education and training (NCHSPCS, 1996a). Rebelling against attitudes and practices that embodied phrases such as 'there is nothing we can do for you' (Clarke, 2000), hospices aimed to specialize in providing excellence in terminal care for those dying of cancer, facilitating the quality rather than the quantity of life (Saunders, 1985, 1987). This involved a growing recognition of the importance of patients' physical, emotional, social and spiritual needs and of addressing any associated distress. Family and carers' needs were specifically incorporated within this framework, as illustrated by Parkes et al.'s (1969) research into bereavement and the provision of supportive care for families after the death of their loved one.

In order to achieve this, hospice teams frequently comprise chaplains, social workers and volunteers as well as nurses and doctors. It seems clear that the modern hospice movement was founded on a model of care that was holistic, one that embodied collaborative multi-disciplinary working. Hospice care increasingly became not just a reference to a specific building or service but instead a philosophy of care. It is this emphasis on the individualized, total care of patients and families by professional and lay hospice workers that has generated the success of hospice care (Copp, 1999) and inspired considerable professional and public support (NCHSPCS, 1995a).

With the establishment of hospices, the contribution of nurses received particular attention. Hospice nursing not only aimed to relieve the distress and symptoms of the dying, but also actively encouraged nurses to build relationships with the dying person and his or her family. Comforting, caring and family care were dominant themes within the palliative nursing literature (Degner et al., 1991), with explicit emphasis on the importance of 'being' with someone as well as 'doing' for them exemplifying caring in hospice nursing. Nurses welcomed this perceived approach to caring, which provided some with an incentive to leave more traditional nursing roles to seek hospice work (Dobratz, 1990). It could be argued that many of the characteristics of hospice nursing are reflected in the work on caring by Leininger (1988) and Watson (1979). The portrayal of the hospice nurse as caring and nurturing is a powerful image exemplified through national advertising campaigns for Macmillan Cancer Relief and the Marie Curie Foundation.

Despite establishing a wide reputation for excellence in the care of the dying, hospices were not without criticism (Harris, 1991; Douglas, 1992). Most lacked scientific evaluation and cared exclusively for those with cancer, few developing links with NHS services or universities (NCHSPCS, 1996a). Hospice terminology itself can be criticized as 'terminal care' appears insensitive, blunt and too narrowly confined to the last days of life (Ahmedzai, 1993; Fisher, 1995). This raises an important point as many people today still believe that hospice care, and thus hospice nurses, are synonymous with imminent death and that hospices are merely places where people go to die. Indeed, there remains a high degree of association between terminal and palliative care, even for community and hospital doctors and nurses (Lowden, 1998).

The term 'palliative care' has therefore been adopted over the past decade or so, although the debate surrounding where palliative care begins is currently highly topical. Palliative medicine became recognized as a medical speciality in 1998, acknowledging the role that doctors have in the study and practice of those with advanced progressive incurable disease (Gilbert, 1996). The Royal College of Nursing (RCN) Palliative Nursing Group (now Forum), set up in 1989, was the first to use the term 'palliative nursing' (Johnston, 1999). Now one of the largest RCN forums, it represents nearly six thousand members (Bridge, 2000). Since then, opportunities for nurses to undertake further study in palliative nursing have progressed from English National Board courses numbers 931 and 285 to include specialist diploma, undergraduate and postgraduate courses throughout the UK.

The year 1991 saw the inception of the National Council for Hospices and Specialist Palliative Care Services (NCHSPCS), an umbrella organization bringing together palliative care workers from the NHS, the voluntary and charitable services, and the professional organizations (NCHSPCS, 1996a).

DEFINITIONS

PALLIATIVE CARE

In 1990, the World Health Organization formed a definition of palliative care that is now widely accepted.

> Palliative care is the active total care of patients whose disease is not responsive to curative treatment. Control of pain, of other symptoms, and of psychological, social and spiritual problems is paramount. The goal of palliative care is the achievement of the best possible quality of life for patients and their families.
>
> Palliative care:
>
> • Affirms life and regards dying as a normal process.
> • Neither hastens nor postpones death.
> • Offers a support system to help patients live as actively as possible until death.
> • Offers a support system to help those close to the patient cope both during the patient's illness and in their own bereavement.

The National Association of Health Authorities and Trusts (NAHAT, 1991) then defined terminal illness as 'active and progressive disease for which curative treatment is not possible, or not appropriate, and from which death can reasonably be expected within twelve months'. Terminal care is therefore incorporated within palliative care. It generally refers to the management of patients in their last few days, weeks or months of life when a progressive state of decline is apparent (NCHSPCS, 1995a).

The NCHSPCS (1995) produced a paper aiming to clarify and distinguish the approaches, attitudes and services involved in palliative care. This asserts that half of all deaths in the UK are anticipated and that these patients have the right to receive palliative care appropriate to their needs. The report identifies the fundamental concept of a palliative care approach, which aims to promote physical and psychological well-being for all those who are dying. This should be provided by all health practitioners and is fundamental to generalist care.

THE PALLIATIVE CARE APPROACH

This is a vital, central feature of all good practice, whatever the illness or its stage, and follows patients wherever they may be. Care is tailored to meet the patients' and carers' constantly changing needs. The key principles are:

- a focus on quality of life, which includes good symptom control;
- a whole-person approach, taking into account the person's past life experience and current situation;
- care that encompasses both the dying person and those who matter to that person;
- a respect for patient autonomy and choice;
- an emphasis on open and sensitive communication, which extends to patients, informal carers and professional colleagues.

NCHSPCS, 1995a

PALLIATIVE PROCEDURES

Palliative procedures and techniques are important adjuncts to palliative care; these include counselling, radiotherapy, chemotherapy and surgical procedures such as stent insertion, tumour debulking and creating stomas. These are undertaken by specialists from disciplines other than palliative medicine (NCHSPCS, 1996a).

SPECIALIST PALLIATIVE CARE

Specialist palliative care is provided by services that have palliative care as their core speciality, these serving a significant minority of people whose death is anticipated (NCHSPCS, 1995a). Care is provided by a multi-professional team that has undergone recognized specialist palliative care training and possesses a broad mix of skills. Practitioners skilled in medicine, nursing, pastoral and spiritual care, social work, physiotherapy and occupational therapy, pharmacy and other related specialities support patients and families with progressive disease and a limited prognosis (NCHSPCS, 1999). Access to specialist palliative services should be based on need rather than life expectancy (Lowden, 1998).

The characteristics of a specialist service are outlined elsewhere (NCHSPCS, 1995b) but further include the provision of recognized bereavement support, volunteer service, education and training opportunities, staff support, quality assurance, audit and research programmes (NCHSPCS, 1995a). The services are staffed to support primary health-care teams and generalist hospitals providing advice, home-care teams, day care, hospice-at-home, hospital support teams and in-patient units (NCHSPCS, 1995a, 1999).

Palliative care nurses recently added to the definition of specialist palliative care, stating that it is grounded in moral and ethical principles and is available in a diversity of settings taking account of cultural needs. It is inclusive and does not discriminate on grounds of age, gender, ethnicity, social class or diagnosis (Royal College of Nursing Palliative Nursing Group, 2000). Figure 13.1 represents the provision of palliative care for patients and those who matter to them.

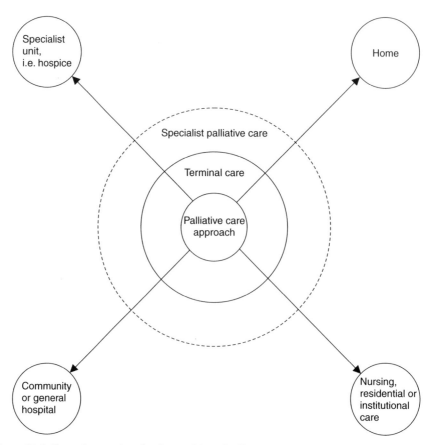

Figure 13.1 The various settings for the provision of palliative care

DESCRIPTIONS OF PALLIATIVE NURSING

Supporting individuals who are dying is a very difficult task requiring a range of skills and qualities, including flexibility, motivation, knowledge, sensitivity, confidence, competence and an ability to be rational and critical in care delivery (Durgahee, 1996). Research into the palliative nursing role is, however, sparse. Readily available literature examining the role varies from descriptive or anecdotal articles and books to a small, albeit growing, number of studies varying in their methodological rigour and quality. Perspectives, anecdotes and research findings on all aspects of palliative care are offered through peer-reviewed journals specific to multi-disciplinary palliative care, palliative medicine and palliative nursing.

The palliative nursing role has been studied using a variety of research methodologies, research into palliative nursing being most frequently viewed from the perspective of the palliative nurse. Some studies question other health-care workers, for example general practitioners or community nurses, about their perceptions of palliative nurses, or elicit the views of the bereaved carer. Only a small body of research directly involves patients and/or carers.

There are clearly practical difficulties in researching the dying: for example, recruiting very ill patients into studies often leads to a poor response rate. The methodological and ethical issues of palliative care research are examined elsewhere by Corner (1996) and Wilson-Barnet and Richardson (1995), but the resulting paucity of studies could affect our understanding of the palliative nurse role. There are no studies examining the role of the nurse working in the hospice setting in the UK (Johnston, 1999). Even in the USA, the majority of hospice care is represented by studies examining community models in which palliative care is delivered in the home setting (Dobratz, 1990). The palliative nursing role to be described in this chapter is largely that of the nurse specializing in palliative care as this appears to have received the most attention in the literature, a small number of studies in both the UK and USA focusing on this role and its development.

One literature review of palliative care in the USA (Dobratz, 1990) describes palliative nursing as 'intensive caring, collaborative sharing, continuous knowing and continuous giving':

- Intensive caring is the management of the physical, psychological, social and spiritual problems of the dying person and his or her family.
- Collaborative sharing refers to the co-ordination of hospice services and collaboration with other colleagues involved in care.
- Continuous knowing recognizes the skills and knowledge required of a hospice nurse in communicating, managing, instructing and caring.
- Continuous giving balances the complexities and intensities of death and dying with the nurse's own self-care needs.

This offers a general view of some main aims of palliative nursing and indicates certain skills or competencies, but it does not account for how the nurse achieves these and what influences nursing interventions.

One Canadian study begins to address the poor understanding of what constitutes expert nursing practice in the care of the dying. Degner et al. (1991) interviewed 10 nurse educators and 10 experienced palliative nurses who were asked to describe situations in which both qualified and student nurses displayed very positive and very negative attitudes to care of the dying. Their findings offer a descriptions of seven positive and negative nursing behaviours that are deemed critical in palliative nursing:

1 responding during the death scene
2 providing comfort
3 responding to anger
4 enhancing personal growth
5 responding to colleagues
6 enhancing the quality of life during dying
7 responding to the family.

Although this small and limited study may not be generalizable to other counties and other settings, especially as it represents the views of only two groups – educators and nurses – it does, however, begin to describe nursing actions and possibly a framework for caring for dying people.

One of the strengths of Degner et al.'s study lies in describing negative nursing behaviours as much of the literature focuses on positive ones, which may not always be reflected in real-life situations. For example, positive nursing behaviours when responding during the death scene include the nurse informing and involving family members and maintaining a sense of calm. Negative behaviour occurs when the nurse shows a fear and horror of the situation, increasing the anxiety of those involved.

In the UK, Cox et al. (1993) used a critical incident technique in their small study to explore the perceptions of 8 patients, 5 carers, 2 general practitioners and 5 district nurses of Macmillan nurses' care. Each respondent was interviewed and asked to recall a meaningful event or happening that encapsulated the effectiveness, or otherwise, of the specialist nurse. A variation in findings arose from the different groups of respondents, but there was an overall positive appreciation in areas such as the provision of psychological and emotional support, specialist knowledge in terminal care and liaison skills. Patients and carers also placed a high value on having time to talk with the nurse, who was viewed as being available and providing continuity of care for patient and carer in a friendly, informal manner. District nurses and general practitioners also valued a flexible, accessible service that integrated service provision and the opportunities for formal teaching and education that the nurses could offer.

In 1992, Graves and Nash adapted a checklist developed from previous research, also to examine the working patterns of Macmillan nurses. Nine nurses each purposively sampled six patients and completed 132 checklists, one for each visit. The analysis of the data revealed information such as the frequency of visits and the amount of time spent by the nurses with patients and carers and in liaison with other health-care workers. Although the checklist provided some useful information, the study identified limitations in using a checklist to examine the purpose and effectiveness of the nursing visits (Graves and Nash, 1992). Although such descriptive research methods are essential to knowledge development (Polit and Hungler, 1995) as they describe facts concerning situations, people and activities, the checklist method does not assist understanding the experiences of the palliative nurse. This may account for the lack of in-depth examination of the content of the visits and the role of the Macmillan nurses in this study.

Arguably one of the most important studies in this area also arose out of a dissatisfaction with using statistical information to capture and describe the role of the supportive nurse in palliative care. Betty Davies and Kathleen Oberle, two Canadian nurse researchers, examined solely the clinical aspect of one palliative liaison nurse working in the hospital and community. This was significant as, for the first time, research aimed deeply to explore and analyse the nurse specialist's clinical interventions and to identify coping strategies to deal with the stress inherent in the role. The previous investigation of stress in hospice workers had identified that stress arises more from work and occupational issues such as staff conflict and job–home interactions than it does from working with dying patients and their families (Vachon, 1987).

Davies and Oberle (1990) used a qualitative grounded theory approach to investigate the palliative nurse role. Using open-ended interviews, one nurse recalled 20 cases, in 10 of which she has shared a good relationship with the patient and family and in 10 of which the relationship had been difficult. Four other palliative nurses then validated the resulting themes, the model of supportive care pictured in Figure 13.2 thus being generated (Davies and Oberle, 1990).

Before exploring the model in detail, it is important to note some limitations of the study. It can be criticized for reflecting only the views of one nurse and her practice within a North American setting, the authors noting that further research with nurses in other settings and other cultures needed to be undertaken in order to determine the applicability of the findings. The methodology used acknowledges however, that the validity of the phenomenon can be measured by the extent to which it 'rings true' with other people's experiences (Polit and Hungler, 1995). In other words, it may be meaningful to others in different contexts (Carr, 1994). This may explain the impact of the study in the UK, where it is studied during some higher education palliative nursing courses, such as that at the Institute of Cancer Research at the Royal Marsden NHS Trust.

Building on the work of Davies and Oberle (1990), a further Canadian study by McWilliam et al. (1993) also examined the experiences of two palliative nurses working within a support team. Using a phenomenological approach, the nurses' audiotaped reflections of their nursing experiences over 1 year were followed by in-depth interviews. The findings are consistent with the model produced by Davies and Oberle (1990), and the authors extend the model (Figure 13.3), illustrating factors that facilitate or impede the nurses' functioning. They identify everyday fundamental work experiences as the 'primary work effort', which, if impeded, demands that the nurse finds ways of overcoming the difficulties

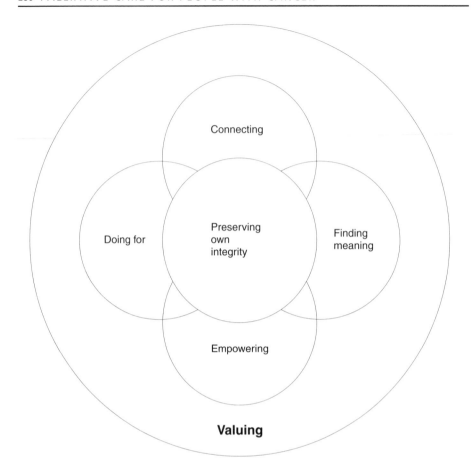

Figure 13.2 Dimensions of the nurse's supportive role (Davies and Oberle, 1990)

Valuing
- Global
- Particular

Preserving integrity
- Looking inward
- Valuing self
- Acknowledging own reaction

Finding meaning
- Focusing on living
- Acknowledging death

Connecting
- Making the connection
  - Establishing credentials
  - Explaining role(s)
  - Getting base line information
  - Explaining how to contact nurse
  - Establishing rapport
- Sustaining the connection
  - Being available
  - Spending time
  - Sharing secrets
  - Giving of self
- Breaking the connection

Empowering
- Facilitating
- Encouraging
- Defusing
- Mending
- Giving information

Doing for
- Taking charge
  - Controlling pain and symptoms
  - Making arrangements
  - Lending a hand
- Team playing

involved. This is described as 'secondary work effort', in which role adaptation and the management of intrapersonal and interprofessional conflicts occur (McWilliam et al., 1993).

A further attempt to address some methodological issues of Davies and Oberle's (1990) research was made by Davis (1995), who replicated the study in the UK

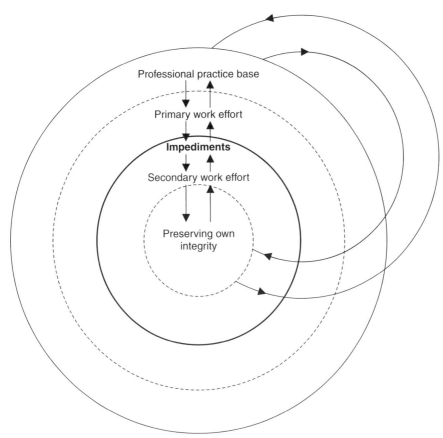

I.   Preserving own integrity
II. Professional practice base
     A. Values
     B. Motives
     C. Expectations
III. Primary work effort
     A. Supportive care to patients and families
          1. Connecting
          2. Empowering
          3. Doing for
          4. Finding meaning
     B. Facilitating the work of other professionals
          1. Supporting
          2. Co-ordinating
          3. Managing
IV. Impediments to preserving own integrity in the primary work effort of palliative care
     support-team nursing
     A. Limitations of the system
     B. Intrapersonal conflict
     C. Interprofessional conflict
     D. Characteristics of palliative care
V.   Secondary work effort
     A. Role adaptation
     B. Intrapersonal conflict management
     C. Interprofessional conflict management

Figure 13.3 Dimensions of the experience of palliative care support – Team Nursing (Mc William et al., 1993)

with five clinical palliative nurse specialists working in hospital/community posts in central London. This unpublished study confirmed that Davies and Oberle's (1990) supportive dimensions are transferable to a UK context, but it also broadened the dimensions, adding to the understanding of this complex role.

Finally, the findings from a study of 15 Australian palliative nurses by Taylor et al. (1997) appear to mirror many of the dimensions of both Davies and Oberle (1990) and McWilliam et al. (1993). Using another qualitative method, story-telling, the nurses describe cases in which they felt they had, or had not, made a difference by their care of patients and families. Both the nature and the effects of palliative nursing are then described.

In light of this support for the model, it has been chosen for further description and exploration using other literature to support, clarify, question and illustrate palliative nursing practice. It should, however, be noted that it may not entirely capture the essence of palliative nursing as Copp (1999) argues that the work of others such as James (1986) and Smith (1992) may also be worthy of doing. Indeed, Copp's (1999) own 4-year research provides further useful insight into the experiences of nurses caring for dying cancer patients.

The Davies and Oberle (1990) model, or theoretical framework, consists of six dimensions: 'valuing', 'preserving own integrity', 'connecting', 'empowering' 'doing for', and 'finding meaning'. Although these dimensions are discrete, they are also interrelated, and progression through the dimensions can be sequential: the nurse has, for example, to connect with the patient before she can empower the patient. Although all are vital to the support process, some dimensions (e.g. doing for) are more task orientated and others (e.g. valuing) more attitudinal (Davies and Oberle, 1990).

VALUING

Valuing can be thought of as the contextual dimension in which support occurs (Oberle and Davies, 1992). This involves nurses' attitudes towards and beliefs in the worth of those they care for, and it is fundamental to the other dimensions of support. Two types of valuing are described (see Figure 13.2 above). 'Global valuing' acknowledges the innate worth of human beings regardless of their individual characteristics, whereas 'particular valuing' refers to the nurse's respect for the unique characteristics and abilities of each individual (Davies and Oberle, 1990).

The dimension of valuing has similarities to what Carl Rogers (1967) calls 'unconditional positive regard'. This involves having a total respect for others and suspending one's judgement on people. Heron (1990) also endorses the humanity behind valuing others, believing that 'helping arises from the grace within the human spirit'. Identifying valuing as a discrete dimension raises an important point as it acknowledges the individuality of nurses, with their own personal values and beliefs, hence supporting Martocchio's (1987) statement that one cannot separate the nurse as professional from the nurse as person.

Valuing others may not necessarily be gained through professional education as it is clearly difficult to teach attitudes and values. One could argue that the concept of valuing may predestine people to become nurses as, without a belief that people as patients are worthy, it is difficult to imagine care occurring. This is perhaps best illustrated by conceiving nursing care devoid of valuing others, in which neglect, ignorance and abuse would be evident.

Although Davies and Oberle (1990) state that valuing involves an attitude or 'mind-set', a person's values and beliefs are, however, more than just an attitude as they are displayed through one's behaviours (Burnard, 1995). People's thinking influences how they act, and how they act influences how they think (Egan, 1990), thus affecting the relationship between nurse and patient. Hopper (2000) supports this and suggests that nurses' conduct, what they do, how they do it and importantly why they do it all contribute to understanding what it means to be a palliative care worker. Certainly, Hockley (1989) finds that nurses' behaviours are linked to their own perceptions of the dying patient's problems.

Two studies illustrate the significance of valuing for the nursing relationship. In her examination of 14 terminally ill patients, Raudonis (1993) describes how patients feel 'affirmed as an individual, a person of value', which is experienced as an empathetic relationship with the hospice nurse. As in Davies and Oberle's work, this empathizing is integral to helping, forming the foundation of a supportive relationship. Nurses displaying negative nursing behaviour such as ignoring patients' attempts to gain information about dying or spiritual issues are, however, viewed by nurses as being disrespectful to the patient (Degner et al., 1991). This could indicate nursing behaviour that does not value patients.

The link between thoughts and behaviour is clear, but what remains undetermined is the extent to which nurses can support when valuing is compromised. What the model fails to address are the potential difficulties for nurses in this situation. This is raised by nurses in Davis's (1995) study, which identifies intrinsic and extrinsic factors that influence or undermine the nurse's intent to value. These UK palliative nurses believed that an obvious tension could arise if the patient's values conflicted with those of the nurse (Davis, 1995). Particular valuing is clearly more difficult if the nurse dislikes the patient, this threatening the supportive relationship. Encountering the disliked patient and managing difficult relationships is discussed by Liaschenko (1994), and is recognized within counselling relationships (Mearns and Thorne, 1988), but it remains poorly explored within palliative nursing. The relationship between liking and valuing is therefore unclear.

At other times, the limitations on health and social services resources in the UK threaten operational valuing, for example if the patient desires a home death yet the nurse knows that this is not practically viable (Davis, 1995). This presents difficulties for the nurse in continuing to provide support, especially if the nurse takes on an advocacy role, for example representing a patient's interest at case meetings. Some palliative nurses view acting as an advocate as an important role aspect (Taylor et al., 1997), which clearly suggests another dilemma for the nurse in supporting. Davies and Oberle do not discuss the potential difficulties for the nurse valuing the patient.

PRESERVING OWN INTEGRITY

This dimension also acknowledges the nurse as a person and, because it is fundamental to the nurse functioning effectively, is the core concept of the Davies and Oberle's (1990) model and ultimately the goal of nursing care (Davies, 1992). In other words, the nurse must be satisfied that he or she is doing the right things for the right reasons (Davies, 1992). The nurse maintains energy by using different strategies, including distancing oneself in order to regain control, using humour and hiding or sharing personal feelings (Davies and Oberle, 1990).

This dimension has three components: 'looking inward', 'valuing self' and 'acknowledging own reaction' (see Figure 13.2). In *'looking inward'*, nurses reflect on and examine their own values and basic beliefs about the world and their philosophy of palliative nursing. Inner strength or energy arises from a number of sources, for example the nurse's spirituality or faith (Davies and Oberle, 1990). Faith and family or colleague support are essential to managing any internal conflict and preserving integrity (McWilliam et al., 1993; Taylor et al., 1997).

'Valuing self' involves the maintenance of feelings of self-worth and self-esteem (Davies and Oberle, 1990). A reinforcement of nurses' wholeness may come from within themselves or from others who acknowledge their worth, for example patients, carers and colleagues. An intrinsic knowledge and valuing of oneself may take considerable courage and time to achieve (Egan, 1990; Burnard, 1995), but there is value in being self-aware as those nurses with a strong sense of worth are more likely to act genuinely, authentically and thus therapeutically (Heron, 1990; Burnard, 1995). This is demonstrated by Wilkinson (1991), whose study reveals that those nurses who are less self-aware are more likely to block effective communication with cancer patients.

The final component, that of *'acknowledging own reaction'*, includes nurses' continual self-assessment and appraisal through examining their own behaviours, feelings, reactions and needs (Davies and Oberle, 1990). This again involves nurses being honest with themselves, learning from mistakes, identifying personal strategies and accepting, for example, their own reaction to grief and loss. The nurses in Davis's (1995) study also describe recognizing their own personal limitations without reproach in order to remain well. Indeed, McWilliam et al. (1993) acknowledge that preserving integrity involves an active, concerted effort on the part of the nurse. They suggest that work effort may involve role adaptation, which could require nurses to modify their expectations and consciously forfeit control in order to remain fulfilled and work effectively with others. The effect of day-to-day contact with the dying may exact an emotional toll on palliative nurses (Dobratz, 1990; Copp, 1999), and although this is explored in more detail by Smith (1992), information on how nurses cope with this aspect is still lacking (Copp, 1999).

Other nursing strategies that help to preserve integrity include making telephone contact outside work, attending case discussions, supervision and debriefing opportunities within work (McWilliam et al., 1993; Davis, 1995).

Although Davies and Oberle (1990) are not explicit about the idea of reflective practice, they suggest that a perspective may be maintained through questioning and identifying feelings associated with situations so that the nurse can then use these insights to set boundaries that will help to preserve integrity. It could be argued that this process of developing and managing self-awareness is indicative of reflective practice as the process of reflection internally examines and explores the nurse's experience. Indeed, McWilliam et al. (1993) state that preserving integrity is achieved through a continuous process of reflecting on personal values, motives and expectations as these comprise professional practice and shape experience.

Reflective learning creates and clarifies meaning in terms of oneself, thereby leading to greater understanding and appreciation in a relationship (Von Klitzing, 1999). Although reflective practice is covered more thoroughly in Chapter 14, the potential for reflection to assist congruent, authentic practice cannot be underestimated. Reflection allows for an assessment of the implications and consequences of actions and beliefs, as well as of the underlying rationale for practice (Goodman, 1984). If, as Copp (1999) suggests, much of palliative nursing knowledge is implicit, this is of particular relevance for palliative nursing, because reflective practice can reveal the hidden aspects of real-life nursing, what Schön (1991) refers to as the 'swampy lowlands' of practice, which may not yet be exposed in the work of the palliative nurse.

CONNECTING

The next dimension is connecting, which involves establishing, maintaining and finishing a relationship. Davies and Oberle (1990) describe this as 'getting in touch with, and getting to know' the patient and family members in order to establish and develop a trusting relationship. Making connections and building relationships are also strong themes in Taylor et al.'s (1997) study.

Connecting has three components, as shown in Figure 13.2. The first, '*making the connection*', establishes the nurse's role through giving information and explanation, often at the initial referral (Davis, 1995). In addition, the nurse aims to 'establish rapport' by 'finding commonality' with the patient and family. Davies and Oberle (1990) cite an example in which the nurse expends considerable effort in establishing a connection with one patient, visiting him several times in hospital and at home. This indicates that active effort and time spent connecting is deemed worthwhile to the nurse.

'*Sustaining the connection*' is concerned with maintaining the trusting relationship. Strategies include 'being available' to respond when needed, either by telephone or in person at any hour of the day or night, and in 'spending time' with the patient and family (Davies and Oberle, 1990). Further strategies acknowledge the role of the nurse as confidant, patients 'sharing secrets' with the nurse, for example talking about feelings and fears they feel unable to express with their family. Similarly, the nurse may also share feelings with the family by crying and laughing with them. This 'giving of self' is viewed as integral to sustaining the connection (Davies and Oberle, 1990).

Finally, with the death of the patient, the process of *'breaking the connection'* begins. This important insight has received little research attention in palliative nursing. Even though the nurse may attend the funeral, the nurse's contacts with the family will diminish. Some families, notably ones with whom a stronger connection has been forged, are obviously more difficult to break from (Davies and Oberle, 1990).

Several points that merit further exploration arise from this dimension. Nurses in the UK study demonstrated some difficulties in making the connection (Davis, 1995). One patient who did not speak English required an interpreter, the interpreter in turn facing difficulties in wishing to withhold information about the patient's diagnosis, stating cultural reasons. Another patient with a lengthy previous involvement with health professionals rejected help, limiting contact with the nurse.

The issue of working with different cultures and languages is not evident in Davies and Oberle's (1990) study, yet Mulhall (1996) reminds us that nursing takes place in a complex social and cultural arena and that nurses are bound by their code of conduct to provide care commensurate to the variety of grief reactions encountered in a multi-racial society. She suggests that nurses must develop a wider, not just Westernized, sociological and anthropological view of death (Mulhall, 1996). Therefore, palliative nurses must again gain good insights into other social and cultural aspects of death, suspending their presuppositions, if they are to respond to individual needs (Becker, cited in Mulhall, 1996).

Connection requires considerable patience and perseverance, and may not be straightforward (Davis, 1995), but the continual encounter between the nurse and patient has a deepening effect on the relationship (Copp, 1999). In addition, a link between connecting and preserving integrity is made in that these UK nurses indicated the need to have clear personal and professional boundaries. In the UK, the sharing of self appears to be individual to the nurse and each relationship (Davis, 1995). The extent to which giving oneself affects the relationship is therefore unclear.

The component of breaking the connection also differs with UK nurses. Limited bereavement care is offered by nurses as part of the formal structure of the service, and referral to other services, or perhaps other professionals who offer continued appropriate bereavement support, eases the breaking of the connection (Davis, 1995). This suggests fewer direct or ongoing relationships with the bereaved than are seen with the nurse in the Canadian study. This may be a benefit of working within a multi-disciplinary team as social workers and clergy have an additional and specific understanding of and training in loss (NCHSPCS, 1996b).

Although the follow-up of bereaved people may be haphazard, depending on locally available resources and practice (Penson, 1995), the palliative nurse must clearly have education in and an understanding of theories of loss and grief; this is required in order to assess any adjustment to the loss, encourage the expression of feelings associated with grief and act as an effective resource (Penson,

1995). Equally, nurses must also be sensitive to their own support needs when working with loss and grief on a daily basis. Another study identifies the potential difficulty for nurses of 'closure' with patients, particularly if they have been involved in managing a difficult, prolonged death (Copp, 1999).

Unlike the Canadian study, the UK study revealed that connections were also broken while the patient was still alive (Davis, 1995). This may indicate differences in service provision as UK nurses manage their caseload flexibly, for example by discharging patients whose symptoms may become controlled following their input. This raises a significant point: as well as these studies having been undertaken in different countries, they were also dated 5 years apart, during which time, considerable changes occurred within palliative care and the NHS.

The Standing Medical Advisory Committee and Standing Nursing and Midwifery Advisory Committee report of 1992 recommended the expansion of palliative care services in the UK to include the care and support of patients with non-cancer life-threatening illness and care from an earlier stage in the disease trajectory. Although this move is generally supported (NCHSPCS, 1997), some services may be stretched not only to deal with a growing number of cancer patients, but also to support patients with human immunodeficiency virus, circulatory and respiratory, and other progressive diseases. This could indicate the potential for a different level of direct and indirect intervention for palliative nurses. This may include longer-term, complex interventions as well as con-sultancy or short-term interventions depending on individuals' needs (Royal College of Nursing Palliative Nursing Group, 2000). Within my own palliative care service in Devon, we have adopted a flexible management approach to caseloads. This may involve admitting, discharging and re-referring those patients with a relatively long prognosis and those in remission.

The potential effects on the nurse–patient relationship of this pattern of making and breaking contacts do not appear to have been researched. Interestingly, Davis (1995) notes that breaking connections with patients is viewed as a joint process and may suggest that patients and carers are ready to accept discharge. A recognition of the need to end the relationship, and the manner in which this is achieved, may help nurses to preserve their integrity (Davis, 1995). This, however, requires further study as the emotional leap from a status as a dying patient to one of a survivor poses different challenges (Copp, 1999). Copp suggests that there may be conflicts for some nurses between a desire to continue supporting patients in case they relapse while struggling to resource the support offered.

Instances from personal experience (Case study 13.1) also call into question the impact of team nursing on the process of connection (Case study 13.1). The type of contact described in the case study appears to be unexplored in palliative literature, yet it is clearly important for nurses working in team environments in which caseloads are shared to provide continuity of care around the clock. This may also be relevant to other settings: patient's symptoms in the hospital setting are, for example, sometimes presented as a crisis, requiring urgent intervention from the palliative nurse (Davis, 1995). The link between connecting and doing

CASE STUDY 13.1

One Sunday evening, I was called to a patient and his wife. My colleague had previously visited this elderly gentleman on several occasions, during which a good relationship had developed. On visiting, he appeared in considerable distress, curled up in his bed, sobbing and asking to die, saying that he 'could no longer fight'. His wife, shocked by this sudden change in his outlook and behaviour, was at a loss to know how to help him. I had never met either of them before, and making the connection in such circumstances takes on a different hue. One could envisage that a connection had been made and sustained with the palliative service through visits from my colleague and preparation for emergency cover, which might have had a bearing on my subsequent visit, but my own relationship with this man and his wife nevertheless started in a moment of despair and crisis. There was little time to establish credentials and build rapport, but this apparently stoical, reserved man very quickly talked openly with me of his fears about taking 'too long a time to die' and of 'feeling worthless' as an individual. Both he and his wife appeared more at ease by the end of my long visit, and I felt that a deep connection had been made within a relatively short time.

for may help to establish trust as the credibility of the nurse may be achieved through effective symptom control, explored below.

Other studies have drawn attention to the nurse–patient relationship (Morse, 1991; Ramos, 1992; Copp, 1999). Like Davis (1995), Morse (1991) suggests that the level of the relationship is related to the duration of contact between nurse and patient. A brief, superficial contact involving quick investigations or treatments that are not usually serious or life-threatening is described as a 'clinical relationship' (Morse, 1991) or one involving nurses working at an 'instrumental level' (Ramos, 1992). Here, there is little personal involvement of or investment on the part of the nurse (Morse, 1991; Ramos, 1992). However, once a relationship has developed over time, the nurse may view the patient first as a person and second as a patient, forming a 'connected relationship' (Morse, 1991). Ramos (1992) describes a connected relationship in which a balanced purposeful, emotional and cognitive connection is made with the patient. Although the nurse tries to understand the patient's perspective at this level of relationship, the nurse retains control of the process (Ramos, 1992).

If trust becomes established within a nursing relationship, which could involve the nurse taking on an advocacy role, a 'therapeutic relationship' may develop (Morse, 1991). A deeper emotional and cognitive bond occurs when the patient and nurse mutually reciprocate beyond a superficial level (Ramos, 1992). Reciprocity, time, courage and honesty also feature as fundamental aspects of a close relationship for palliative nurses (Rasmussen et al., 1995). Nurses who are able to relate at a cognitive, emotional and practical level derive the most benefit from their relationships, but not all nurses are able, or choose, to do this (Ramos, 1992). In deciding to become a hospice nurse, there is a hoped-for expectation that the relationships formed with patients will be close ones (Rasmussen et al., 1995).

Finally, an 'overinvolved relationship' occurs when the professional relationship is compromised and the nurse, committed to the patient as a person, overrides decisions and responsibilities made by others involved in caring (Morse, 1991).

There appears to be a strong link between connecting and other dimensions in the supportive model, notably the ability of nurses to connect while preserving their own integrity. Even if relationships are based on compassion, there remains a risk that co-dependency can arise from an intimate relationship (Nebauer et al., 1996).

Connection is clearly a strong and important theme in the relationships that nurses develop with dying patients, leading to, and influencing, other aspects of support such as empowering and finding meaning (Davies and Oberle, 1990). Connecting may not, however, be straightforward but may require considerable energy and skill on the part of the nurse to overcome language barriers and caseload and resource difficulties and to maintain appropriate individual personal boundaries. Both James and Smith (cited in Copp, 1999) identify the emotional and physical labour involved in such caring work. Nevertheless, building, maintaining and leaving relationships with patients and their families may be necessary in order for other aspects of support to occur (Oberle and Davies, 1992), and the relationship may in itself be energizing, rewarding and worthwhile for the nurse.

EMPOWERING

Davies and Oberle (1990) identify empowering as a further dimension in the role of the supportive nurse. This is helping the patient and family to find their own ways of meeting their own needs, drawing on their unique intrinsic resources. It involves the nurse using the less tangible or task-orientated skills of encouraging, facilitating, providing information, mending and defusing (see Figure 13.2 above).

'Facilitating' involves the nurse recognizing and acknowledging individual and family strengths, abilities and limitations by helping, suggesting and planning strategies that enable them to make decisions or encourage them to continue (Davies and Oberle, 1990). An example is cited in which the sister of a patient became estranged as her brother deteriorated. The nurse, recognizing this, telephoned the sister, who stated she could not cope with being in the house watching her brother die and expressed guilt. The nurse suggested that undertaking practical tasks such as shopping, cooking and cleaning might be another way to help, so the sister re-emerged into the caring network.

'Encouraging' refers to situations in which nurses openly support choices, give approval and note special abilities that encourage patients to do what they want (Davies and Oberle, 1990).

'Defusing' involves dealing with negative feelings and is vital to empowering (Davies and Oberle, 1990). The nurse encourages the expression of feelings of anger and guilt, giving permission for others to ventilate and deal with such emotions. The nurse also listens undefensively to those who need to express such feelings (Davies and Oberle, 1990).

'*Mending*' concerns aspects aimed at unifying the family or care-giving group. Overcoming rifts in order to continue care is achieved by helping the proponents to see each other's points of view (Davies and Oberle, 1990). The nurse therefore acts as a kind of mediator.

'*Giving information*' is seen as empowering and is a constant attempt to help others to understand what is happening. This may involve the nurse explaining about changes in a patient's condition or describing tests or medication usage (Davies and Oberle, 1990).

The concept of empowerment has been highlighted and explored in the nursing literature. It is suggested that empowerment brings about positive changes in health through a dynamic process arising from a relationship that values others (Gibson, 1991; Chavasse, 1992; Rodwell, 1996). The importance of giving information, as identified by Davies and Oberle (1990), is consistent with the view of Gibson (1991), who suggests that nurses may empower patients by using teaching and communication skills. The nursing behaviours of facilitating and encouraging described by Davies and Oberle (1990) are empowering and can assist people's capacity for growth and change, helping them to develop and use resources for themselves (Rodwell, 1996). Patients state that 'receiving information' and 'a knowledge of the facts' are among the most helpful nursing-related factors involved in reassuring patients (Fareed, 1996).

Empowerment is 'best understood by its absence: powerlessness, helplessness, hopelessness, alienation, victimisation, subordination, oppression, paternalism, loss of control over one's life and dependency' (Gibson, 1991). In situations involving those whose lives are limited and threatened by illness, it is easy to conceive that empowerment may offer considerable benefit in managing that which remains. However, despite the overtly positive connotations of empowerment referred to in Davies and Oberle's (1990) research, there may also be difficulties.

The first of these, highlighted by Davis (1995), occurs when there is a mismatch between the wishes of the patient and those of the family, carer or palliative nurse. Examples may include disclosing information on the diagnosis when asked to by a patient even though the partner has explicitly requested that the patient should not be told (Davis, 1995). Alternatively, a considerable care package may be required for the dependent patient to be cared for at home, but all care is declined and refused by the patient or carer and thus risks failing (Davis, 1995).

I can recall personal difficulty in empowering when visiting a patient who, despite severe cachexia, pain and vomiting at the very end of her life, continued to request chemotherapy against the oncologist's advice. Although the patient wanted me actively to encourage her decision to continue chemotherapy, I felt that it would not be congruent with my own values and beliefs had I done so; this caused considerable personal distress.

These examples raise many thought-provoking debates as some would argue that, in order truly to empower others, nurses must give up their own power (Gibson, 1991; Malin and Teasdale, 1991; Pyne, 1994). If this is so, nurses may decrease patients' dependence on them for care and support. Hopper (2000) suggests that the life of a professional involves the reconciliation of competing values in choosing the 'higher' good for each individual while recognizing the individual's place in the wider social context.

A further point to raise here is the notion that patients actually wish to determine their care choices and decisions themselves. If the nature of empowerment depends on individual patients, and is defined by them rather than the nurse (Davies and Oberle, 1990), it is also possible that patients may wish to remain passive and dependent, choosing to avoid making decisions for themselves. It may therefore be argued that, although nurses can offer patients the opportunity for self-empowerment, they must recognize that not all patients will accept or wish this. This may also be apparent, for example, if patients feel too ill to take charge of themselves. People's information needs are obviously also variable: although some require a large amount of information, searching the Internet for the latest details on cancer management, others need very little or even none at all.

Defusing is interesting and clearly links with the views of Kübler-Ross (1970) and Buckman (1995) in that the dying person may express feelings of anger and guilt. There is little reference in the palliative nursing literature to help nurses dealing with this normal reaction to anticipated loss. When it is described as part of the role, the experienced palliative nurse is viewed as showing respect and empathy for the anger expressed by the person, understanding that the source of anger or abuse reflects the other person's situation and is not to be taken personally (Degner et al., 1991). Nurses who cry, respond harshly showing frustration and refuse to accept patients' apologies are, however, deemed inexperienced and undeveloped in their philosophical approach to anger management (Degner et al., 1991). This clearly appears to be somewhat simplistic and may even place the nurse at risk in some situations, as although anger may be energizing, it may also be destructive, and physical violence is never acceptable (Sheldon, 1997). Intractable emotional responses and aggressiveness clearly affect palliative nursing work and may make it less satisfying for some (Taylor et al., 1997).

Equally, empowerment through the component of mending may not be possible when family rifts are too entrenched and reconciliation is neither desired nor expected (Davis, 1995; Taylor et al., 1997). This latter point reflects the insight by Gibson (1991) that one cannot empower someone – people can only empower themselves.

Finally, Davies and Oberle (1990) also state that empowerment involves harnessing and building on the intrinsic strengths of the patient and family. In order for nurses to assist the patient in this way, they must first empower themselves (Chavasse, 1992), only then possessing expertise and knowledge that can be passed on to the patient. Again, difficulties may arise when the nurse is unprepared or inexperienced. For example, a less-experienced clinical nurse specialist empowered a patient with motor neurone disease to believe that continuing to be supported at home was possible; when this failed, the patient was angry with the nurse, and the nurse felt that she had betrayed the patient (Davis, 1995).

The concept of empowerment therefore raises potential difficulties for the palliative nurse. Moral and ethical dilemmas of truth-telling and collusion, practical difficulties in terms of care resources and restraints, and the individual's and family preferences to be information-seeking and self-directing all affect the nurse's ability to truly empower. Furthermore, nurses' own abilities in the area of empowerment are tested through experience and attitude, if giving up power is indeed vital to empowerment.

DOING FOR

The dimension 'doing for' illustrated in Figure 13.2 involves the two components of taking charge of situations and negotiating the system for patients and families. It focuses on the physical care of the patient and, unlike empowerment, draws on help that is extrinsic to the patient and family (Davies and Oberle, 1990).

'*Taking charge*' involves the consistent and important aspect of palliative nursing of 'controlling pain and symptoms'. Davies and Oberle (1990) describe how the nurse organizes and administers the appropriate medication to relieve severe pain and teaches the family to give morphine injections. The nurse is also able to provide hands-on care, for example in performing last offices following the patient's death and in dealing with any incontinence or removing catheters. This usually occurs when families can no longer cope. Taking charge also involves 'making arrangements' for the home loan and installation of equipment such as hospital beds (Davies and Oberle, 1990).

The second component of taking charge is that of '*team-playing*'. The nurse often finds herself negotiating the system on behalf of the patient, for example by arranging admission to hospital or a palliative care unit. It also illustrates the liaison aspect of the role in sharing and consulting with other team members on the care of individual patients and families. This could involve mediating between different care-givers and institutions, explaining, encouraging and even pleading on behalf of the patient (Davies and Oberle, 1990).

Davis (1995) finds evidence to support the dimension of doing for in the UK and again also finds distinctions within the dimension. There is strong support for the nurse's role in pain and symptom control. UK nurses describe this as the least time-consuming and least complicated aspect of the role (Davis, 1995). Similarly, others identify that often complex symptom management forms a significant part, or primary activity, of the palliative nurses' role (Dobratz, 1990; Irvine, 1993; Nebauer et al., 1996). In a study of 705 London general practitioners, 96 per cent stated that they would refer patients with difficult symptoms to specialist home-care teams (Boyd, 1995). Similarly, 97 per cent of general practitioners and 100 per cent of community nurses studied in Exeter, UK are aware that help with symptom control is offered by the palliative care service (Seamark et al., 1993).

Although nurses may identify symptom control as a most satisfying part of the role (Davis, 1995), neither this study, nor that of Davies and Oberle (1990), identifies the potential effect on the nurse and patient if the symptoms cannot be successfully controlled. Being unable to help with symptoms is briefly referred to in the findings of a small study of Macmillan nurses by Graves and Nash

(1992). Despite the best efforts by all those involved in caring, I can also recall situations from my own practice in which symptoms such as pain, nausea, breathlessness, anorexia and fatigue remained persistent and unrelieved.

Some of these difficult symptoms have more recently received important research attention, especially in examining non-pharmacological nursing interventions for managing breathlessness (Corner et al., 1995, 1996) and in recognizing and supporting patients complaining of fatigue (Richardson, 1995). Nevertheless, given that others also perceive symptom control to be integral to the role, the effect of a failure to achieve the relief anticipated deserves more research attention. This may be especially pertinent when palliative nurses have high expectations in their desire to relieve all suffering and in generating breakthroughs with patients (McKee, 1995; Taylor et al., 1997). This may cause the individual nurse considerable stress (Vachon, 1987).

Davis (1995) confirms the component of 'making arrangements'. Lending equipment importantly promotes a successful discharge for patients dying at home. In another example, one nurse describes how she helped to arrange a holiday by the seaside for a patient and her husband. This aspect is also demonstrated by Taylor et al. (1997), who describe the loaning or 'stealing' of equipment as being part of the nurse's advocacy role.

Although neither study refers to the nurse helping with the person's financial affairs, making arrangements could also cover obtaining financial help or information. This could involve referral to the local authority social services, social security department or hospice social worker. In my own practice, however, it is common for the nurse to instigate applications for appropriate benefits such as Attendance Allowance, Disability Living Allowance or charity grants. The nurse must certainly have an awareness of the implications of life-threatening illness on the finances of an individual or a family, and have a knowledge and understanding of the benefit system and the organizations that can offer advice or financial aid.

One difference between Davies and Oberle's (1990) study and that of Davis (1995) in 'doing for' arises in the aspect 'lending a hand'. The UK nurses did not describe hands-on care except in one instance where a nurse helped to lay out a body (Davis, 1995). Indeed, they described strong demarcations between themselves and the community and hospital nursing teams or volunteers in assisting patients with physical care. This is reflected in my own practice, as like the nurses in Davis's (1995) study, hands-on nursing care is not part of my job description. This finding could suggest differences in the interpretation of the clinical nurse specialist role in different countries or within different services.

Although the clinical nurse specialism is not explored in any depth in this chapter, it is relevant to illustrate areas that can influence the understanding and practice of palliative nursing. Such practitioners first being used in the USA in the early 1960s, Davis (1995) states that clinical nurse specialists are prepared at a high level for a particular area of clinical nursing. In the UK, the model for the palliative clinical nurse specialist was strongly influenced and developed by the charity Cancer Relief Macmillan Fund (now Macmillan Cancer Relief) (Johnston, 1999). In 1975, the first Macmillan home-care service began, resulting in a steady increase in the number of nursing posts throughout the UK, initially funded in the main by the charity. Indeed, Davis (1995) notes that the appeal of the clinical nurse specialist in this field is so influential that palliative nurses now form the largest group of nurse specialists in the UK. There are about 1800 Macmillan nurses in the UK working for different national and local charities and NHS Trusts in hospitals and in the community (Hospice Information Service, 2000).

Descriptions of the palliative clinical nurse specialist role appear in the literature, most of which identify the advisory, complementary, educational or resource nature of the role (Sloan and Grant, 1989; Nash, 1990; Graves and Nash, 1992; Johnston, 1999). Clinical nurse specialists use their expertise in helping generalist colleagues with particular clinical situations (Graves and Nash, 1992), acting more as a resource for others and ensuring that the skills, knowledge and expertise of palliative care are widely available (Webber, 1994). This is illustrated by Bullen's (1995) description and interpretation of her role as a clinical nurse specialist in palliative care, in which she identifies six aspects of her role.

The first, 'professionalism', is described as having legal and moral account-ability, responsibility and autonomy. The clinical nurse specialist collaborates with others, utilizing palliative care knowledge and practice for all patients. He or she also has a critical role in 'providing a challenge' and 'providing a structured approach to care' for other professionals. The clinical nurse specialist identifies and develops practice, ideas, procedures, policies and protocols through direct leadership or by working collaboratively, for example using clinical multi-professional audits (Bullen, 1995). 'Maintaining nursing standards' and having a 'balance of view' are important in maintaining quality and identifying areas for improvement. Finally, the clinical nurse specialist aids 'communication' through educational responsibilities and teaching opportunities.

Although this description is anecdotal, it would appear that practical, hands-on nursing care is not generally considered to be part of the clinical nurse specialist role in the UK, which supports Davis's (1995) findings. It is worth noting that both Davies and Oberle (1990) and Davis (1995) use nurse specialists as the subjects of their enquiry: lending a hand may be less significant in these nursing roles, whereas nurses working within palliative care in other settings, for example day care, in-patient units, hospice-at-home and night nursing services such as that of Marie Curie nurses, will deliver practical, hands-on care. Within the general setting of acute management, nurses regard physical care as an important aspect of terminal care, which can be easier to carry out than the less tangible aspect of 'being there' (Hockley, 1989).

The final component of 'doing for', that of 'team-playing', has greater significance for the nurses in the UK study (Davis, 1995) and is implicit in the descriptions of the clinical nurse specialist role. Nurses find themselves working within two teams, described as an 'inner team' of palliative care colleagues and an 'outer team' of other professionals including the hospital, primary health-care and social services teams.

Sharing with colleagues in teams could reduce stress or could, conversely, create stress for the nurse (Davis, 1995). Again, communicating, co-ordinating and collaborating with other team members was seen to take up considerable time, both physically and emotionally (Dobratz, 1990; Davis, 1995). Sometimes, the effort expended team-playing did not pay off: time spent by one UK palliative nurse negotiating and orchestrating one patient's discharge did not achieve the desired outcome as, in the end, funding was not available to care for her at home (Davis, 1995). Thus, the emergence of a political interface between the nurse and the health-care system affects the outcome of supportive care (Davis, 1995). This has not previously been raised in studies examining the role.

McWilliam et al. (1993) recognize that interprofessional conflict may arise that impacts upon nursing goals and presents problems of symptom relief for the patient (Dobratz, 1990). Issues such as role overlap in multi-disciplinary teams when working with patients and families with complex physical and psychosocial needs can be difficult and impede the progress of the work (McWilliam et al., 1993).

In one study of 58 community nurses in Devon, UK, one-third felt that they had difficulty knowing who had overall responsibility for patient care, and over a quarter felt their own contribution to be underrated when hospice nurses were involved (Seamark et al., 1993). Similarly, in a study of 99 community nurses and 84 health visitors in Scotland, territorial issues emerged when home-care nurses were perceived to encroach on other nursing roles (Kindlen, cited in Davis, 1995). This could be explained by the fact that each team individual is striving to excel in his or her care and may be oblivious to the others also committed to the patient (McWilliam et al., 1993), or it may characterize genuine issues of role threat. Nevertheless, the palliative nurse may have to work hard to generate effective, co-operative team-working in terms of keeping the channels of communication open and exercising maturity in understanding someone else's perspective (McWilliam et al., 1993; Davis, 1995).

Greater complexities and responsibilities within nursing practice have encouraged the growth of highly experienced, specialised expert nurses. In her review of hospice literature, Dobratz (1990) suggests that expert hospice nursing arises from the ability and skill of the nurse to judge and decide which decisions can be made independently and which require a collaborative interchange with other team members. This is especially apparent in times of crisis and when care is required out of hours, and is a particular competency in line with Benner's (1984) research.

Managing personal and professional conflict requires considerable effort, skill, expertise and personal maturity, which may not be recognized as part of the palliative nursing role (McWilliam et al., 1993) yet is, in some studies, evident within the lived experiences of nurses.

FINDING MEANING

The final dimension of the model of supportive care is 'finding meaning' (Davies and Oberle, 1990). The nurse has the ability, and the opportunity, to both 'focus on living' and 'acknowledge death' (see Figure 13.2). This frequently means having open, perhaps difficult, conversations with patients about their lives, beliefs and hopes, and helping them to make sense of their situation (Davies and Oberle, 1990). As in 'empowering', the nurse encourages the patient to draw on intrinsic reserves to gather mental fortitude (Davis, 1995).

In '*Focusing on living*', the nurse helps patients to live until they die, talking about what they would like from the time remaining and in reflecting on life. In discovering one paralysed patient's wish to see her baby daughter baptized, the nurse arranged for this to take place at home as the mother's condition meant that she could not attend the church (Davies and Oberle, 1990).

'*Acknowledging death*' means that the nurse talks about painful issues such as death and is prepared to give or reiterate bad news in helping people come to terms with dying (Davies and Oberle, 1990). This aspect is clearly fundamental to the speciality of palliative nursing.

The importance of communication in palliative care is well documented (Maguire and Faukner, 1988; Buckman, 1992, 1995; Anstey, 1995) and is explored further in this book. It is clear that, in order to help the patient to find meaning, the nurse must enter into a dialogue that can potentiate this important aspect. It is vital to remember that the nurse's actions and behaviours are influential in patients' own constructions of their death and dying (Copp, 1999).

Focusing on life is empowering (Davies and Oberle, 1990) so nurses adopt different approaches to assist the patients and their families in finding meaning (Davis, 1995). Strategies may include the nurse helping to set realistic goals for the person to look forward to, or to adapt to different or even new priorities in order to gain pleasure in his or her remaining life (Davis, 1995). Finding meaning through having a sense of direction is one aspect that influences a patient's perception of hope (Herth, 1990). Despite being close to death, hope can be increased if patients feel valued, have meaningful relationships, are symptom controlled and set realistic goals (Herth, 1990). This may be easier for the nurse when there is an established rapport with the patient (Davis, 1995) and thus links with the dimension of 'connecting'.

Communicating about painful subjects can nevertheless be difficult. Some nurses actively avoid communicating at a deep level with patients and their families (Bond, 1982; Wilkinson, 1991). In one study nurses' reasons for avoiding discussions about the diagnosis and prognosis of cancer included the belief that nurses wished to protect themselves from hurt (Wilkinson, 1991). This is also demonstrated in studies examining non-verbal behaviours such as touch. Withdrawal from using touch can indicate that the nurse is trying to protect herself from, be it perceived or real, physical or emotional harm or overinvolvement (Estabrooks, 1989; Bottorff, 1993; Routasalo and Isola, 1996). Once more, there are clear links with the core dimension of preserving integrity, illustrating the potential for nursing interventions to be influenced by the nurse's own sense of wholeness (Davies, 1992) and personal well-being. If, however, an avoidance of meaningful communication with patients is, as Tschudin (1988) suggests, directed by nurses' fear, it can prevent nurses helping others in difficulty.

Another identified reason for avoiding honest discussions is the concern that nurses may inflict more distress on patients (Wilkinson, 1992). Although it is true that one cannot turn bad news into good, and cannot therefore soften the impact (Maguire and Faulkner, 1988), this should not be a panacea for avoiding difficult conversations.

Truth-telling is but one of the many particular ethical issues that palliative nurses may face in their daily work; others arise from areas such as consent, research, advance directives, patient autonomy and euthanasia (NCHSPCS, 1996b). Despite the fact that there is little educational provision in ethics for health-care workers (NCHSPCS, 1996b), it is probable that the palliative nurse will encounter a number of dilemmas when caring for the dying (Kendall, 1995). It is therefore important that nurses have both the opportunity and support to understand and ethically explore dilemmas as they relate to their practice.

Finding meaning is such an important concept in palliative care. Anstey (1995) and Holmes (1988) argue that 'effective' or 'meaningful' communication between patient and staff has a role in improving or maintaining an acceptable quality of life. Frankl (1987), a Jewish psychiatrist imprisoned in a concentration camp, his entire family perishing in camps during the Second World War, brilliantly illustrates this point. He found meaning during that time in remembering the love of his wife and in imagining his future life beyond the camp. He offers many insights into suffering and the meaning of life, stating that no human being can relieve another of his or her suffering, and that to do so denies individuals their spiritual freedom, which gives purpose and meaning to life.

Although the nature of spiritual care is explored elsewhere in this book, helping patients and families to make sense of their situation may involve the nurse helping a person to explore his or her spirituality. Sheldon (1997) remarks that palliative care literature on spirituality makes great effort to remind us that spirituality and religion are not necessarily the same.

Although spiritual and religious care can be an elusive concept for palliative nurses, Hopper (2000) argues that spiritual care is inherent within everyday holistic palliative care practice, in not just what is said, but also in what is done for the person. She suggests that, in coming to the end of life, a person's uniqueness and relatedness with others in his or her life is brought starkly into view. She cites Lunn, a hospice chaplain, who remarks that although practitioners are regularly asked questions that are unanswerable or even unidentifiable, that is not the same as having no response. Palliative nurses must, at the very least, provide the opportunities for patients and their loved ones to explore their lives and their thoughts and feelings about death and loss. Not everyone will wish to talk openly, and even if they do, they may be unable to find meaning in their situation. Nevertheless, cues in patients' conversations should not be ignored or avoided (Degner et al., 1991; Wilkinson, 1991).

Being with, or alongside, a patient in distress, and helping patients to find meaning from their situation, is integral to the role of palliative nurses (Davies and Oberle, 1990; Degner et al., 1991; Anstey, 1995; Nebauer et al., 1996). Although communicating at a deep level may be difficult for some nurses (Bond, 1982; Hockley, 1989), and positively avoided by others (Wilkinson, 1991), such avoidance may deny patients the opportunity to explore the meaning of their situation and limit their spiritual freedom (Frankl, 1987).

EDUCATION

The educative role of the palliative nurse is implicit within the model of supportive care that Davies and Oberle (1990) propose: empowering, for example, involves giving information, explaining and teaching about medication, changes and pain. This largely involves teaching patients and their carers. Other literature, however, makes explicit the palliative nurse's responsibility to share knowledge and experience through educating others, notably health professionals, volunteers and the lay public (Sloan and Grant, 1989; NCHSPCS, 1995a; Lindop et al., 1997). This educative role appears to be well received and understood by others (Cox et al., 1993; Seamark et al., 1993; Boyd, 1995).

There is support for using the underpinning holistic model of palliative care to inform and generate further knowledge in nursing generally, for example to form an integral part of general nurse training (Herring et al., 1995). In addition, the NCHSPCS states that it is vital for there to be the provision of a coherent and comprehensive framework for education relating to death for all professionals beyond registration (NCHSPCS, 1996b). An examination of education in palliative care needs to occur at all levels – from students through those working in community and hospice settings to those in advanced practice roles, such as clinical nurse specialists (Corner, 1995). The notion of lifelong learning is not new to nurses, who currently are required to undertake a minimum of 5 days study or their equivalent every 3 years and to maintain a personal professional profile for registration with the United Kingdom Central Council for Nursing, Midwifery and Health Visiting.

This emphasis on the importance of disseminating good practice and research, advocated by Cicely Saunders, historically has resulted in visits to hospices, in-service training and a variety of short course or study days on various aspects of palliative care for a whole range of practitioners (Smith 1996). A large variety and number of themes in educational subject matter are offered. In a review of advertised conferences and short courses over 1 year, the subjects most frequently included loss and bereavement, symptom control, holistic palliative care, communication skills, complementary therapies and ethical, religious and spiritual issues (Smith, 1996). Again, with the explosion in the provision of palliative care diploma, undergraduate, postgraduate and Master's degree courses, there are more opportunities for nurses both to educate others and to be educated. Despite this, palliative nurses may themselves feel educationally unprepared for their role (Corner, 1995).

The question of how best to educate others is a huge topic inappropriate for exploration here. It has, however, received the attention of palliative educators, the spotlight again being turned on multi-professional education in palliative care (NCHSPCS, 1996b). Sheldon and Smith (1996) note that one focus of palliative care education, and thus practice, is to understand the concept that palliative care is done 'with' and 'for' people rather than 'on' them.

The practice of palliative nursing demands a high level of clinical competency and quality assurance, assimilated into formal education and built on firm theoretical foundations (Dobratz, 1990). Dobratz describes the process of supporting people through the complexities of their dying as 'continuous knowing'. As the demands on the developing role of nurse specialists require in-depth knowledge and expertise (Dicks, 1990), palliative nurses are challenged to demonstrate flexibility and adaptability in updating their skills and knowledge, especially in light of current social, political and technological change (Frost, 1996).

In order to educate and prepare others, palliative nurses must be clear that their teaching is both appropriate and effective, yet there has been little research and academic scrutiny into palliative care education (Sheldon, 1995). This is ever more challenging with today's increasing emphasis on delivering and teaching evidence-based care, especially if, as Copp (1999) suggests, much of the expertise of palliative knowledge still remains implicit.

Educating others in palliative care means grappling with the emotional content of the work (Sheldon, 1995). Faulkner and O'Neill (1994) suggest that most practitioners are left to learn the necessary skills through personal experiences that may not produce the best results. Just as the dying face uncertainty over when, where and how they may die, or whether there is an afterlife (Degner and Gow, 1988), so too nurses face uncertainties surrounding how they will respond, relate and behave. There is considerable anxiety with regard to death, especially among inexperienced or junior nurses and doctors (Hurtig and Stewin, 1990; Boyle and Carter, 1998); it is suggested that palliative nurses have a clear role in supporting learners risking uncertainty (Sheldon and Smith, 1996) if, as with patients confronting fear, this can help to create meaning and understanding for the individual (Frankl, 1987).

Palliative care is a dynamic process, one that is active rather than passive (NCHSPCS, 1996b). Confronting and reconciling one's own fears and anxieties concerning death and dying is necessary in helping others to meet death with dignity (Hurtig and Stewin, 1990) and in delivering a high quality of nursing care (Boyle and Carter, 1998); palliative care education should not shrink from facing death and all its implications (NCHSPCS, 1996b).

RESEARCH

Measuring and demonstrating efficacy in palliative nursing and palliative education is challenging, but the imperative to find solutions to such difficulties is there. Palliative nurses today have a professional, ethical and political requirement to use and apply research and evidence within their practice, but, despite the growing professional and political insistence on increasing the research base of nursing, research utilization remains poor (Polit and Hungler, 1995; Camiah, 1997).

Nurses are not fully prepared for using research (Dunn et al., 1998) and lack basic skills in research awareness (Camiah, 1997). Consequently, research is neither meaningful nor significant to these nurses, so its findings are not utilized (Camiah, 1997). Research that offers realistic solutions to problems is required if nurses are to implement research findings (Corner, 1991) since, if nurses are not influenced, innovations will not benefit the patient (Cullum, 1996).

A recent UK study showed that the top 10 barriers to research use include the poor preparation of nurses for research, insufficient time and facilities, and a lack of support in implementing findings (Dunn et al., 1998). Previous research has revealed similar obstacles (Hunt, 1981; Walczak et al., 1994). This lack of support may have a bearing on nurses publishing their findings in palliative care. In reviewing the literature for this chapter, it is worth noting that some regularly cited research about the specialist and palliative nursing roles remains unpublished. Work by Castledine (1982), Lunt and Yardley (1986), James (1986), Kindlen (1987), Bunn (1988), Davis (1995) and Macnish (1998), usually completed for first or Master's level degree programmes, remain in university libraries around the UK, gaining general access to these being more difficult. This could indicate that nurses need more encouragement to publish as there are arguably now more opportunities to do so given the number of publications relating to palliative care. The breadth of publications available, and initiatives such as the NHS Review and Dissemination Centre at York, also means that poor access to research can no longer be a justified barrier to its utilization (Corner, 1991).

But the palliative nurse must also find time to read the literature: Webb and Mackenzie showed that, in 1993, few nurses regularly read journals, although this situation may now have improved. Walczak et al.'s (1994) study of oncology nurses similarly showed that a lack of time within work to access the data was a significant barrier to their usage. This illustrates the complexity of personal and managerial responsibility for research in practice and suggests that opportunities for and access to study should be available within working hours.

Skilled time management may be a significant competency for today's palliative nurse in balancing clinical, educational and research activity, this again appearing to have eluded research interest. This may be especially important if, in order to be successful in achieving time management, undertaking and utilizing research requires nurses and managers to use a set of core values different from those associated with caring and nurturing (Hicks, 1996).

Resistance to reading and using research for practice may also arise from a fear of change as care based on traditional beliefs, values, common sense, intuition and personal experience remains highly valued, especially among senior clinical staff (Camiah, 1997). This may be pertinent within palliative nursing – as previously stated there is little research into the role, especially early on in the developing hospice movement. Furthermore, a positive research culture has previously been lacking in palliative care (Twycross and Dunn, 1994; NCHSPCS, 1997). Maybe hospice nurses, like other UK nurses, are more comfortable in applying knowledge based on experience rather than derived from systematic empirical study (Closs and Cheater, 1994). Nevertheless, although nursing that does not have a research base may be skilful, it may also be dangerous (Akinsanya, 1994). Corner (1996) suggests that development of a responsive research strategy for palliative care is now required.

The relationship between nursing research and practice is a multi-factorial phenomenon (Pearcey, 1995). Cultural, historical and organizational factors are strongly influential in developing a positive research culture within organizations (Cullum, 1996), and researchers, managers, nurses and educationalists must take both individual and collective responsibility for removing the barriers to research-based practice (Polit and Hungler, 1995).

Most importantly, research can assist palliative nurses to understand the core of what they do, to help to reveal the 'hidden' aspects of palliative nursing. Furthermore, although the experience of nurses is valuable, research into the care of the dying will test and validate both experiences and theory so that practice can be effective. MacGuire (1991) makes this point well when he says that, by fostering research, the practice of nursing can become therapeutic by intent rather than by chance.

The role of the nurse in palliative care is complex and demanding, involving active effort on the part of the nurse in maintaining personal well-being, knowledge and expertise, and in generating effective or meaningful professional and patient relationships. The research used in this chapter illustrates many similarities in – and a few differences between – how palliative nurses view their role. This role is influenced by a host of variables such as culture, context, politics and organizational structures, research, education, resources and the individual nurse, patient and family or supportive caring network. It is perhaps travelling with and negotiating these challenges and complexities that leads to the inevitable joys and satisfaction that this work can bring. Understanding and nurturing oneself seems, however, to be the fundamental element in supporting the dying.

This chapter is dedicated in recognition of all the patients and families who have gone before us and helped us to understand what it means to be dying and to lose those whom we love. In the words of Mother Teresa, we can do no great things, only small things with great love.

REFERENCES

Ahmedzai, S. 1993: The medicalisation of dying. In: Clarke D. (ed.) *The Future for Palliative Care*. Buckingham: Open University Press.

Akinsanya, J. 1994: Making research useful to the practice of nursing. *Journal of Advanced Nursing* 19, 174–9.

Anstey, S. 1995: Communication. In: Penson, J. and Fisher, R. (eds) *Palliative Care for People with Cancer*, 2nd edn. London: Edward Arnold.

Benner, P. 1984: *From Novice to Expert*. Menlo Park, CA: Addison-Wesley.

Bond, S. 1982: Communicating with families of cancer patients. 2. The nurses. *Nursing Times* (Jun 16), 1027–9.

Bottorff, J. 1993: The use and meaning of touch in caring for patients with cancer. *Oncology Nursing Forum* 20(10), 1531–8.

Boyd, K. 1995: The role of specialist home care teams: the views of general practitioners in south London. *Palliative Medicine* 9, 138–44.

Boyle, M. and Carter, D. (1998) Death anxiety amongst nurses. *International Journal of Palliative Nursing* 4(1), 37–43.

Bridge, C. 2000: Editorial. *Contact* (summer).

Buckman, R. 1992: *How To Break Bad News: A Guide for Health Care Professionals*. London: Papermac.

Buckman, R. 1995: Communication in palliative care: a practical guide. In: Doyle, D., Hanks, G. and MacDonald, N. (eds) *The Oxford Textbook of Palliative Medicine*. Oxford: Oxford University Press.

Bullen, M. 1995: The role of the specialist nurse in palliative care. *Professional Nurse* 10(12), 755–6.

Bunn, F. 1988: An Exploratory Study of the Role of the Macmillan Nurse. Unpublished BSc project, Kings College, University of London.

Burnard, P. 1995: *Learning Human Skills*, 3rd edn. Oxford: Butterworth-Heinemann.

Camiah, S. 1997: Utilization of nursing research in practice and application strategies to raise research awareness amongst nurse practitioners: a model for success. *Journal of Advanced Nursing* 26, 1193–202.

Carr, L. 1994: The strengths and weaknesses of quantitative and qualitative research: what method for nursing? *Journal of Advanced Nursing* 20, 716–21.

Castledine, G. 1982: The Role and Function of Clinical Nurse Specialists in England and Wales. Unpublished MSc thesis, University of Manchester.

Chavasse, J. 1992: New dimensions of empowerment in nursing – and challenges. *Journal of Advanced Nursing* 17(1), 1–2.

Clarke, D. 1993a: *The Sociology of Death*. Oxford: Blackwell.

Clarke, D. 1993b: *The Future for Palliative Care*. Buckingham: Open University Press.

Clarke, D. 2000: Palliative care history: a ritual process? *European Journal of Palliative Care* 7(2), 50–5.

Closs, J. and Cheater, F. 1994: Utilization of nursing research: culture, interest and support. *Journal of Advanced Nursing* 19, 762–73.

Copp, G. 1999: *Facing Impending Death*. London: Nursing Times Books.

Corner, J. 1991: Cancer nursing research. *Nursing Times* 87(37), 42–4.

Corner, J. 1995: The nursing perspective. In: Doyle, D., Hanks G. and MacDonald, N. (eds) *The Oxford Textbook of Palliative Medicine*. Oxford: Oxford University Press.

Corner, J. 1996: Is there a research paradigm for palliative care? *Palliative Medicine* **10**, 201–8.

Corner, J., Plant, H. and Warner, L. 1995: Developing a nursing approach to managing dyspnoea in lung cancer. *International Journal of Palliative Nursing* **1**(1), 5–11.

Corner, J., Plant, H., A'Hern, R. and Bailer, C. 1996: Non-pharmacological intervention for breathlessness in lung cancer. *Palliative Medicine* **10**, 299–305.

Cox, K., Bergen, A. and Norman, I. 1993: Exploring consumer views of care provided by the Macmillan nurse using the critical incident technique. *Journal of Advanced Nursing* **18**, 408–15.

Cullum, N. 1996: Networking for research dissemination. *Nursing Times Research* **1**(2), 119.

Davies, B. 1992: The dimensions of the supportive role of the nurse in palliative care. *Proceedings of the Palliative Care Symposium, 7th International Conference on Cancer Nursing*, Vienna, August.

Davies, B. and Oberle, K. 1990: Dimensions of the supportive role of the nurse in palliative care. *Oncology Nursing Forum* **17**(1), 87–94.

Davis, C. 1995: Dimensions of the Supportive Role of the Clinical Nurse Specialist in Palliative Care: A UK Replication. Unpublished MSc thesis, Institute of Cancer Research Library, London.

Degner, L. and Gow, C 1988: Preparing nurses for care of the dying. *Cancer Nursing* **11**(3), 160–9.

Degner, L., Gow, C. and Thompson, L. 1991: Critical nursing behaviour in care for the dying. *Cancer Nursing* **14**(5), 246–53.

Dicks, B. 1990: The contribution of nursing to palliative care. *Palliative Medicine* **4**, 197–203.

Dobratz, M. 1990: Hospice nursing: present perspectives and future directives. *Cancer Nursing* **13**(2), 116–22.

Douglas, C. 1992: For all the saints. *British Medical Journal* **304**, 579.

Doyle, D., Hanks, G. and MacDonald, N. 1995: Introduction. In: *The Oxford Textbook of Palliative Medicine*. Oxford: Oxford University Press.

Dunn, V., Crichton, N., Roe, B., Seers, K. and Williams, K. 1998: Using research for practice: a UK experience of the BARRIERS scale. *Journal of Advanced Nursing* **27**, 1203–10.

Durgahee, T. 1996: Facilitation: the concepts in use in palliative care nursing. *International Journal of Palliative Nursing* **2**(3), 158–61.

Egan, G. 1990: *The Skilled Helper: A Systematic Approach to Effective Helping*, 4th edn. Belmont, California: Brooks/Cole.

Estabrooks, C. 1989: Touch: a nursing strategy in the intensive care unit. *Heart and Lung* **18**(4), 392–401.

Fareed, A. 1996: The experience of reassurance: patients' perspectives. *Journal of Advanced Nursing* **23**, 272–9.

Faulkner, A. and O'Neill, W. 1994: Bedside manner revisited: teaching effective interaction. *European Journal of Palliative Care* **1**(2), 92–5.

Fisher, R. 1995: Introduction: palliative care – a rediscovery. In: Penson, J. and Fisher, R. (eds) *Palliative Care for People with Cancer*, 2nd edn. London: Arnold, 1–7.

Frankl, V. 1987: *Man's Search for Meaning*. London: Hodder & Stoughton.

Frost, M. 1996: An analysis of the scope and value of problem based learning in the education of health care professionals. *Journal of Advanced Nursing* **24**, 1047–53.

Gibson, C. 1991: A concept analysis of empowerment. *Journal of Advanced Nursing* **16**, 354–61.

Gilbert, J. 1996: Palliative medicine: a new specialty changes an old debate. *British Medical Bulletin* **52**(2), 8.1–8.12.

Goodman, J. 1984: Reflection and teacher education: a case study and theoretical analysis. *Interchange* **15**(3), 9–26.

Graves, D. and Nash, A. 1992: A friendship that inspires hope. *Professional Nurse* **9**, 478–85.

Harris, L. 1991: The disadvantaged dying. *Nursing Times* **86**, 26–9.

Heron, J. 1990: *Helping the Client*, 3rd edn. London: Sage.

Herring, R., Wilson-Barnett, J. and Ball, S. 1995: The role of Macmillan nurse tutors: an interview study with postholders. *International Journal of Palliative Nursing* **1**(4), 217–25.

Herth, K. 1990: Fostering hope in terminally ill people. *Journal of Advanced Nursing* **15**, 1250–9.

Hicks, C. 1996: A study of nurses' attitudes toward research: a factor analytic approach. *Journal of Advanced Nursing* **23**, 373–9.

Hockley, J. 1989: Caring for the dying in acute hospitals. *Nursing Times* **85**(7), 47–50.

Holmes, S. 1988: 'Meaningful communication': can it enhance quality of life? *Holistic Medicine* **3**, 195–203.

Hopper, A. 2000: Meeting the spiritual needs of patients through holistic practice. *European Journal of Palliative Care* **7**(2), 60–2.

Hospice Information Service 2000: *Directory of Hospice Services in the UK and Republic of Ireland*. Sydenham: St Christopher's Hospice.

Hunt, J. 1981: Indicators for nursing practice: the use of research findings. *Journal of Advanced Nursing* **6**, 189–94.

Hurtig, W. and Stewin, L. 1990: The effect of death education and experience on nursing students' attitude toward death. *Journal of Advanced Nursing* **15**, 29–34.

Irvine, B. 1993: Developments in palliative nursing in and out of the hospital setting. *British Journal of Palliative Nursing* **2**(4), 218–24.

James, N. 1986: Care and Work in Nursing the Dying: A Participant Study in a Continuing Care Unit. PhD thesis, University of Aberdeen.

Johnston, B. 1999: Overview of nursing developments in palliative care. In: Lugton J. and Kindlen, M. (eds) *Palliative Care: The Nursing Role*. Edinburgh: Churchill Livingstone.

Kendall, M. 1995: Truth telling and collusion: the ethical dilemmas of palliative nursing. *International Journal of Palliative Nursing* **1**(3), 160–4.

Kindlen, M. 1987: The Role of the Hospice Nurse as Perceived by Macmillan Nurses, District Nursing Sisters and Health Visitors. Unpublished MPhil thesis, University of Edinburgh.

Kübler-Ross, E. 1970: *On Death and Dying*. London: Tavistock.

Leininger, M. 1988: *Care: The Essence of Nursing and Health*. Detroit: Wayne State University Press.

Levine, S. 1988: *Who Dies?* Bath: Gateway.

Liaschenko, J. 1994: Making a bridge: the moral work with patients we do not like. *Journal of Palliative Care* **10**(3), 83–9.

Lindop, E., Beach, R. and Read, S. 1997: A composite model of palliative care for the UK. *International Journal of Palliative Nursing* **3**(5), 287–92.

Lowden, B. 1998: Introducing palliative care: health professionals' perceptions. *International Journal of Palliative Nursing* **4**(3), 135–42.

Lunt, B. and Yardley, J. 1986: A Survey of Home Care Teams and Hospital Support Teams for the Terminally Ill. Unpublished document. Cancer Care Research Unit, Royal South Hants Hospital, Southampton.

MacGuire, J. 1991: Tailoring research for advanced nursing practice. In: McMahon R. and Pearson, A. (eds) *Nursing as Therapy*. London: Chapman & Hall.

McKee, E. 1995: Stress and staff support in hospice: a review of the literature. *International Journal of Palliative Nursing* **1**(3), 155–9.

Macnish, K. 1998: An Exploration of Nursing Touch: What Is the Role of Touch for the Palliative Nurse Specialist? Unpublished BSc (Hons) dissertation, University of Manchester/Institute of Cancer Research Royal Marsden NHS Trust.

McWilliam, C., Burdock, J. and Wamsley, J. 1993: The challenging experience of palliative care support-team nursing. *Oncology Nursing Forum* **20**(5), 779–85.

Maguire, P. and Faulkner, A. 1988: How to do it: communicate with cancer patients. 1. Handling bad news and difficult questions. *British Medical Journal* **297**, 907–9.

Malin, N. and Teasdale, K. 1991: Caring versus empowerment: considerations for nursing practice. *Journal of Advanced Nursing* **16**(3), 657–62.

Martocchio, B. 1987: Authenticity, belonging, emotional closeness and self representation. *Oncology Nursing Forum* **14**(4), 23–7.

Mearns, D. and Thorne, B. 1988: *Person-centred Counselling in Action*. London: Sage.

Morse, J. 1991: Negotiating commitment and involvement in the nurse–patient relationship. *Journal of Advanced Nursing* **16**(4), 455–68.

Mulhall, A. 1996: The cultural context of death: what nurses need to know. *Nursing Times* **92**(34), 38–40.

Nash, A. 1990: The role of the Macmillan nurse. *Nursing Standard* **5**(13): 33–7.

National Association of Health Authorities and Trusts 1991: *Care of People with Terminal Illness*. Birmingham: NAHAT.

National Council for Hospices and Specialist Palliative Care Services 1995a: *Specialist Palliative Care: A Statement of Definitions*. Occasional Paper No. 8. London: NCHSPCS.

National Council for Hospices and Specialist Palliative Care Services 1995b: *Information for Purchasers*. London: NCHSPCS.

National Council for Hospices and Specialist Palliative Care Services 1996a: *Working Together, Dilemmas and Directions: The Future of Specialist Palliative Care. A Draft Discussion Paper*. London: NCHSPCS.

National Council for Hospices and Specialist Palliative Care Services 1996b: *Education in Palliative Care*. Occasional Paper No.9: London: NCHSPCS.

National Council for Hospices and Specialist Palliative Care Services 1997: *Dilemmas and Directions: The Future of Specialist Palliative Care: A Discussion Paper*. London: NCHSPCS.

National Council for Hospices and Specialist Palliative Care Services 1999: *Palliative Care 2000: Commissioning through Partnership*. London: NCHSPCS.

Nebauer, M., Prior, D., Berggren, L. et al. 1996: Nurses' perceptions of palliative care nursing. *International Journal of Palliative Nursing* **2**(1), 26–34.

Oberle, K. and Davies, B. 1992: Support and caring: exploring the concepts. *Oncology Nursing Forum* **19**(5), 763–7.

Parkes, C., Benjamin, B. and Fitzgerald, R. 1969: Broken heart: a statistical study of increased mortality among widowers. *British Medical Journal* **1**, 740–3.

Pearoey, P. 1995: Achieving research based practice. *Journal of Advanced Nursing* **22**, 33–9.

Penson, J. 1995: Caring for bereaved relatives. In: Penson, J. and Fisher, R. (eds) *Palliative Care for People with Cancer*, 2nd edn. London: Arnold.

Polit, D. and Hungler, B. 1995: *Nursing Research: Principles and Methods*, 5th edn. J.B. Philadelphia: Lippincott.

Pyne, R. 1994: Empowerment through use of the code of professional conduct. *British Journal of Nursing* **3**(12), 631–4.

Ramos, M. 1992: The nurse–patient relationship: themes and variations. *Journal of Advanced Nursing* **17**, 496–506.

Rasmussen, B., Norberg, A. and Sandman, P. 1995: Stories about becoming a hospice nurse. *Cancer Nursing* **18**(5), 344–5.

Raudonis, B. 1993: The meaning and impact of empathetic relationships in hospice nursing. *Cancer Nursing* **16**(4), 304–9.

Richardson, A. 1995: Fatigue in cancer patients: a review of the literature. *European Journal of Cancer Care* **4**(1), 20–32.

Rodwell, C. 1996: An analysis of the concept of empowerment. *Journal of Advanced Nursing* **23**, 305–13.

Rogers, C. 1967: *On Becoming a Person*. London: Constable.

Routasalo, P. and Isola, A. 1996: The right to touch and be touched. *Nursing Ethics* **3**(2), 165–76.

Royal College of Nursing Palliative Nursing Group 2000: *Contact* (summer).

Saunders, C. 1985: *The Management of Terminal Illness*, 2nd edn. London: Edward Arnold.

Saunders, C. 1987: What's in a name? *Palliative Medicine* **1**, 57–61.

Saunders, C. 1995: Foreword. In: Doyle, D., Hanks, G. and MacDonald, N. (eds) *The Oxford Textbook of Palliative Medicine*. Oxford: Oxford University Press.

Schön D. 1991: *The Reflective Practitioner*, 2nd edn. San Fransisco: Jossey Bass.

Seamark, D., Thorne, C., Jones, R., Pereira Gray, D. and Searle, J. 1993: Knowledge and perceptions of a domicillary hospice service among general practitioners and community nurses. *British Journal of General Practice* **43**, 57–59.

Sheldon, F. 1995: Education for palliative professionals – the future. *European Journal of Palliative Care* **2**(1), 4.

Sheldon, F. 1997: *Psychosocial Palliative Care*. Cheltenham: Stanley Thornes.

Sheldon, F. and Smith, P. 1996: The life so short, the craft so hard to learn: a model for post-basic education in palliative care. *Palliative Medicine* **16**, 99–104.

Sloan, D. and Grant, M. 1982: Evaluating a Macmillan nursing service: the benefits of care. *Senior Nurse* **9**(5), 20–1.

Smith, A. 1996: Continuing education and short courses. *Palliative Medicine* **10**: 105–11.

Smith, P. 1992: *The Emotional Labour of Nursing*. London: Macmillan.

Standing Medical Advisory Committee and Standing Nursing and Midwifery Advisory Committee 1992: *The Principles and Provision of Palliative Care*. London: HMSO.

Taylor, B., Glass, N., McFarlane, J. and Stirling, C. 1997: Palliative nurses' perceptions of the nature and effects of their work. *International Journal of Palliative Nursing* **3**(5), 253–8.

Tschudin, V. 1988: Counselling. In: Tschudin, V. (ed) *Nursing the Patient with Cancer*. London: Prentice Hall.

Twycross, R. and Dunn, V. 1994: *Research in Palliative Care: The Pursuit of Reliable Knowledge*. London: NCHSPCS.

Vachon, M. 1987: *Occupational Stress in the Care of the Critically Ill, the Dying, and the Bereaved*. New York: Hemisphere.

Von Klitzing, W. 1999: Evaluation of reflective learning in a psychodynamic group of nurses caring for terminally ill patients. *Journal of Advanced Nursing* 30(5), 1213–21.

Walczak, J., McGuire, D., Haisfield, M. and Beezley, A. 1994: A survey of research-related activities and perceived barriers to research utilization among professional oncology nurses. *Oncology Nursing Forum* 21(4), 710–15.

Watson, J. 1979: *Nursing: The Philosophy and Science of Caring*. Boston: Little, Brown.

Webb, C. and Mackenzie, J. 1993: Where are we now? Research mindedness in the 1990s. *Journal of Clinical Nursing* 2, 129–33.

Webber, J. 1994: The evolving role of the Macmillan nurse. *Nursing Times* 90(25), 66.

Wilkinson, S. 1991: Factors which influence how nurses communicate with cancer patients. *Journal of Advanced Nursing* 16, 677–88.

Wilkinson, S. 1992: Good communication in cancer nursing. *Nursing Standard* 7(9), 35–9.

Wilson-Barnett, J. and Richardson, A. 1995: Nursing research and palliative care. In: Doyle, D., Hanks, G. and MacDonald, N. (eds) *Oxford Textbook of Palliative Medicine*. Oxford: Oxford University Press.

World Health Organisation 1990: *Cancer Pain Relief and Palliative Care*. Technical Report Series No. 804. Geneva: WHO.

FURTHER READING

Brown, J., Kitson, A. and McKnight, T. 1992: *Challenges in Caring: Explorations in Nursing and Ethics*. London: Chapman & Hall.

Burnard, P. 1989: *Teaching Interpersonal Skills*. London: Chapman & Hall.

Lawler, J. 1991: *Behind the Screens*. Melbourne: Churchill Livingstone.

McMahon, R. and Pearson, A. 1992: *Nursing as Therapy*. London: Chapman & Hall.

Walter, T. 1994: *The Revival of Death*. London: Routledge.

chapter 14

REFLECTIVE PRACTICE IN PALLIATIVE CARE

Ann Hopper

> I have this that I must do one day;
> Overdraw my balance of air,
> And breaking the surface of water
> Go down into the green
> Darkness to search for the door
> To myself...
> R.S. Thomas

There are numerous definitions and interpretations of what is meant by reflective practice, all having in common the purpose of improving practice and all recognizing that practice is best improved by individual practitioners coming to understand themselves and their practice afresh. Reflection is essentially learning through the experience of practice. This chapter identifies several ways of cultivating the skills of reflection on action in order to develop different perspectives on individual palliative care practice and to see the context of palliative care in fresh, illuminating ways. One particular approach, reflective writing about palliative care, is used in the analysis of a significant event, a critical incident. This worked example is used to identify the characteristics of reflective writing, some practical advice being offered on how to get started on the path to writing about palliative care practice in critical and analytical ways.

THE IMPORTANCE OF LEARNING TO REFLECT

Learning through experience goes beyond turning to the textbooks to learn new facts to help in new situations, although that may well be part of the process. What we learn through reflection on experience is more about *ourselves* and about the *context* in which we work.

The challenge of learning through the experience of palliative care rests in the recognition of aspects of ourselves that we need to change. This is because it is the whole of our self that we bring to the practice of palliative care. This self extends beyond the intellect. It is of course vital to engage the intellect in order to act rationally and safely, but, to lay claim to offering holistic palliative care, it is necessary to engage more than the intellect. In the practice of palliative care, how we act and what we say derives from more than intellectual thought – it derives from who we are and why we have become who we are.

How we approach our professional work is influenced by past experience in ways that we may not fully understand. We are all inclined to reinforce existing patterns of behaviour and to take for granted, without questioning them, the routines of the working day. In order to make a lasting change in either ourselves or the way in which we practise palliative care, we must consciously set out to view both ourselves and the world of practice in new ways. Working in the context of palliative care causes practitioners to draw deeply from the well of their own integrity and humanity. Caring for people with advanced incurable disease inevitably confronts palliative care practitioners with questions about life and death, fundamental questions with which all human beings struggle. Having no solution or answer to those questions is not the same as having no response (Lunn, 1990), palliative care being of itself one such response, the caring action of its practitioners another. To respond palliatively to suffering magnifies the need to understand our own values and purposes in so doing. Reflection is a means to such understanding.

CULTIVATING THE WAYS AND MEANS OF REFLECTION IN PALLIATIVE CARE

It is possible to cultivate and develop the skills of reflection that are necessary to learn from experience in various ways. Although this chapter focuses on writing about practice, there are several other ways based on reading and talking about practice.

Reading the literature helps us to bring practical affairs into a relationship with theory and to see our own perspective on practice objectified as only one of various ways in which it might be understood (Smith, 1992). Talking about practice to a 'critical friend', a supervisor or a mentor (Fish and Twinn, 1997), as well as listening to others talking about practice (Schön, 1991), brings similar rewards. What a respected, critical friend can do is to challenge and press us about our practice, asking questions rather than making statements, using our experiences rather than their own in the process of helping us to restructure or re-see experience.

'Clinical supervision' is a term used to describe the more formal process of support and learning that enables individual practitioners to develop knowledge and competence and to assume responsibility for their own practice. Clinical supervision 'has been seen as central to the process of learning through practice and as a means of encouraging analytic and reflective skills' (Department of Health, 1993).

UNCOVERING THE INFLUENCES ON CURRENT PRACTICE

However analytical and reflective processes are facilitated, the first step towards reflective practice is to become self-critical: to explore the values and beliefs to which we are committed, where they have come from and how they influence the way in which we conduct ourselves in the world of work. To learn through experience, we need from time to time to unravel aspects of our own biography that lie hidden from others and often from ourselves. Some writers (e.g. Fish and Coles, 1998) have used the metaphor of an iceberg to identify how some aspects of our personalities that deeply influence the way in which we act are hidden below the surface. We either ignore this personal history or take it for granted, but these are the depths that we need to plumb if the experiences we have in practice are to be used as meaningful learning.

THE CONTEXT OF PALLIATIVE CARE AND ITS RELEVANCE TO CURRENT PRACTICE

In order to learn from the experience of palliative care, rather than uncritically drift through it, is also important to unravel aspects of the context of care in which we practise as this vitally effects what we are able to do and the manner in which we do it. These contextual aspects of care include the history of the profession for which we work and how members of that profession have in the past cared for people with a life-threatening disease. The care of people with a life-limiting illness has a rich social, political, medical and religious history that still influences it. Understanding the history of a situation helps us to throw light on current events. Similarly, we need to understand how contemporary health-care policies and practices influence everyday practice. Many of these influences we cannot change, the important thing being, as St Francis of Assisi knew, to accept what cannot be changed, to change what should be changed and to be able to distinguish the one from the other.

THE STRUGGLE TO UNDERSTAND OURSELVES

The complex analysis of the beliefs and assumptions that underlie our everyday practice in palliative care is not something that can be achieved rapidly, or even accomplished daily. The unpacking of a single incident in a truly reflective way involves thoughts, attitudes and feelings built up over a lifetime. A consultant in palliative medicine identified this struggle in his reflective writing about teamwork in palliative care: 'To struggle with dilemmas that have been con-sciously of half-consciously with you for years…is not easy' (Hillier, 1998). This is nevertheless the struggle in which we are called to engage if we are to learn through life experience and the experience of practice rather than just gain experience.

So how are we to uncover the influences of the past on current practice in order to learn through an ongoing experience of practice? The place to start on this journey is something that has actually happened in practice. Something had occurred in Hillier's everyday work in palliative care that had jolted him into thinking about it more deeply. Such a jolt may arise from something that happens that pleases us, appals us or in some way or another leads to pause for thought because our normal equilibrium has been disturbed by it.

THE USE OF CRITICAL INCIDENTS IN REFLECTION ON PRACTICE

I recently completed a doctoral thesis about the complexity of professional judgement within interprofessional hospice care (Hopper, 2000a). A critical incident from my days as a student nurse became a rich source of thought and inspiration that I now see as leading directly to the reasons why I chose to study within the context of palliative care. I have since learnt ways of analysing what was for me at the time a distressing incident, the impact of which remains with me, as I hope the following example of reflective writing illustrates.

RESEARCHING IN THE CONTEXT OF PALLIATIVE CARE

Why I chose hospice care as the setting for my research is only just becoming clear to me now that it is finished. This gradual dawning of understanding and the way in which we learn through the experience of practice was in part the subject of the research itself. I shall try to set out here why I believe that researching and writing about palliative care professionals led me to question how and what I was learning myself through the experience of researching. Inseparable from this learning was my need to rethink my whole approach to life and to death.

At the outset of the study, I was extremely vague about what I wanted to research and why. Two things, however, fascinated me: how people work together as interprofessional teams, and how health-care professionals learn through experience to hone the judgements that they need to make in the ever-changing world of clinical practice. What I needed was a context in which to study these. During the autumn of 1996, I was searching through libraries for information about interprofessional care when I happened upon some of the books and papers written by Dame Cicely Saunders. Since interprofessional care was one of the founding principles of the modern hospice movement, I thought, why not study it now, in action? I remember being excited by this idea but hesitant as I had no experience of palliative care. In fact, as a midwife and teacher of midwives, a school nurse and a leader in curriculum in a school of nursing, my career had kept me at some distance from it.

CONFRONTING MY OWN PROBLEMS

All my reasons for choosing to work in palliative care can be expressed intellectually. I can give a string of rational answers to questions concerning why I chose to study interprofessional work and learning through the experience of practice in the hospice context. Slowly, I began to acknowledge during the writing of the thesis that the work was, as well as an academic exercise, part of a long, laborious and challenging journey that has forced me to confront many of my own vulnerabilities related to death and dying.

I was fortunate that the educational environment in which I was based at the university encouraged the acknowledgement of the autobiography of the researcher in any research. I was not encouraged to work in a value-neutral manner that would exclude reflection on 'who' it was I took into the field of research and why. One of the scholars whose work I read, Donald Schön (1991), discussed how we need to be conscious of our own underlying stories and values in order to search out the sources of our own blindness and bias. It seemed important that I set out my sensibilities to death and from where I thought those sensibilities had originated. *Not* to be clear about this risks the inability to resist on the one hand being overintellectual about the subject and on the other hand emotionally swamped by it.

As well as childhood encounters with grief and loss, there remain unresolved dilemmas from incidents that I know I handled ineptly during my years of practice as a nurse and midwife. I am beginning to recognize that this ineptitude stemmed from my early socialization and from experiences that shaped my beliefs and values long before my professional training. Some, like the death of my father, were buried in the mists of early childhood.

One event I particularly remember from my training as a student nurse. This incident concerns the story of a dying man being transferred to a hospice (Case study 14.1). Like all health service stories, it is contextualized by the social and economic factors that influenced the situation. It also demonstrates the problematic nature of handling power and knowledge in health care. It is an incident in which I was given a very simple technical task to perform, but this led me into ethical conflict.

RETROSPECTIVE REFLECTIONS

For reasons that were not at all clear to me at the time, I was uneasy about the undignified and dishonest shuffling of the man from the ward that is described in Case study 14.1. I knew from ward reports that this man was expected to die very soon and that he was going to St Joseph's Hospice. Had he and I known about the work undertaken by the nursing order of nuns at the hospice, we would both have been less despairing about his going there.

At the time I knew little about myself or about the complexities of health care. There was nothing to alleviate my sense of unease and helplessness; all I could feel was a sense of naked pity for the man himself and an impotence to act in any helpful way. I knew that something was happening that was beyond my power to influence as a student, but it felt dishonest and uncomfortable to be part of it. My values were affronted in a way that I did not understand. This man was looking to me as someone to be trusted, but I felt untrustworthy by professional association with what the patient was and was not being told. I held important knowledge about him that he did not hold about himself. The

CASE STUDY 14.1

As a student nurse in the East End of London during the 1960s, I was asked to help to discharge a dying man from the medical ward in which I was then learning and working. I vividly remember the facial expression and the posture of this particular patient. His body was hunched, his colour a yellowing grey. His diagnosis is long forgotten, but the expression of despair and helplessness on his face still remains with me.

What I recall is a sense of this man's trusting gentleness and quiet humanity, as well as the appeal for help unspoken but undeniable in his sad eyes. Those eyes followed me as I worked, desperately needing someone, something to comfort him. His gaze was heavy, with a naked, almost cowering fear. I was afraid too. Afraid of saying anything, afraid of saying nothing, fearful for him and fearful for myself. This was a test of emotional strength far greater than the fear of seeing a dead body, a fear that was understood by the hospital culture and freely discussed. More-senior nurses took care of us when we experienced death for the first time as students, but the process of dying was not discussed. Dying patients were carefully nursed like other very sick patients, but the process of dying, the pain and fear of dying, was ignored.

The subject of dying was taboo, and my fear of it rendered me speechless. As I packed his few belongings and prepared for this patient to leave the ward, a doctor appeared through the curtains and told this dying man that he was being transferred to a convalescent home for a few weeks 'to get better'. I have been haunted by this incident. It has come to mind on many occasions since when, in the early hours of the morning, a patient has asked, 'Am I dying?' and my answer has been at best evasive – 'We need to talk to the doctor in the morning' – or at worst dishonest: 'No' or 'I don't know.'

fact that my knowledge was vague and I understood little of what was happening only served to magnify my discomfort.

Like the patient, I had no help immediately available to me. I had a ward assessor, who would tick the blue practical assessment book to say that I could discharge a patient, but nothing in the tradition at that time would have invited or encouraged me to explore the incident as problematic and therefore a source of personal learning. My tutor, whom I would see on a study day the following week, was, not unnaturally, concerned to cover the syllabus and to translate for us the content of the doctors' lectures that comprised the main focus of the course. We were thus given a watered-down medical curriculum of anatomy and physiology, and the signs, symptoms and treatments of various diseases. Dying was, as far as I remember, not part of the syllabus, although the laying out of a dead body was one of the tasks to be ticked off in the blue practical assessment book.

SOME PERSPECTIVES ON THIS INCIDENT FROM THE LITERATURE

Cicely Saunders (1984) suggested that medical education needs to teach not only how to diagnose and treat, but also how those who do not recover from a given disease may suffer, and the ways in which to alleviate their suffering. Her need to say this highlights a yawning gap in the medical textbooks. If death and dying were not part of medical students' syllabus in the 1960s, they were unlikely to feature in the nursing syllabus, although both were an everyday occurrence for us in large teaching hospitals and therefore certainly part of our informal curriculum. They were, however, an unexplored part of our learning.

Unknown to us then as students, attempts were being made at just about the time of this incident to explode some of the taboos surrounding death and dying. The sociologists, Glaser and Strauss, were disturbed by their own experiences of the American hospitals in which their parents died. Their book *Awareness of Dying* (1965) developed explanations of what was going on in relation to patients' and their families' awareness of dying. Glaser and Strauss studied the perceptions and interactions of dying people, their families and their professional carers. Their work took the form of a long research process later to be set out as their book on grounded theory (Glaser and Strauss, 1967). What they learned from the actual study was that, despite training and working with the dying, much of the professionals' demeanour towards death and dying resembled that of a layman. 'Personnel in contact with terminal patients are always somewhat disturbed by their own ineptness in handling the dying' (Glaser and Strauss, 1965).

The early socialization that shaped the experiences, beliefs and values of the professionals who were dealing with the dying in hospital wards in Glaser and Strauss' study would have been shaped by much the same cultural patterns as those of their patients, patterns of thinking laid down long before their professional training, many of them emanating from childhood. The same ineradicable effects of early conditioning clearly apply to me as well as to the patient and the doctor in my story (Case study 14.2).

LEARNING AS A WHOLE PERSON

There is much to be learned from the experiences set out above, learning that is inseparable from the learner that is me, inseparable too from an openness or preparedness to learn. Is it from such troubling experiences that professionals best learn? Is confronting our own values, assumptions and personal biographies an essential and integral part of this? The experience of reconsidering this incident has certainly reminded me that when I learn from experience, all of me learns; it is as if my whole personality, and not just some disembodied intellect, is learning. There is no neat parcel of knowledge for me to take and apply like a poultice to another situation. What emerges is a fresh understanding that I shall not be the same person entering a new situation as the one who practised before the experience set out above and the thinking to which it led me.

This is reflection: learning that occurs in response to some kind of jolt. This may be an affront to one's values, a gap in one's knowledge and understanding or a sense of surprise. It can also be the recognition that some of life's painful experiences and apparent failures need to be confronted before new learning can occur. This can happen long after the event, when fresh insights bring a

CASE STUDY 14.2

In my own lower middle-class upbringing, I had been protected from death and dying, and expected not to grieve but to be brave at all costs. Three grandparents and my own father died during my early childhood. One grandmother actually died in my bedroom, out of which I had been moved so that she could be nursed in her son's house. Beyond an explanation of this disturbance of my sleeping arrangements, there was no discussion of my grandmother's illness or death.

My father died during the night in a local cottage hospital after a series of heart attacks at home. I was 11 years old at the time, attending a direct grant school some 15 miles from home. My brother and I made the journey to school by bicycle, train and bus. We normally caught a train at 8 a.m., but the morning after our father died, our mother made the concession of allowing us to catch the next train, at 10 a.m. I arrived at school with a note for the teacher excusing my late arrival. She read the note and asked me one question: 'Did your father know that he was dying?' I remember declaring with some certainty that he did not, guessing somehow that this was the answer that she most wanted to hear, but for me a whole new horror gaped. The thought that Dad perhaps *knew* that he was going to die was far more awful to me than the thought that he was dead. Now he could not suffer, then he must have done so…if he knew…

Explanations of death in my family had always been couched in terms of 'falling asleep'. I didn't know when I was going to sleep, so how could Dad have possibly known that he was going to die? But suppose it was possible to know? I was in a classroom full of watching eyes. I hid behind the lid of my desk and cried for a moment, then remembered that my mum and the school would expect me to be brave.

different slant to the memory of the experience. Writing about this was an important part of learning where my attitudes and beliefs about death had originated and why I had been so inept as a practitioner nursing patients with life-threatening illness.

Some analysis of why this experience was, for me, jolting can be unpacked or unthreaded by applying questioning, critical and self-critical reflection to aspects of the practice in which learning occurs. These threads of practice are personal, social, historical, economic, political and ethical. Having located the incident above in my own biography, I will unravel some of the other contextualizing threads.

CONTEXTUAL INFLUENCES ON PRACTICE

Every practical event has a history. It is not difficult to see, in the incident described in Case study 14.1 above, the social history of the relationship between doctors and nurses and the patriarchal and matriarchal stances traditionally taken by those two professions, both in their turn located within the historical relationship between men and women. The doctor had the knowledge to give or withhold; I had the task of being with the patient and helping him to do the things he could not do for himself. These two professional traditions and the dissonant situations to which they give rise are thoroughly explored in the work of Salvage (1985) and Mackay (1993).

Politics and economics play their inevitable part in the context of the story. It is tempting to look back at a golden age without the pressures and economies of present-day health care. If ever there was such a time, it was before 1960. Part of the pressure that I have no doubt the doctor in my story was experiencing was the fact that there was already another patient waiting to be admitted to the ward. The continuing care of those unresponsive to cure was then, and remains now, a low priority for large hospitals. Since the Community Care Act 1990 (Department of Health, 1989), there has been the added complication that continuing care is an area of conflict between the health and social services in respect of funding. Klein (1989) Ham (1992) and James (1994) set out these political and economic dilemmas.

ETHICAL AND MORAL ISSUES IN PALLIATIVE CARE

The ethics of the incident remain the focus of an ongoing 'conversation' between myself and the situation in which I was involved so long ago. What to tell patients about their prognosis is an example of the exercise of professional judgement, to be worked out in every new situation through 'principled understanding' and the exercise of 'moral wisdom' consistent with the 'challenges of the situation' (Carr, 1995).

Every situation will be as different as the people involved in it. There are many levels of knowing for the practitioner, as exemplified in the critical incident analysed in Case study 14.1 above. I must have had some little tacit knowledge, knowledge from experience, even at this stage of training, but it would have been concerned with what *not* to do or say and tied up with fear of doing the wrong thing. Some knowledge might have been articulate ('I had knowledge about him he did not have himself') and some pre-articulate ('The fact that my knowledge was vague and I understood little of what was happening only served to magnify my discomfort'). Some new knowledge was gained at the time; other new knowledge would have involved understandings for which I was not ready. Some of that knowledge could only be articulated or verbalized in ways that I would not, at the time, have understood even had someone else tried to teach me.

Patients trying to understand the enormity of life-threatening illness must respond to the new knowledge of their condition in similar ways. Acceptance is not something that an individual can choose to do; it is not some light that can be switched on at will. 'Acceptance is like the settling of silt in a troubled pond' (Kearney, 1996). Some people may wish to know and will fully understand the knowledge and be able to deal with it. Others may not wish to know, or at least not wish to have the knowledge verbalized in ways for which they are not yet ready. Rarely will such understandings emerge at any level without anxiety and fear. There is also a powerful counter-argument to telling the patient about impending death, which is of course the possibility of destroying any hope of possible remission or recovery.

There are, then, delicate ethical decisions for the professionals involved in giving knowledge to patients. These are decisions in which the technical and the ethical cannot be separated. The moral issue embedded in the dilemma of what to tell a patient was sharply exposed by Glaser and Strauss (1965) in the following way:

> From one point of view the problem of awareness is a technical one: should the patient be told he is dying and what is to be done if he knows, does not know, or only suspects? But the problem is also a moral one, involving professional ethics, social issues, and personal values. Is it really proper, some people have asked, to deny a dying person the opportunity to make his peace with his God, to settle his affairs and to provide for the future of his family, and to control his style of dying, much as he controlled his style of living? Does anyone, the physician included, have the right to withhold such information?

There seem to me to be 'profound questions here about the moral end and goals of human life' (Carr, 1995), the sorts of question in which, as health professionals and teachers of other health professionals, we are all implicated.

These questions are particularly important in the context of contemporary health care. When more people were taken into hospital, both to be treated and to die, a certain amount of ambiguity could remain concerning the boundary between possible recovery and inevitable death. In keeping such knowledge to themselves resided some of the power of the physicians and surgeons. When, however, the first modern hospices for patients with intractable cancer were established during the late 1960s, a boundary was more clearly set between the possibility of curative medical intervention with its supporting hospital services and palliative intervention. Palliative care depends less on medicine and more on the values and skills of a whole team of people, not all of whom come from a hospital background. This team of people – social workers, clergy, doctors, therapists, nurses and volunteers – unite their efforts in an approach that connects facets of a personal, technical, practical, moral, social, emotional and spiritual kind (MacLeod and James, 1994).

THE UNCERTAINTIES OF PRACTICE

To practise health care is to be constantly confronted by uncertainty. Each encounter with a person who is suffering in whatever way is a unique encounter. Practitioners have to act rationally and ethically in the face of this uncertainty and not be paralysed by it, which is never easy. To act in the best interest of another means exploring the values to which we are committed and which we try to live out through the activities of care (Hopper, 2000b). To practise reflectively means exploring these values.

There can be no set rules on how to reflect on the individual practice of palliative care in order to learn from it, although various models and frame-works have been suggested (Boud et al., 1985). Reflection needs to be eclectic, employing all the forms of enquiry available to shed light on the situation as it is uncovered. Using an example from my own experience, I have set down in this chapter an approach to learning through experience that has been facilitated by reflective writing.

HOW TO GET STARTED ON THE PATH TO REFLECTIVE WRITING

Writing, especially that which incorporates the struggle to make some sense of experience, is rarely easy. Be gentle with yourself, and take comfort from the fact that all the contributors to this book have had to confront the spectre of an empty page; all will have found it hard to make a beginning and will then have drafted and re-drafted their writing many times. The important thing is to make a start. Begin as I did with an incident, an event, something that actually happened that was meaningful to you. A discussion of the event with a trusted colleague (a critical friend) may be useful in helping to set your thought processes in action.

The practice of palliative care will almost certainly confront you at some time or another with an experience that in some way 'disturbs' you. It may make you happy, or sad, or puzzled, or angry. Try to write about it as if you were writing a letter to an interested friend or colleague. (While doing this, confidentiality must of course be maintained: as with any writing or talking about practice, no harm must come to anyone as a result.)

Just write. Begin with your feelings, your anxiety, your puzzled thoughts. It is not necessary to wait for a fully formed paragraph or even a coherent sentence. Nor is it necessary to worry about the beginning, the middle and the end of the story; all that comes much later. At first, just describe the incident. In this situ-ation, a situation in which you are trying to learn, and essentially to learn more about yourself, description is an essential part of the writing form. Description is sometimes frowned upon in intellectual work, but reflective writing is an exer-cise from which to learn. An assessment of parts of it for a course of study might follow, but that is not your primary reason for writing.

Table 14.1 sets out the characteristics of reflective writing, but what matters most is not the quality of the writing but the depth of the learning that it brings about.

CONCLUSION

To be reflective in palliative care is to engage in the process of learning through the experience of one's own practice. Reflection promotes the recognition that practice is complex and shot through with ethical issues that demand the

Table 14.1 Characteristics of reflective writing

- Deals with concrete situations
- Uses the first person singular
- Exists 'in the moment'
- Studies an action that includes intention and context
- Describes the whole and the relationship between the whole and the parts
- Narrative in style
- Shows evidence of learning or deepening understanding
- Sometimes metaphorical
- Identifies factors that contribute to the situation, which may be historical, political, economic, social, ethical, autobiographical and psychological
- Draws attention to what might previously have been taken for granted, rendering the familiar strange
- Objectifies experience by the acquisition of new perspectives
- Seeks relationships to wider theory and general principles

exercise of wise professional judgement on the part of individual practitioners. Working reflectively helps practitioners to 'think palliatively' (Coles, 1996) and to develop an interest in the wider theory that surrounds palliative care. The personal and professional development of the practitioner is thus considered in relation to this literature. The attempt to write about the insights derived from reflective activities provides the means through which ideas can be shared with a wider audience, both in palliative care and beyond it.

REFERENCES

Boud, D., Keogh, R. and Walker, M. 1985: *Reflection: Turning Experience into Learning*. London: Kogan Page.

Carr, D. 1995: Is understanding the professional knowledge of teachers a theory–practice problem? *Journal of Philosophy of Education* 29(3), 311–31.

Coles, C. 1996: Undergraduate education and palliative care. *Palliative Medicine* 10, 93–8.

Department of Health 1989: *Caring for People: Community Care in the Next Decade and Beyond*. Cmd 849. London: HMSO.

Department of Health 1993: *The Vision of the Future: Nursing, Midwifery and Health Visiting's Contribution to Health Care*. London: HMSO.

Fish, D. and Coles, C. 1998: *Developing Professional Judgement in Health Care*. Oxford: Butterworth-Heinemann.

Fish, D. and Twinn, S. 1997: *Quality Clinical Supervision in the Health Care Professions: Principled Approaches to Practice*. Oxford: Butterworth-Heinemann.

Glaser, B.G. and Strauss, A.L. 1965: *Awareness of Dying*. New York: Aldine.

Glaser, B.G. and Strauss, A.L. 1967: *The Discovery of Grounded Theory: Strategies for Qualitative Research*. Chicago: Aldine.

Ham, C. 1992: *Health Policy in Britain*. London: Macmillan.

Hillier, R. 1998: Good practice: lessons in working together, in Fish, D. and Coles, C. (eds) *Developing Professional Judgement in Health Care*. Oxford: Butterworth-Heinemann.

Hopper, A. 2000a: *Dying Values: A Study of Professional Knowledge and Values in Health Care Practice*. Unpublished PhD thesis, University of Exeter.

Hopper, A. 2000b: Spiritual care: the primacy of holistic practice. *European Journal of Palliative Care* 7(2), 60–2.

James, A. 1994: *Managing to Care: Public Services and the Market*. London: Macmillan.

Kearney, M. 1996: *Mortally Wounded*. Dublin: Marino.

Klein, R. 1989: *The Politics of the National Health Service*. Harlow: Longman.

Lunn, L. 1990: Having no answer. In Saunders C. (ed.) *Hospice and Palliative Care: An Inter-disciplinary Approach*. London: Edward Arnold.

Mackay, L. 1993: *Conflicts in Care: Medicine and Nursing*. London: Chapman & Hall.

MacLeod, R. and James, C. 1994: *Teaching Palliative Care: Issues and Implications*. Penzance: Patten Press.

Salvage, J. 1985: *The Politics of Nursing*. London: Heinemann.

Saunders, C. 1984: On dying well. *Cambridge Review* (Feb), 49–52.

Schön, D. 1991: *The Reflective Turn*. New York: Teachers' College Press.

Smith, R. 1992: Theory: an entitlement to understand. *Cambridge Journal of Education* 22(3), 387–98.

FURTHER READING

Brookfield, S.D. 1987: *Developing Critical Thinkers*. Milton Keynes: Open University Press.

Field, D. 1984: We didn't want him to die alone – nurses' accounts of nursing dying patients. *Journal of Advanced Nursing* 9, 59–70.

Golby, M. and Appleby, R. 1995: Reflective practice through critical friendship: some possibilities. *Cambridge Journal of Education* 25(2), 149–60.

Langrebe, B. and Winter, R. 1994: Reflective writing on practice: professional support for the dying. *Educational Action Research* 2(1), 227–38.

chapter 15

MANAGING CHANGE/SETTING STANDARDS

Suzanne Mace

Change is not made without inconvenience, even from worse to better.

Richard Hooker

The modern hospice movement began in 1967 when St Christopher's Hospice in Sydenham was founded by Dame Cecily Saunders; by her action, she launched the palliative care movement as we know it today. The key issue underpinning this development was one of quality, and Dame Cecily addressed the complex issue of how quality of life could be measured, recognizing that it involves a variety of physical, emotional, social and cultural components that can change through the course of a disease.

The purpose of this chapter is therefore to explore how this philosophy can be put into practice in our continual quest to seek ways of improving the quality of palliative care we offer our patients. Achieving this requires change, the chapter examining some of the many change theories before moving on to the process of change and some strategies that may be adopted. It acknowledges that there may be potential blockages to suggested changes in practice and suggests ways of minimizing or eliminating such barriers. We will then consider quality, offering some definitions, dimensions and systems, and conclude with how palliative care can be evaluated through standard-setting, touching briefly on audit.

CHANGE

Change is a normal and inevitable fact of life, affecting everyone, whether professionally or personally. Without change, there would never be any progress. Change within health-care is constant, and one could be forgiven for feeling that there is little or no time to effect one change before others are presented. One such example was general practitioner fund-holding, which was quickly replaced by primary care groups and trusts. The Patient's Charter, the Health of the Nation strategy and the focus on public and consumer involvement all necessitated change. In addition, health-care practice is rapidly altering, nurses now working in very different ways and at higher levels of practice. Many nurses now run services, make complex patient-related decisions and lead programmes of care. The government is committed to these developments so they are likely to continue (Department of Health, 1999).

Faced with the inevitability of change, any person or organization ignoring the concept of change does so at their own peril. It is imperative to recognize that change occurs continuously, that it has numerous causes and that it needs to be addressed all the time. This applies as much to the organizations and staff concerned with palliative care as it does to those working in any other speciality. Consider how diagnostic procedures and cancer treatments have evolved and developed, and how day hospice facilities have grown over the last decade or so.

According to Oldcorn (1982), change is generally introduced because someone inside the organization is dissatisfied with the status quo. Houle (1980), on the other hand, suggests that everyone must expect constant change and, with it, new goals to be achieved and new understanding and skills to be mastered. The United Kingdom Central Council for Nursing, Midwifery and Health Visiting (UKCC, 1991) report of the Post-Registration Education and Practice Project (PREPP) concluded that there was a need to strengthen the structure, raise the standards of post-registration education and reflect the changing environment of health-care delivery.

Introducing change is not just the prerogative of managers: anyone may, possibly as the result of attending a post-registration course in palliative care, have felt encouraged to introduce innovation into the workplace. Examples of change that might be considered include the introduction of high-quality evidence-based information to assist patients to make informed choices, introducing a formal way of gaining feedback from patients and carers through the introduction of a consumer council, and reducing the risk of back injuries to staff and volunteers through an alteration in working practice.

THE PROCESS OF CHANGE

Before considering process, it may be helpful to examine some of the many change theories. The origin of classical change theory is accredited to Lewin (1951), who described three steps in the change process:

1 unfreezing
2 moving to a new level
3 refreezing.

Unfreezing includes motivating participants in the direction of readiness for change by 'thawing them out'. During this phase, participants recognize the need for change, work to diagnose the problem and generate a solution by making a selection from a number of alternative approaches.

Lewin (1951) also introduced the concepts of driving and restraining forces that either help or hinder the change process. Driving forces are those which

Table 15.1 Ways of altering the status quo, in order of effectiveness

Increasing driving forces	Decreasing restraining forces
Using a model or demonstration on one unit	Maintaining a forum for open discussion, meetings and conferences
Providing continuous support and encouragement throughout the change process	Providing essential information at the appropriate time and level of cognition of the participants
Using the change as an example when it works well	Using a problem-solving approach

facilitate the change process by moving the participants in the direction desired by the change agent. In contrast, restraining forces impede the change cycle. When the driving and restraining forces are equal, the status quo is maintained. Change occurs when one set of forces outweighs the other. Lewin (1951) found that it was far easier to remove restraining forces than it was to generate more driving forces – in doing the latter, the resisting forces increase in strength to compensate. Olson (1979), on the other hand, lists, in order of effectiveness, three factors that will increase the strength of the driving forces and three that can be used to decrease the restraining forces (Table 15.1).

Rogers (1962) expanded on Lewin's three phases of change by emphasizing both the background of those participating in the change process and the environment in which the change takes place. He described five phases in the change cycle: awareness, interest, evaluation, trial and adoption. Rogers believed, in essence, that the process of adopting any change was more complex than the three steps discussed by Lewin. In Roger's view, each participant in the change process could initially accept the change or reject it. He further maintained that the effectiveness of change depends on whether the participants are keenly interested in the change and show a commitment to implementing it.

Taking a rationalist approach, Lippitt (1973) defined change as 'any planned or unplanned alteration to the status quo in an organisation, situation or process' and planned change as 'an intended, designed or purposive attempt by an individual, group, organisation, or a situation'. He contended that no-one can escape change, the question being, 'How do we handle the change?' Lippitt suggested that the key to dealing with change was to develop a thorough and carefully thought-out strategy for intervention, identifying seven steps in the change process (Table 15.2).

In managing change, care needs to be taken in the selection of an appropriate strategy and in recognizing its strengths and weaknesses. Lancaster (1982) put forward a variety of strategies for change:

- The *empirical–rational strategy* suggests that it is rational for people to find outcomes that offer maximum value to the individual when faced with the possibility of risk. Unfortunately, not all people are prepared to face the possibility of risk, even for what appears to be a rational suggestion of change.
- The *power–coercive strategy* assumes a sense of control and recognizes that those people with less power will always comply with the orders from the leader.
- With the *normative–re-educative approach*, the emphasis is on the values of staff and their attitudes to the proposed change.
- The *eclectic approach* considers the other three strategies and forms a combination of strategies rather than isolating one. The reason for the change may clearly dictate the choice of strategy, but the coercive strategy is generally best left as the last resort.

Table 15.2 Seven steps in the change process

---

1 Diagnosis of the problem
2 Assessment of the motivation and capacity for change
3 Assessment of the change agent's motivation and resources
4 Selection of progressive change objectives
5 Choosing an appropriate role for the change agent
6 Maintenance of the change once it has started
7 Termination of a helping relationship

BARRIERS TO CHANGE

Improvements in quality of care require, among other things, knowledge-led innovation. This approach is likely to require a change in practice, and there will inevitably be potential blockages to such changes. There are, however, ways of eliminating, or at least minimizing, such barriers.

Polit and Hungler (1993) highlighted four main factors that can slow or block the process of knowledge-led innovation:

1 the characteristics of the research itself;
2 the attitudes and backgrounds of the individual practitioners;
3 the organizational setting;
4 the barriers between the professions.

Hunt (1981) suggested several reasons why nurses do not use research findings:

- they do not know about them;
- they do not understand them;
- they do not believe them;
- they do not apply them;
- they are not allowed to use them.

McIntosh (1995), in looking at barriers to research implementation, concluded that Hunt's observations still applied some 14 years later.

Lacey (1994) in her small study of 20 hospital nurses, found that barriers included uncooperative doctors, older nursing auxiliaries and second-level nurses, a lack of time to read research findings and a lack of resources.

A useful tool for identifying potential blockages to knowledge-led innovation is the Barriers to Research Utilisation Scale, an instrument developed by Funk et al. (1991). Using this tool to find out the potential blockages within our own organization, I invited the members of the care team to complete the utilization scale. From the completed forms, 12 barriers emerged, four potentially blocking research to a great extent and eight blocking it to a moderate extent. The four most powerful blockages were:

1 research reports and articles not being readily available;
2 that the nurse did not have time to read research;
3 the relevant literature not being held in one place;
4 that the amount of research information was overwhelming.

These results had many similarities with those identified by the researchers previously discussed, which suggests that barriers have remained virtually unchanged for the past two decades.

So, having identified the barriers, what can be done to eliminate or minimize them? As Funk et al. (1991) suggest, it is only when specific barriers are identified that we can effectively intervene to reduce or eliminate them or alter professionals' perceptions of them. The elimination, or at least reduction, of barriers is an important step towards improving nursing practice through research and, as a consequence, quality of care.

Carroll et al. (1997), in their study to explore the nurse's perception of the barriers to and facilitators of using research findings in nursing practice, employed the Barriers Scale (Funk et al., 1991) and grouped the top 10 barriers into three types, those of the adopter (nurse), the organization and communication.

The *'adopter'* (nurse) encompasses the identified blockage that the nurse is unaware of the research. Deacon (1986) suggested that, once qualified, nurses tend to read very little literature related to their work, which could imply that they lack the knowledge of research that is available to inform their practice. This view is not, however, supported in the findings of a study by Luckenbill-Brett (1987), which showed that, of 216 qualified nurses questioned, 70 per cent were aware of research findings and 58 per cent were persuaded of their value. What may be the problem with regard to nurses not knowing about research findings is that these are often printed in large, not easy to digest tomes that are not widely read by clinical nurses. If research findings were to be published in the more popular nursing press, which nurses tend to prefer to read, their awareness of research findings might increase.

The *'organization'* covers the nurse's lack of time to read the research, the feeling that the benefit of changing practice will be minimized and the beliefs that other staff are not supportive in their implementation and clinicians will not co-operate with it. There will also inevitably be a resistance to change, but the implementation of knowledge-led innovation does mean that change will occur. MacGuire (1990) and Robinson (1987) among others have identified the difficulties associated with trying to make changes based on research findings. We are arguably creatures of habit, there existing, both personally and professionally, a 'why change?' mentality. Holland (1993) holds the view that nurses in the UK have a deeply ingrained sense of the history of nursing and its traditions, to the extent that traditional knowledge and practice have become part of the nurse's cultural inheritance, which has made cultural change difficult to achieve. Traditional practices can create a sense of stability and familiarity, allowing people to feel at ease and confident in terms of what to expect.

'Communication' encompasses such blockages as the fact that research reports and articles are not readily available, that the relevant literature is not compiled in one place and that statistical analyses are not understandable. Ford and Walsh (1994) lament the fact that history has left us with a significant number of nurses who do not have the academic skills to appreciate the significance of research findings, and although this is being addressed in today's nurse education, it does seem to remain an unfortunate fact.

In light of the above, it would seem especially important that research findings are presented in a clear and acceptable way without, as Ford and Walsh (1994) suggest, recourse to 'pseudoscientific jargon'. Parahoo (1997) cautions that being aware of research findings and the need for research is only the first step towards fulfilling the research role of nurses, utilizing research to underpin practice being the ultimate aim. Parahoo and Reid (1988) draw attention to the need for nurses to be able to critically evaluate research findings, as the naïve adoption of every new idea is as damaging to the profession as a refusal to consider change. Hunt (1987) suggests that the only lasting capabilities that teachers can help nurses to acquire are self-directed learning skills, which are dependent on their ability to find and evaluate information. The nature of specialist palliative care moves it very much into the realms of education, and it is important that practitioners' knowledge and skills develop and expand without their feeling threatened by changes in practice.

So what can be done to eliminate or minimize blockages to knowledge-led innovation? Rogers (1983) described five conceptual stages commonly passed through when research findings are successfully adopted:

- knowledge
- persuasion
- decision
- implementation
- information.

Knowledge is an essential pre-requisite to the adoption of innovation so it is therefore important that findings are disseminated in the most accessible form. One way of achieving this is to hold regular (monthly) team meetings for educational purposes, to be used specifically to examine and discuss a relevant piece of research. It may be useful for such meetings to be facilitated by the tutor or education manager.

In addition, any identified resistance to change, either within or outside the organization, needs to be addressed. As the *Health Pickup Workbook* (National Health Service Training Division, 1995) suggests, this requires a certain degree of mutual trust and respect, as well as clear and frequent communication. Managers, educators and nurses all need to work together in effecting any change.

It is also useful to find ways of increasing individuals' exposure to research findings, perhaps by undertaking a literature search on an aspect related to specialist palliative care and sharing the information found with colleagues.

QUALITY

A quality specialist palliative care unit or service delivers appropriate, acceptable and effective care to patients and those close to them, making the most efficient possible use of resources and having regard, when appropriate, to equity and accessibility of provision. The palliative care approach emphasizes the importance of quality of life and focuses on the needs of patients and their families and carers as individuals. Palliative care has been defined as:

> the active total care offered to a patient with progressive disease and their family when it is recognised that the illness is no longer curable, in order to concentrate on the quality of life and the alleviation of distressing symptoms within the framework of a co-ordinated service.
>
> Standing Medical Advisory Committee (1992)

Quality is notoriously hard to define, definitions for it abounding. Perhaps the one which we should be striving towards in the palliative care approach is to be found in the *Collins English Dictionary* (1979): 'A degree or standard of excellence, especially high standard'.

Quality is multi-dimensional, one of the best known theoretical models in this area being Maxwell's (1984) six dimensions of effectiveness, efficiency, equity, acceptability, accessibility and appropriateness. This model provides a useful checklist but, as a complete approach, is quite difficult to implement because the six dimensions are not distinct, sometimes overlapping and even at times being at variance with each other. Higginson (1993) has applied some of these dimensions to palliative care and concluded that evaluations have tended to centre on the effectiveness and acceptability of care, there having been few published studies considering equity, accessibility and efficiency.

Equally, the quality of care a patient receives on any one occasion is the end result of a complex system of activities. The 'systems' view of health care is reflected in the simple but influential categorization by Donabedian (1980) of indicators of quality under the headings of structure, process and outcome. To improve the service, it is necessary to pay attention to all three since structure and process are ultimately important only in terms of the outcomes they produce, whereas outcomes can only be changed via the structure and processes that produce them.

Quality and standards are being addressed in all walks of life and, if we believe in promoting excellence in nursing practice, we need to have standards and audit systems in order to identify shortcomings and ways for continuous improvement.

Definitions of palliative care are plentiful, all including reference to quality; the World Health Organization (1990) describes it as 'the active, total care of patients whose disease no longer responds to curative treatment and for whom the goal must be the *best quality* of life for them and their families and carers'. We all have expectations, individuals, families and other carers experiencing a life-threatening illness being no exception. They can expect and require access to comprehensive, co-ordinated and multi-agency care; Table 15.3 provides some suggestions for how this might be achieved.

The Calman-Hine Report (Department of Health, 1995) reinforces the need for all cancer patients to have access to a uniformly high standard of care and for palliative care to be integrated in a seamless way with all cancer treatment, serving to provide the best possible quality of life for the patients and their families. Much is talked about quality systems, a quality system being one which ensures and demonstrates that services conform to the specified requirements (NCHSPCS, 1992). Quality assurance – the definition of standards, the measurement of their achievement and the mechanisms to improve performance – is also widely discussed (Shaw, 1989). More simply, the following steps need to be taken:

- define the standard;
- measure the level of achievement;
- introduce mechanisms to improve performance.

SETTING STANDARDS

The process thus starts with defining and setting the standards, the process by which they are set and the way in which they are written contributing to their effectiveness as a means of promoting quality care. Standards come in many

Table 15.3 How access to comprehensive, co-ordinated, multi-agency care may be achieved

- Standard setting at local and organizational level
- Customer satisfaction surveys
- Clinical audit involving all staff
- Peer review
- External audit
- Effective complaints procedure
- Comprehensive education programmes and support systems for all staff

guises and serve a variety of purposes. They sometimes represent requirements that *must* be met for the service to be acceptable (minimum standards). In palliative care, however, standards should be ideals of best practice to aim for (optimum standards). Optimum standards to promote better care:

- are realistic, with motivating aims;
- do not represent an unattainable ideal;
- do not represent something too easily achieved.

But should nurses write their own standards or adopt published ones that have been tried and tested? As with most things, there are pros and cons to both approaches (Table 15.4). If the decision is taken to write one's own standards, the following may be of help in getting started. The first step is to decide the subject of the standard, for example a source of concern, an area of interest, an area identified as requiring improvement or a new idea to be checked out. The decision-making process should also include asking the following questions:

- Is the problem within your sphere of responsibility, can you *really* do anything about it?
- Is it a situation that can be improved within a *reasonable* amount of time, with a *reasonable* amount of effort?
- Will the standard result in a *direct improvement* of patient care?
- Will you be able to *demonstrate* an improvement?
- Do other staff share *similar* views about the need to look at the chosen area?
- Do you have or can you find enough *information* and *expertise* to deal with the topic?
- Do you have enough *support* to go ahead?

Table 15.4 The pros and cons of using published standards or writing one's own

Pros	Cons
Using published standards	
More economical in terms of time and effort	May reduce involvement
	May lack relevance to local circumstances
Avoids reinventing the wheel	Potentially less credible
May be well tried and of recognized value	Reduced staff commitment
Writing one's own standards	
Develop naturally from the organization's values and aims	Time-consuming
	Lack of expertise
Reflect local circumstances and preferences	Failure to reach a consensus
Written with the active participation of the staff	
Appreciation of relevance to own work	

It is important to involve a wide range of people in this decision-making process so it may be appropriate to consider involving some or all of the following:

- staff at all levels
- trustees
- volunteers
- patients
- families and carers
- local health professionals.

Whoever is involved, it is essential that the production of any standard should be preceded by consultation and communication to ensure its validity and to gain the total support of everyone involved in its use.

Adopting the approach categorized by Donabedian (1980), the standard is usually written as a statement of a desired outcome, for example 'The patient and his/her carer(s) have access, in confidence, to expertise in counselling, psychological and spiritual care, to provide emotional support'. Then follow the structure, process and outcome.

The *structure* derives from the human, physical and financial resources that provide health care. Its characteristics are stable and include the providers of care, the tools and resources they have at their disposal, and the physical and organizational settings in which they work. Resources include:

- staffing – mix and grades
- finance
- home care, hospital and hospice services
- drugs
- equipment.

The *process* is the activity that goes on with and between the practitioner and the patient, in other words how the resources are used. The use of resources include:

- the number of visits
- the time taken during a visit
- throughput
- procedures carried out
- drugs prescribed
- equipment given out.

The *outcome* is the result of the intervention that has taken place between practitioner and patient, that is, the change in a patient's current and future health status. The results of interventions include:

- symptoms alleviated
- pain relieved
- anxiety allayed

- needs met
- fears, grief and anger resolved
- choices respected
- satisfaction.

An example of a standard statement, together with its structure, process and outcome criteria, is shown in Box 15.1.

An example of ready-published standards is that of the Trent Hospice Audit Group (1992), who have produced seven palliative care core standards that consider the overall palliative care service. Developed as a regional audit collaboration by a group of senior medical and nursing staff, the Trent standards take the form of seven principles and their corresponding structure, process and outcome statements, also combining the measurement of several standards into logical audit packages.

The standard-setting process would not be complete without the inclusion of a review process, and this is where audit comes into its own. In palliative care, audit can benefit patients and families, it can benefit the services providing palliative care, it can be of benefit for education and training, and it is important for the purchasers of health care. Much has been written about audit and measurement tools, but it is useful to remember three mnemonics, compiled by Higginson (1993) based on audit experience (both good and bad) and building on guidelines from Shaw (1989, 1992).

Start your audit with a SPREE:

- Small – begin small and then grow when the audit is more established.
- Plan – there needs to be a clear plan of audit and commitment to it on the part of the staff.
- Regular – audit meetings, the collection of information and a review of the results must occur regularly.
- Exchange ideas within audit group and other audit groups, learning from your mistakes and successes.
- Enjoy it! It should not be seen as a threat.

BOX 15.1 EXAMPLE OF A STANDARD STATEMENT

The patient and his/her carer(s) have the information they seek relating to the diagnosis, prognosis and progress of the illness and the care options available to enable them to make informed choices.

Structure criteria	Process criteria	Outcome criteria
The patient has access to qualified and competent members of a multi-disciplinary team	Team members discuss with the patient and carer(s) their information needs	The patient understands as much as he/she wants about his/her illness

When choosing methods of audit, be BRAVE:

- Borrow methods and measures from others.
- Reliable measures or criteria are necessary if more than one person will be assessing the standards.
- Appropriate standards and measures are needed.
- Valid measures and criteria are important to achieve an improvement in the care of the patient and family.
- Easy – the methods must be simple enough to understand and to apply to routine practice.

Finally, when some information has been collected and the difficult stage in the audit cycle of feedback and review has been reached, don't abandon it but ARISE:

- Analyse often so that the results are considered early.
- Review the audit results.
- Instigate change, however small, before the audit cycle is repeated.
- Set new standards to be monitored in a new audit cycle.
- Effect a new cycle, building on the result of the previous audit.

CONCLUSION

By continually questioning, reviewing, changing and repeating the cycle, there will be ongoing improvements in the quality of palliative care we offer. This chapter has hopefully provided the necessary stimulation and impetus to encourage readers to initiate a change – however small – that will enhance quality of care.

REFERENCES

Carroll, D.L., Greenwood, R., Lynch, K.E., Sullivan, J.K., Ready, C.H. and Fitzmaurice, J.B. 1997: Barriers and facilitators to the utilisation of nursing research. *Clinical Nurse Specialist* **11**(5), 207–12.

Deacon, L. 1986: Does anyone read research? *Nursing Times* **82**(32), 58–9.

Department of Health 1995: *A Policy Framework for Commissioning Cancer Services.* Calman Hine Report, London: D.H.

Department of Health 1999: *Making a difference: strengthening the nursing, midwifery and health visiting contribution to health and health care.* London: DoH.

Donabedian, A. 1980: *The definition of quality and approaches to its assessment.* Michigan: Health Administration Press.

Ford, P. and Walsh, M. 1994: *New rituals for old – nursing through the looking glass.* London: Butterworth-Heinemann.

Funk, S.G. Champagne, M.T., Wiese, R.A. and Tornquist, E.M. 1991: Barriers: The barriers research utilisation scale. *Applied Nursing Research* **4**(1), 39–45.

Higginson, I. 1993: Quality costs and contracts. In: Clark, D.(ed.) *The future for palliative care*. Buckingham: Open University Press.

Holland, K.C. 1993: An ethnographic study of nursing culture as an exploration for determining the existence of a system of ritual. *Journal of Advanced Nursing* **18**(9), 1461–70.

Houle, C. 1980: *Continuing learning in the profession*. London: Jossey-Bass.

Hunt, J. 1981: Indicators for nursing practice: the use of research findings. *Journal of Advanced Nursing* **6**, 189–94.

Hunt, M. 1987: Process of translating research findings into nursing practice. *Journal of Advanced Nursing* **12**(1), 101–10.

Lacey, A. 1994: Research utilisation in nursing practice: a pilot study. *Journal of Advanced Nursing* **19**, 987–97.

Lancaster, J. 1982: Change theory: an essential aspect of nursing practice. In: Lancaster, J. and Lancaster, W. (eds) *Concept for advanced nursing practice: the nurse as a change agent*. London: C.V. Mosby.

Lewin, K. 1951: *Field theory in social science*. New York: Harper & Row.

Lippitt, G.L. 1973: *Visualising change: model building and the change process*. San Diego, CA: University Associates.

Luckenbill-Brett, J.L. 1987: Use of practice research findings. *Nursing Research* **36**(6), 344–9.

MacGuire, J.M. 1990: Putting nursing research findings into practice: research utilisation as an aspect of the management of change. *Journal of Advanced Nursing* **15**, 614–20.

McIntosh, J. 1995: Barriers to research implementation. *Nurse Researcher* **2**(4), 83–91.

Maxwell, R. 1984: Quality assessment in health. *British Medical Journal* **288**, 1470–2.

National Council for Hospice and Specialist Palliative Care Services 1992: *Quality, standards, organisational and clinical audit for hospice and palliative care services*. Occasional Paper No. 2. London: NCHSPCS.

National Health Service Training Division 1995: *Health pickup workbook. Using research at work: towards informed practice*. NHSTD.

Oldcorn, R. 1982: *Management. A fresh approach*. Suffolk: Chaucer Press.

Olson, E.M. 1979: Strategies and techniques for the nurse change agent. *Nursing Clinics of North America* **14**, 323–36.

Parahoo, K. 1997: *Nursing research principles, process and issues*. Basingstoke: Macmillan.

Parahoo, K. and Reid, N. 1988: Research skills number 5 – Critical reading of research. *Nursing Times* **84**(43), 69–72.

Polit, D.F. and Hungler, B.P. 1993: *Essentials of nursing research: methods, appraisal and utilisation*, 3rd edn. Philadelphia: J.B. Lippincott.

Robinson, J. 1987: The relevance of research to the ward sister. *Journal of Advanced Nursing* **12**, 421–9.

Rogers, E. 1962: *Diffusion of innovation*. New York: Free Press of Glencoe.

Rogers, E. 1983: *Diffusion of innovation*, 3rd edn. New York: Free Press.

Shaw, C. 1989: *Medical audit – a hospital handbook*. London: King's Fund Centre.

Shaw, C. 1992: *Speciality medical audit*. London: King's Fund Centre.

Standing Medical Advisory Committee 1992: *The principles and provision of palliative care*. Joint report of the Standing Medical Advisory Committee and Standing Nursing and Midwifery Advisory Committee. London: SMAC.

Trent Hospice Audit Group 1992: *Palliative care core standards. A multi-disciplinary approach*. Sheffield: Trent Hospice Audit Group.

United Kingdom Central Council for Nursing, Midwifery and Health Visiting 1991: *The report of the post-registration education and practice project*. London: UKCC.

World Health Organization 1990: *Cancer pain relief and palliative care*. Technical Report Series No. 804. Geneva: WHO.

FURTHER READING

Buchanan, D. and Boddy, D. 1992: *The expertise of the change agent*. Hemel Hempstead: Prentice Hall.

Higginson, I. 1993: *Clinical audit in palliative care*. Oxford: Radcliffe Medical Press.

Kemp, N. and Richardson, E. 1994: *The nursing process and quality care*. London: Arnold.

Plant, R. 1987: *Managing change and making it stick*. London: Fontana.

Robbins, M. 1998: *Evaluating palliative care. Establishing the evidence base*. Oxford: Oxford University Press.

chapter 16

THE SPECIAL NEEDS OF CHILDREN AND ADOLESCENTS

Denise Hodson

> To cure sometimes, to relieve often, to comfort always.
> M. Strauss

The past 25 years have seen great advances in the diagnosis, treatment and survival of children with cancer. Each year, approximately 1500 children and adolescents in the UK are diagnosed as having a malignant disease. Childhood malignancies differ from adult cancers: childhood tumours are commonly sarcomas or blastomas, unlike those of adults, which are principally carcinomas. The most commonly treated childhood cancers are lymphoblastic leukaemia and brain tumours. Childhood cancer is, however, rare, only 1 child in 10 000 per year under 15 years of age developing a malignant disease. The rarity of these diseases led to the development in the UK of regionally based paediatric oncology units in the 1970s to facilitate the research, diagnosis, treatment and evaluation necessary in order to provide the optimal chance of cure for this small group of children. Over 80 per cent of children with malignant disease receive all or part of their therapy in these units, and over 65 per cent are now expected to survive.

The intensive treatment regimes necessitate repeated hospitalization for many children, with their parents, sometimes for lengthy periods. For most children, frequent out-patient visits are necessary, travelling to an oncology unit that may be many miles away. Oncology units may 'share care' with district general hospitals to alleviate some of the problems caused by distance, to promote communication and to establish confidence in the care-givers in the patient's own community.

Paediatric oncology units employ a multi-disciplinary team approach, involving health visitors/liaison nurses, social workers, psychologists, dietitians and others in caring for the child and the family. Spinetta and Deasey-Spinetta (1981) have shown that the whole family is affected when a diagnosis of cancer is made in a child. The unit's aim is to help families in whatever way they feel appropriate to be able to understand and cope with their child's illness, enabling them to continue their natural role as primary care-givers and support them through the treatment and the uncertainty of the eventual outcome (Koocher and O'Malley, 1981). It is the aim of units to adopt an honest and realistic approach from the time of diagnosis, an approach that facilitates discussion and understanding between parents, children and staff.

Although the outlook for most children is encouraging, there remain approximately one-third for whom a cure will not be achieved. A small number of these will die in the earlier stages of the treatment, from their disease, from infection or from complications of the drug therapy, usually in hospital. For others, relapse or failure to achieve a remission may mean further treatment programmes. Advancement of the disease necessitates a reassessment of aims and values, as well as a change in expectations to realize that a cure will not be achieved and a period of palliative care is beginning.

DECISION TO END CURATIVE TREATMENT

The decision to end attempts at curative therapy is not one made lightly. Where there is a progression of disease, or the adverse effects of further treatment outweigh the benefits that can realistically be achieved, ongoing open communication between the parents, the child if he or she is old enough and the oncology unit is essential. It is important that all aspects of the treatment and progression of disease are discussed so that the subsequent decision that active therapy has no further value is understood and made jointly with the professional carers. Over recent years, easy access to the Internet has seen many searching for new or innovative treatments that might help their child, and it is important that the value of these is fully explored with families. Open communication allows older children or teenagers to participate in these discussions so that they too can be helped to decide whether they want to try new drug treatments or whether they wish to set their own agenda in making new goals for their future. No family should be left to make the decision alone.

Children and parents develop close ties and relationships with the carers in the oncology units over many months, often years. Once the decision to end therapy has been made, there is a real need for the assurance of continuing support and an expression of the carers' concern for the child's continuing quality of life. Fears of being 'abandoned' or no longer being part of the unit's immediate priorities are real anxieties experienced by many parents, with fears of what the future will hold and worries about their ability to cope. The goals set for future care will involve re-establishing and making new contacts at home, symptom control and helping the family resume some normality of family life. There is a need to help them make plans and to 'invest' in the time left, making this final time of caring a positive one for living.

Regional oncology units encompass many districts and health authorities, and families may live in densely populated industrial areas or rural districts. It is the practice of oncology centres to establish communication with community carers at an early stage of treatment, contact with the general practitioner being made at the time of initial diagnosis, by telephone and letter. Links will also have been made by the unit's health visitor or liaison nurse to those already involved with the family at home – the health visitor or school nurse and the teachers. The first contact is important not only to establish a link, but also to allow the exchange of relevant information. The rarity of childhood malignancies means that most general practitioners will only see one or two cases of cancer in a child throughout their career. Thus opportunities to meet and discuss cases are usually welcomed by both hospital and community staff.

It is at the time of relapse of the disease and the decision to end attempts at curative therapy that the framework of contact made at diagnosis establishes its importance. By building on the lines of communication, the feasibility of care that is needed can realistically be offered. Martinson et al. (1986) and Chambers et al. (1989) have demonstrated that, by working together, the hospital and community carers can establish a plan of joint care to support the child and family in any way the family deems appropriate to enable them to care for their child.

The availability of carers and facilities differs widely from district to district. Health visitors, district nurses, paediatric community nurses and Macmillan and Marie Curie nurses are but a few of the appropriate professionals whose skills may be sought, but of course not all are available as a resource in any given area. The resources of oncology units also differ. Most can offer visits from liaison nurses/health visitors and social workers; hospital doctors may also visit. With some units, distance may mean that the majority of contact with families and home carers is made by telephone. The most important factor is that appropriate care and support is given by those most acceptable to the family.

ESTABLISHING THE PATTERN OF CARE

Where the needs of the dying child and his or family are best met has been the subject of much discussion and research (Wilson, 1985; Vickers and Carlisle, 2000). At the turn of the twentieth century, home was the natural and obvious place to be born and to die, with family and friends around. Medical advances over the years changed expectations as treatments were developed for many previously life-threatening illnesses. The specialist care centres for children with cancer were presumed to be the most appropriate place for these children to be. Now, however, options other than the acute, busy hospital setting are considered. Dying children especially want to be cared for at home (Vickers and Carlisle, 2000), and care can be given by their parents in familiar surroundings if they are helped by nursing and medical staff, even though they are living with the knowledge that their child will soon die (Martinson et al., 1984).

Many factors can influence the decision: the duration of terminal illness, the distance from the hospital, the availability of local support and the immediate medical and nursing needs of the child are but a few. There may be anxieties expressed by parents about their own ability to deliver adequate care, about the response of other children and about uncontrolled symptoms, especially pain. Parents may be reticent to discuss these fears unless specifically given the opportunity to do so. Parents and children who choose to remain in or return to hospital should not be left with feelings of failure – it may be right for them.

Whatever the outcome, parents should know that no decision is irreversible and that an open-door policy is maintained so that children can be cared for in the most appropriate way and place at any given time. For most families, home is preferable, family, friends and familiar surroundings providing comfort and support throughout this difficult time.

For some children, hospice care may provide the alternative to home or hospital care. The concept of hospice care for adults is well established, the emphasis being on the quality of life and symptom control to enable individuals to live their life with dignity, control and fulfilment. There are an increasing number of children's hospices in Britain, the first to be established to care for children who were dying being Helen House in Oxford.

A retrospective study of 25 families who attended the hospice examined their perceptions of the care offered and of the impact of a life-threatening disease on the family (Stein et al., 1989). Most families felt that they were greatly helped by the individualized family-orientated care and atmosphere, but the fact that the care was delivered in a setting solely for terminally ill children was considered to be a drawback. The home-from-home atmosphere in which all the family could be together was deemed particularly appropriate for those whose child or children suffered a degenerative condition and for whom periods of respite care could be offered. The impact on families as a result of the illness was substantial and felt by all their members. It included psychological difficulties, worries about symptom control, emotional and behavioural difficulties in siblings and financial and employment problems.

Figures show that the largest group of children to benefit from the care of Helen House in its first year were those with central nervous disorders, followed by those with mucopolysaccharidosis (Burne et al., 1984). Children with a malignant disease formed a much smaller group. Most of the children were admitted for respite care, either as a planned admission or as a crisis-situation intervention. The duration of terminal illness in children with malignant disease differs widely from those with degenerative disorders. For most, the time-span can be measured in weeks to short months, establishing care at home as a feasible option. The role of the children's hospice should remain an option to be considered and offered to all families when care for a child is being planned.

Caring for a dying child is one of the most difficult and emotional situations in which professional carers can be involved (Pfund, 1998). The previous experience of nurses and practitioners in the community will probably be limited, and many have expressed their feelings of anxiety in caring for a child and in their ability to deliver appropriate care and symptom control. The initial reaction is often that children are 'different' and that they lack the necessary expertise. The actual principles of caring for the terminally ill are similar no matter what the age of the patient; although the practices may differ when the patient is a child, community carers still have a wealth of experience and skills to offer.

Over long months or years, the parents have become 'specialists' in their child's disease and treatment, and have usually actively participated in general procedures, treatments and care. Their dependence on the oncology unit has already been described. The feelings of inadequacy experienced by some carers are understandable as families may bypass their general practitioner or nurse and contact the hospital unit directly. This can lead to feelings of 'exclusiveness' and make involvement seem difficult. If pathways of communication are kept open and contact is freely made by both hospital and home carers, some of these difficulties can be minimized through active discussion and the sharing of problems.

PRINCIPLES OF CARE

The principles of palliative care remain constant whatever the situation.

TO CONTINUE MEANINGFUL COMMUNICATION WITH THE CHILD AND FAMILY

Research has shown that the majority of time spent in the child's home is spent listening to the worries, fears and feelings expressed by families, and providing a 'listening' support (Martinson, 1980; Norman and Bennet, 1986). To be able to sit and listen is probably the most valuable contribution any carer can make. It asks carers to question their own attitudes to the process of dying and death, and to acknowledge the grief felt within the family.

SYMPTOM CONTROL WHEN NECESSARY

As symptoms arise through the progression of the disease, it is important that they are not considered in isolation but that the physical and emotional needs of the child as a whole are considered. There may be more than one specific cause, and younger children may have difficulty explaining how they feel. Various tools (Wong and Baker, 1988; Carsol, 1993) are available to assist in assessing symptoms, especially pain. Parents will also describe changes in physical or emotional needs or abilities, which often provides a valuable guide.

TO RESPOND APPROPRIATELY TO THEIR ONGOING NEEDS

The needs of the child and family can change quickly as palliative care evolves. The duration of care is variable, input in practical terms depending on the advance of the disease and the symptoms experienced. Subjects discussed may relate to other family members or friends or to practical issues such as finance, heating, bills or other needs. It may be appropriate to draw on the particular skills of other carers in the hospital or community in order to address specific problems.

EFFECTIVE LIAISON AND THE SHARING OF INFORMATION BETWEEN HOSPITAL AND COMMUNITY CARERS

Throughout this time and after death, the oncology unit will maintain contact by telephone calls and visits to the child and family. Joint visits with community carers can reassure parents that everyone is working in close co-operation for their child's comfort and support, and maintaining contact between the hospital and community can lessen the feelings of isolation for staff and families alike.

COMMUNICATING WITH PARENTS

The families of dying children are generally more extended than those of adults in similar circumstances, including grandparents, relatives, close friends and the child's peers in their family unit. Younger members may not have experienced death before, the experience being made more intense and felt more strongly when the death is that of a child (Wilson, 1988). The needs of the family and their child have been identified as being similar, but not identical, to those of dying adults and their families (Wilson, 1985).

Parents may again feel all the emotions that surrounded the time of initial diagnosis, those of shock, anger and of disbelief: 'Perhaps the doctors have made a mistake, perhaps the scan is wrong, or not my child's'. For many, these feelings are entwined with a deeper knowledge gained by living with the child's disease and its treatment over many months or years, and with an acknowledgement that the grief began at diagnosis and has only been suppressed.

Parents are individuals in their own right, and their needs will differ throughout this time. They may find it difficult to relate to one another as the impact of their differing emotions falls on the person they are closest to. They need to be given time to talk freely together, and individually with carers. A common reaction is to blame either themselves for not preventing the disease or the impending death, or others for not diagnosing the disease earlier.

Their hopes and expectations are forced to change direction, from the hope of a cure to being able to give their child a peaceful, happy and pain-free time to come. In a study to try to identify the needs of families with a terminally ill relative, O'Brian (1983) noted, first, their need for information, and second, their need to be assured of their relative's comfort and their receipt of appropriate care. The same opportunities to talk to medical and nursing staff should be open to the child's siblings and relatives as they may have questions that they feel are inappropriate to ask of the parents at this time.

In conversation with parents, some have said that their relatives make the situation more difficult to cope with. They seem entwined in their own grief and their need to 'put things right', as well as in expressing false hopes with newspaper and Internet articles about the latest miracle cures around the world. Repeated explanations about changes in the child's condition and treatment become tiresome in the battle of maintaining some normality of family life. Parents express a need to talk to people who understand what is happening and for whom explanations are not necessary.

All parents will ask when their child will die – 'How long do we have with him?' – a question that is impossible to answer in absolute terms. We can only answer in the very broadest sense in light of our past experiences. No one can answer in definitive terms of weeks or months, except maybe in the final hours.

Other questions will explore the way in which death will occur: 'Will it be sudden?' and, most importantly, 'Will he be in pain?' The professional carer is more able to discuss the answers to these questions at length, having a knowledge of the most likely developments of the child's particular disease. It is difficult to describe these developments as options that may or may not happen to families, but parents feel better prepared to deal with symptoms or situations such as fits or bleeding as they arise. They know that individual possibilities have been anticipated and that measures that will ensure their child's comfort have been planned.

COMMUNICATING WITH THE PATIENT

Childhood encompasses a wide age range, from babies up to adolescents. The individual's age, development, both physically and psychologically, and experiences are important factors to be considered. During illness and hospitalization, children's need for their parents increases as they fear separation from the people and places they know best. Children are happiest in their own home, the normality of family life providing a secure environment. Concepts of death are directly related to age and personal experience, and one needs to know about children's understanding of death to be able to hold a meaningful discussion with them.

CHILDREN

For healthy children aged 0–3 years, the word 'death' has little meaning. The most frightening thought is that of separation from their parents and of being left alone. Between 3 and 5 years, a curiosity about death and 'being dead' develops. Seeing birds or animals who have died promotes the idea of not moving, or eating, maybe sleeping? But whatever it is, it is not permanent. Children feel invincible, acting out Superman and other heroes. They will associate death with heaven, which seems a real place where dead people go to be with others. The concept of not being able to visit, or of those who have died not returning at some time, seems strange. Young children are egocentric, believing that they cause events, both good and bad, to happen by what they say or do.

From 6 years of age, there is a gradual understanding that being dead is permanent, although for many, games played or television programmes watched reiterate the fact that their heroes recover to fight another battle next week, or that they can 'begin again' in a different game. Death can be thought of as a 'ghost' or as being associated with acts of violence or being 'bad'. 'Wishing' is a powerful tool of thought that can 'make' good or bad things happen.

The development of children from 10 years upwards and the wider experiences they have gained leads them towards a more adult reasoning of dying and death, and an awareness that one day they too will die and that it will be permanent.

The above outline is very broad and generalized as children will vary widely in their understanding of death, as they do in their physical development and intellectual ability at any age. Children who are very ill and have experienced repeated hospitalization, traumatic procedures and possibly the loss of a friend through death will experience a much greater awareness of its meaning, possibly at a younger age than most of their peers.

It was once thought that ill young children had little or no concept of their own death, but research has shown that they possess a much higher anxiety level and feelings of isolation (Spinetta et al., 1974), possibly as their parents seek to protect them by avoiding addressing the issue or by changes in their normal attitude towards the child. Parents may have prepared themselves, however subconsciously, for the time when curative treatment ends. This preparation has been defined as anticipatory mourning, a set of processes that are directly related to the awareness of impending loss, to the emotional impact and to the adaptive mechanisms whereby emotional attachment to the child is relinquished over time (Futterman and Hoffman, 1973). The depth and degree of this mourning period will vary in intensity between families and between the individuals involved.

Difficulties arise when a child dies suddenly in the early stages of his or her disease or during treatment, when parents have not had this time to prepare themselves and their families. Research has shown that more long-term psychological, behavioural and physical problems are experienced by parents and siblings following the sudden death of their child. Children can also demonstrate this distancing from those around from a young age. They want to protect their parents from answers or situations they perceive will cause distress.

It is not unusual for children to choose a person with whom they will discuss what is happening to them, their fears and thoughts, and then deny the reality with others by their silence. Not all children feel the need to have their impending death confirmed. What is important is that children are listened to, that it is recognized that the statements they make may be questions to be answered and that they are answered as honestly, sensitively and openly as possible. A lie or concealment will prevent further open communication and increase feelings of loneliness and isolation.

Parents and carers express their anxieties about what and when to tell a child. They are understandably frightened about saying the wrong thing or not being able to answer because of their own emotions. Children once did not commonly ask outright whether they were going to die, but this has changed over recent years, possibly as children have become more involved and more knowledgeable about their own illness and treatment. They may make a statement, draw pictures that can be discussed or ask a series of questions over a period of time that will provide a telling picture of their knowledge of their disease and of dying. When answering children, one need only answer what is being asked. If one is unsure of the question, a simple return of the question to the child may clarify the thoughts behind it. It is better to say an honest 'I don't know' to a question than to avoid the issue or make up what appears to be a suitable answer.

It should be remembered that children are most concerned with living. When they feel well, however weak, they want to resume their normal activities. For some, this may mean a return to school for all or part of the week. They need to have their siblings and friends to play – or just be – with. They also need the discipline that is the norm within their family unit. When acceptable boundaries of behaviour are lifted, the child becomes more uncertain of his role and limits within the family and feels insecure.

ADOLESCENTS

It is difficult to define an age range that totally encompasses the adolescent years; for most, it includes the ages of 12–20 years. This is a time of great change in the physiological, psychological and social development of the individual. 'No two individuals are alike and at no age are these differences more apparent than during the adolescent years' (Crow and Crow, 1965). Individuals are not yet adults, but neither can they be treated as dependent children.

Life for teenagers becomes a challenge. It is a time of questioning the limits enforced by parents, schools and society in an effort to establish their place and identity. Their appearance assumes great importance as they become heavily dependent on the approval and acceptance of their peer group, and as new personal relationships are formed. In the process of establishing their identity and independence, their mood swings to extremes. They can be sad, happy, uncertain, confident, kind, rebellious and argumentative (McCallum and Carr-Gregg, 1987).

Cancer and its treatment have an enormous impact on teenagers' self-image, identity and relationships within the family and with their peers. The necessity for repeated hospitalization increases their dependence on parents when they would normally be moving away from this. Their education is interrupted frequently, often when the most important study programmes for examinations are to be undertaken. Long or frequent spells in hospital result in a loss of their place in the peer group. This is enhanced by changes in appearance: alopecia and weight gain or loss all reinforce feelings of worthlessness.

Some teenagers regress emotionally and display more childish behaviour; others may exhibit maturity and a more adult understanding. Many want to take on new experiences and opportunities 'to put themselves on an accelerated track for experiencing life. Denial can be part of this race with time' (Johansen, 1988).

Carers especially come face to face with their own attitudes towards death and dying, when faced with a teenager who is dying. 'For health professionals to successfully work with dying adolescents they must first confront their own mortality' (Blum, 1984). Knowing that adolescent dreams and ambitions for the future will not be fulfilled, life seems unfair and unjust. Carers may be close to the patient in age or have teenage relatives, and the situation can become more personal.

'Dying adolescents grieve not only for the life they have lived but also for the life they have not lived. Grieving over their lack of future involves a process of discarding their unfulfilled dreams, expectations and goals' (Papadatou, 1989). Questions such as 'Why me?', 'What did I do?' and 'Why can't I...?.' be can be bitter and painful, and have no answers. Anger and resentment for lost opportunities may follow. Very ill adolescents know that they are dying but will fluctuate between acknowledging this, to either themselves or others, and denial. Their knowledge does not mean that they accept the situation, but, by being able to express their worries to a chosen person, they may gain a freedom to live their lives and reassert their independence (Papadatou, 1989). Box 16.1 demonstrates how two teenagers chose to describe their feelings in writing, in a letter and a poem.

BOX 16.1 LETTER AND POEM BY TWO TEENAGERS

I am writing about this because I daren't talk about it. My tumour had gone – the Chemo had killed it off, but what if my new tumour doesn't respond to treatment and grows. I keep thinking about Tracy and then about this tumour. I might die as well. I know I shouldn't think about this but I just can't help it.

Lynne

REACHING THE LIMIT
Got to go fast,
Head for the hill,
Don't seem to move,
Feeling ill.

Want to drop,
Feet do ache,
Have to stop,
Just can't wait.

Getting close,
Nearly there,
Reached the limit,
People stare.

John

Adolescents especially need to be involved in open discussions about their disease, symptoms and care, to be given control and to share in decision-making. Free communication between family members may be difficult to facilitate where parents try to protect their child (and themselves), a conspiracy of silence and isolation sometimes developing. Opportunities for communication that is honest and caring allow adolescents to express their anxieties and concerns. Research shows that many of their concerns are with the actuality of dying: 'Will I be in pain; for how long?', 'When will it be?' These questions are most likely to be asked of medical or nursing carers, with their professional knowledge, than of their family.

Again, these questions will be asked only where there is the trust and confidence that an honest answer will be given. Opportunities for the teenager to talk alone with medical staff should be made. This can sometimes be difficult to achieve as parental wishes must also be acknowledged, but sensitive exchanges can help them to understand their child's need for independent discussions. Individuals may have certain tasks they wish to complete: saying goodbye to friends, giving presents, making a will or coming to decisions about their funeral. Adolescents need reassurance that they will not be forgotten by their friends and that their life has made an impact on others.

COMMUNICATING WITH OTHER FAMILY MEMBERS

SIBLINGS

Many parents describe real difficulty in approaching the subject of death with their child and his or her siblings. They may be anxious not to say too much too soon, or of leaving explanations and the chance to talk until too late. One can only offer the advice to answer questions honestly as and when they arise. Teenage brothers and sisters will be more aware and involved than younger children and may choose to talk about their feelings with their family or friends. When siblings are encouraged to participate in their brother's or sister's care, questions may arise more naturally over time.

Questions may be asked more than once by siblings. This may relate directly to their age, understanding and concepts of death. There may also be changes in their emotional and behavioural responses relating to the perceived anxieties of their parents. If the sick child becomes the focus of their parents' attentions, and his or her needs and wishes seem paramount, siblings may feel left out, unimportant and isolated. Their behaviour may change so that they became clingy, attention-seeking or withdrawn. In promoting a more normal family life, one can encourage parents to include siblings in care-giving and in planning treats or visits for the whole family to participate in and enjoy.

GRANDPARENTS

The needs of grandparents should not be forgotten when caring for the family as their grief encompasses many losses. They grieve for the impending loss of their grandchild's life, as well as for their own child's sadness. One does not expect one's child to die first, and certainly not one's grandchild, who should have many years left. There is a loss of hope and investment in their future. Many will have played an active role during the hospitalization and treatment of their grandchild, either in relieving parents by the bedside or in caring for other children at home. The relationship of grandparents and grandchildren can also be a very special, close one.

It should not be assumed that returning home and re-establishing day-to-day living when a child is dying is always fraught with difficulties and communication problems. The belief of health professionals that open communication about dying was an essential task for the family has been challenged (Northouse, 1984). 'Not all families need to communicate about death, especially those who have comfortable, agreed upon patterns of not discussing feelings within the family system' (Lewandowski and Jones, 1988).

The families who are identified as needing help are those who want to talk but are uncertain of how to approach the subject, or families in which the needs of one member are at variance with those of the rest of the family. This should not, however, provide an excuse for carers not to explore the need to talk as the palliative care stage progresses. Over time and as symptoms change, carers may become aware of changes in the needs of individuals in the family.

The long periods in hospital or throughout treatment may have felt safe with support from other parents and professionals around, but when therapy has ended, home, with its comforts and familiar belongings, can offer its own respite for many parents.

SYMPTOM CONTROL

IDENTIFICATION AND ASSESSMENT OF PAIN

There have in the past been many myths and misconceptions relating to a child's ability to feel pain. Many assumed that it was not experienced with the same intensity as that perceived by adults. Subsequent research shows this assumption to be unfounded, no evidence being available to substantiate it (Reape, 1990). The child's age, development, behaviour and ability to express feelings are some of the factors that must be taken into consideration when assessing and managing pain control (Twycross, 1998).

Various age-related tools are available to assist in this management. One of the most reliable is the Eland colour tool, in which children use different coloured pens to draw on a body outline (Figure 16.1), choosing their own colours to describe the different intensities of pain felt in different parts of the body. Other scales utilize colours, a range of 'smiling' to 'sad' faces, numbers,

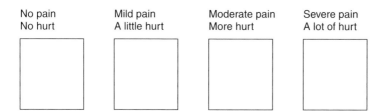

| No pain
No hurt | Mild pain
A little hurt | Moderate pain
More hurt | Severe pain
A lot of hurt |

Pick the colours that mean <u>No hurt</u>, <u>A little hurt</u>, <u>More hurt</u>, and <u>A lot of hurt</u> to you and colour in the boxes. Now, using those colours, colour in the body to show how you feel. Where you have no hurt, use the <u>No hurt</u> colour to colour in your body. If you have hurt or pain, use the colour that tells how much hurt you have.

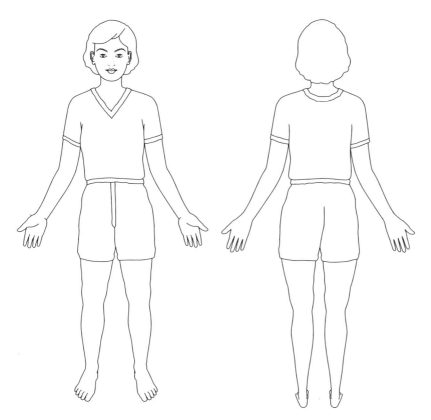

Figure 16.1 Body outline tool used to help children to describe the sites and intensity of their pain

thermometers and linear visual analogue scales in which points are drawn on a straight line indicating 'least' pain at one end and 'worst' pain at the other. Results have shown varying degrees of reliability associated with the age and development of the child when using some of these methods (Wong and Baker, 1988).

The language employed by children to describe pain varies considerably with their age. The actual word 'pain' may not be understood by over half of all children aged between 5 and 8 years so it is important that the specific words used by the child and family are known in order to help to communicate at the child's level of understanding. Some of the words more commonly used include 'sore', 'little hurts' and 'big hurts', specific noises also being made by some children. Mothers naturally identify cries made by their babies or toddlers as denoting 'hunger', 'tiredness' or 'pain'. Studies show us that children can and do express pain but in their own way (Carrol, 1993). They do not imagine or pretend to have pain, but difficulties can sometimes arise in identifying its intensity.

The behavioural changes of young children often described by parents, such as sleeplessness, irritability, anorexia and general unhappiness at being moved or touched, may all indicate that the child is in pain. These symptoms may also of course be described in older children and teenagers. The parents of a child receiving palliative care may not always recognize pain in the child. They know that their child will die and usually have no previous experiences to which to relate this situation. They are experiencing their own pain and may feel that the child's current condition is only to be expected. One must always listen carefully to what is being said as issues that cause them concern may be indicative of pain in their child. Professional carers should also be aware that older children and adolescents can be reluctant to say that they are in pain if they are anticipating a return to hospital as a consequence. When the decision of where palliative care is to be given is being taken, the major cause of anxiety for parents is the fear of uncontrollable symptoms, especially pain (Kohler and Radford, 1985).

Not all children who are terminally ill experience severe pain, and not all require strong opiates. Experience has shown, for example, that many children who have brain tumours require less opiate treatment, although other symptom control is necessary. This contrasts sharply with some children who have bone or soft tissue tumours, for whom opiate drugs are usually needed in large doses for long periods of time along with co-analgesics. If the care of these children is to ensure their comfort effectively, the professional carer must learn to listen, recognize the symptoms then treat them appropriately and quickly (Twycross, 1997).

The principles of assessing pain are well known. Pain may be related directly or indirectly to the disease or to previous anti-cancer therapy, and can be experienced in more than one site. The difference between these pains can be difficult to describe especially for a child. It is possible to anticipate some of the types of pain that can be directly attributed to the nature and progression of disease (Miser and Miser, 1989). Severe headaches, with nausea and vomiting especially on rising, are, for example, most often seen in children with brain tumours and in leukaemia patients who have infiltration of the cerebrospinal fluid by blasts cells, both giving rise to raised intracranial pressure.

Bone pains are commonly experienced by children with leukaemia or metastatic neuroblastoma. The pain results from the invasion of bone and bone marrow, and may be described as dull, aching, constant and progressively increasing in severity. Invasion of the bone and bone marrow also occurs in Ewing's sarcoma and osteosarcoma, occasionally leading to a pathological fracture. Very sharp, severe pain may be indicative of a rapidly growing tumour or an intratumour bleed. The spread of tumour from soft tissue into adjacent nervous tissue results in a localized pain, described as sharp or burning, or in a more diffuse pain along the affected nerve pathways.

TREATMENT OF PAIN

Each pain requires the separate consideration and assessment of its history, severity and nature before a diagnosis can be made. Any treatment previously prescribed and its efficacy must also be noted. When treating the pain, it is vital that an adequate dose is prescribed for the individual child. Most drugs for children are prescribed on a 'milligram per kilogram' basis, but it must be stressed that, when opiates are prescribed, this guide provides only a baseline. Drug dosages may need to be increased quickly to maintain pain control. This increase should also be appropriate, a rise of 50 per cent or more sometimes being necessary to regain control of the symptoms. When the pain is constant, analgesia must be regularly prescribed: there is no place for 'as required' doses for any patient in pain. Co-analgesics will often be necessary and will be described briefly below.

The most careful assessment, diagnosis and treatment are of little value if they are not frequently monitored and reviewed, with empathy and understanding. This may initially necessitate return visits to the home after a short time has elapsed, or regular telephone calls, to establish the effectiveness of the treatment. Such contact, no matter how brief, is always reassuring and welcomed by the family. If an immediate control of symptoms is necessary, contact that occurs once or twice weekly is insufficient and may result in panic calls or return visits to hospital that could be avoided. This can be a very demanding time for community nurses and practitioners.

The decision of which analgesic agent is most appropriate should not be difficult if pain control is commenced early and in an effective dosage. There is a wide choice of drugs available, but a useful recommendation is that one should restrict one's choice to a limited number and become familiar with these (Oakhill, 1988). The widely used 'analgesic ladder' provides a useful reminder that when one form of analgesia fails, changing from one non-opiate drug to another will not regain pain control, progress to a weak opiate being the next logical step.

The practice in our unit is initially to obtain pain control in younger children by prescribing paracetamol elixir, usually in one of the well-known proprietary forms such as Calpol or Calpol 6 plus. These are more acceptably flavoured and usually well known to the child. Where stronger analgesics are needed, progression may be made to dihydrocodeine and then to morphine elixir 4-hourly. Care should be taken when flavouring any medications that favourite acceptable foods or drinks are not used in an attempt to disguise the taste – this may only make the foods unpalatable, with the result that they are totally rejected. Tablets should not be discounted by physicians because of the age of the child. Many children prefer from a young age to take tablets, either whole or crushed, and have become accustomed to doing so throughout their chemotherapy regimes.

Many children aged 5 years and upwards who require strong opiate therapy find MST Continuous (controlled-release morphine) tablets more acceptable. If this is prescribed, morphine elixir should also be available to control any breakthrough pain until the appropriate MST Continuous dose is achieved as there is a delay of up to 4 hours before the peak plasma concentration occurs. It is our experience that MST Continuous tablets need to be prescribed 8-hourly for children of less than 10 years of age and 12-hourly for older children and teenagers: the drug appears to be metabolized more quickly in the younger age group. For children receiving relatively long-term opioid therapy, this can significantly simplify drug-taking and allow for longer periods of rest between doses, especially through the night, for both child and parents. MST granules are now available in a range of strengths in sachets. These are mixed into a suspension in water and provide slow-release pain control, without the need for tablets; these prove useful for many children.

For the majority of children, oral morphine preparations provide good pain control throughout their palliative care, but there are a number of children for whom the oral route becomes inappropriate or insufficient. An alternative method may be necessary if the child's level of consciousness deteriorates, when there is difficulty in swallowing for other reasons, with uncontrolled pain or persistent vomiting, or when large, repeated doses of oral drugs become difficult to tolerate. Failure to comply with any form of oral medication by the child is also a possibility.

Pain relief may be obtained by administering morphine as a suppository. With the exception of a few drugs, such as anticonvulsants, the rectal route is one not commonly used in the UK, being rarely employed in palliative care. It is effective but requires careful explanation for the child and parents for it to be accepted. The child's diagnosis and the condition must be taken into account if this method is to be used. Thrombocytopenia in a child with leukaemia, especially when episodes of bleeding have already occurred, may demand an alternative method of drug delivery. Morphine suppositories are available in 15 mg and 30 mg strengths, but pharmacies may be able to prepare other strengths should they be necessary.

Fentanyl, a synthetic opioid analgesic agent used in anaesthesia, can be used in the form of a skin patch to provide effective pain control for those children who have relatively stable, controlled pain. Patches are not appropriate for children who bruise or bleed easily, or who do not tolerate plasters and their removal (Miser et al., 1989).

In the past, a lack of adequate pain control necessitated a return to hospital for intravenous analgesia for many children, and their families, usually hours or short days before the child's death. Anxiety at the child's condition, the urgency of the situation and a failure to comply with the child's and parents' wishes to remain at home have all led to feelings of helplessness, lack of control, anger and extreme sadness on the part of parents and carers at this already stressful time.

In more recent years, the parental administration of opiates at home via the subcutaneous or venous route has become more widely used. This method of drug delivery has been employed for many years for adult patients, and the principles for care remain the same with children. Some of the children for whom this method is appropriate will already have a venous access device in situ. Skin-tunnelled catheters such as Hickman or Broviac lines, or implanted devices, for example a Portacath or Implant-a-port, are widely used in oncology centres for the administration of chemotherapy, blood products, antibiotics and parental feeding, and for blood sampling, thus negating the need for repeated venepuncture and the resiting of infusions (Sepion, 1990; Tweddle et al., 1997).

A strictly aseptic procedure is essential if such devices are to be accessed. Parents are taught how to clean, dress and flush, with heparinized saline, the skin-tunnelled catheter at home in order to maintain its patency between uses (Clarke and Cox, 1988). When chemotherapy is discontinued, the lines are usually left in situ to provide immediate access should some supportive intravenous therapy be needed.

The administration of diamorphine via the central venous line and a battery-operated syringe driver is very effective in controlling pain. Despite the very slow delivery of the drug, it is rare for these lines to occlude. Should this occur, advice should be sought from the oncology unit. When changing from oral morphine to intravenous diamorphine, the dosage should initially be titrated to one-third of the oral daily dose, although personal experience has shown that a subsequent increase in dosage is often quickly required. It may be more appropriate to titrate opiates to at least half the oral daily dose, especially if there is increased pain.

When introducing new and more technical methods of drug administration, the health professional must always be aware of the increased stress this brings to families. In our experience, with the support of the hospital and, most especially, the community carers, parents can increasingly take over much of the care associated with drug preparation and changing syringes. It is of course essential that parents and community nurses have a full knowledge of and confidence in the equipment and techniques used. Sharing information and resources between oncology units and community carers can only increase this knowledge and thus benefit the child.

Where a central venous line is not available, subcutaneous diamorphine by infusion is a viable alternative, using a Sof-set or fine-gauge 'butterfly' needle. To help to allay anxiety relating to the use of needles in hospital, children are accustomed to (and demand) the application of a local anaesthetic cream (EMLA) (Arts et al., 1994) under an occlusive dressing, applied an hour before the needle is inserted. This practice is recommended prior to needle insertion into subcutaneous sites, the sites most commonly used being the abdomen, arm and chest wall. A transparent dressing over the needle can then be applied to secure the needle and provide easy observation of the site. The site should immediately be changed if there is any sign of inflammation or if the child complains of any discomfort.

Most children and teenagers will tolerate the use of syringe drivers well if the need for this method of administration has been fully explained. It is not unusual to see a child or teenager who has previously appeared withdrawn, uncomfortable or in obvious acute pain become alert and interested in his or her surroundings. Syringe drivers that have a 'boost' control of a preset bolus dose allow the child or parent to administer an isolated increased dose should there be an acute episode of pain (Bray et al., 1996). For children less able to participate in family life, it is comforting for them and for their family to be held and cuddled without this causing signs of distress. There is no need or reason for the repeated, painful intramuscular injections of opiates when other methods of drug administration are available. Figures 16.2 and 16.3 depict the different needs of two children and the ways in which pain control was achieved for them.

Figure 16.2 Pain control in S.H., a child with a neuroblastoma

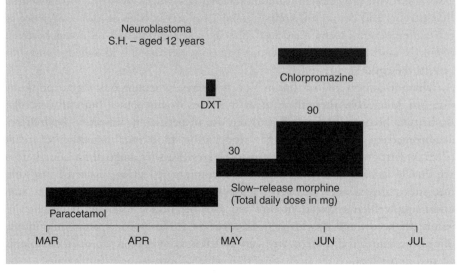

CASE STUDY

S.H. was diagnosed as having stage III neuroblastoma at the age of 8 years. After receiving chemotherapy and surgery, he remained well for 2 years before relapsing twice and was being treated with chemotherapy and radiotherapy. His tumour failed to respond to the second relapse treatment, and a joint decision was made to end attempts at curative therapy. At this time, S.H. had extensive lymph node disease and two areas of bony metastasis. Paracetamol controlled his pain well for some weeks, but towards the end of April he developed pain associated with one of the bony metastases. He was given a short course of radiotherapy and commenced morphine sulphate controlled-release tablets. Throughout this time, S.H. had been mobile and able to attend school on a part-time basis, but as his symptoms of tiredness and lethargy increased, he was less able to go out. He required an increased dose of analgesia, which caused some nausea. This was well controlled by chlorpromazine and he remained pain-free until his death a few weeks later.

Neuroblastoma
S.H. – aged 12 years

DXT

Chlorpromazine

90

30

Slow–release morphine
(Total daily dose in mg)

Paracetamol

MAR   APR   MAY   JUN   JUL

Figure 16.3 Pain control C.K., a child with a Ewing's sarcoma

CASE STUDY

C.K. was a 10-year-old girl who presented with a Ewings sarcoma of her femur. Originally treated with systemic chemotherapy and radiotherapy to the primary tumour, she suffered an extensive local relapse, 2 years after completing treatment. The question of further therapy was discussed, but, after consideration, the decision was made to adopt a palliative approach. She was started on oral parac-etamol, but this failed to control her pain for more than a few weeks so morphine elixir was com-menced. Her localized pain was well controlled by a relatively small dose of morphine, and she remained mobile, attending school, with a relatively good quality of life. During late October and early November, C.K.'s tumour grew and began to encase her pelvis. This required a very close monitoring of the situation, periods of relative stability being followed by fairly sharp increases in her analgesic dose. She became anorexic, cachectic and immobilized by her tumour, refused to take oral medication and preferred changing to a subcutaneous diamorphine infusion with close monitoring and appropri-ate dose increases. Her pain appeared to be well controlled for a further 5 months, until her death.

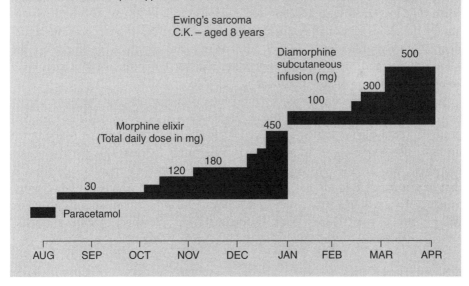

Pain control using opiate therapy is ineffective when the symptoms are not recognized or there is a failure to prescribe an adequate dosage. The question of addiction to these drugs does not arise if pain exists, but children, like adults, will become tolerant of the drugs over a period of time, the dosage therefore being increased to achieve the same level of good pain control as before. A reluctance to prescribe large doses may be expressed by some practitioners who are concerned about depression of the respiratory centre, especially if lung metastases are present. This is not a problem as tolerance develops in the same way as the analgesic effect. Parents may also be concerned about increasing the treatment, sometimes by a substantial amount. Children can tolerate high doses of opiates, and it is a difficult and very different concept for parents that there is no real upper limit to the dose, only that which controls their child's pain.

Time should be spent by nurses and physicians in explaining how opioid drugs work and by what amounts they should be increased at a time. The social and media implications of opiate drug-taking have great impact on the general public so parents may have to be reassured that these drugs are the most effective and appropriate for their child.

Adverse effects of opiate therapy

A side-effect of opiate therapy that is to be anticipated in all patients, is constipation so appropriate laxatives, for example lactulose, Senokot or co-danthramer, should be prescribed in conjunction with opiate drugs. Advice should be given to parents about active measures they can take involving diet and fluids.

Most children and teenagers become drowsy at the start of opiate therapy if they have not previously taken weak opioids. This is usually temporary, lessening after a few days as they become more tolerant to the drug. It is essential that children who are old enough and all parents be advised of this. It can be frightening for parents who are not informed as death may seem to be more imminent when they are faced with a sleepy, less-responsive child. It can also be frightening for the child, who may relate it to his or her own death or to previous experiences of chemotherapy in which antiemetics and sedatives gave rise to the same feelings and memories of impending nausea. For both reasons, they may be reluctant to start opiate treatment.

Nausea and vomiting caused by morphine preparations may be experienced by some children. If these are directly related to opiates, drugs such as metoclopramide and cyclizine can be effective in relieving the symptoms. A retention of urine is also experienced by some, especially after increases in the dosage of morphine; this usually resolves after a few hours. Another common side-effect is that of pruritus. Children may complain of severe itching, which can be very distressing. This will again last only a few days, and prescribing an antihistamine will offer relief over the first days. Unfortunately, a side-effect of some antihistamines is drowsiness.

Adjuvant therapy

Analgesic agents form the basis of pain control, but other drugs may also be used for specific symptoms.

Corticosteroids such as dexamethasone are frequently used to reduce cerebral oedema and thus relieve the raised intracranial pressure caused by a tumour. The reduction in pressure may relieve headaches, nausea and vomiting, and may also cause a raising of the child's level of consciousness. Corticosteroids are also effective when nerve pressure or soft tissue involvement gives rise to 'burning' symptoms. These drugs should be prescribed with care, as the features of Cushing's syndrome and overt weight gain are distressing and disfiguring, and increase nursing problems. The dosage should be maintained at the lowest possible level at which the drug is effective for the child. Non-steroidal anti-inflammatory drugs such as naproxen and ibuprofen may be indicated when bone pain or soft tissue infiltration exists.

Nerve pain may be experienced as 'burning and tingling' or as sharp, shooting pains. Where this pain is opioid resistant, ketamine has been shown to have a therapeutic effect in controlling difficult cancer pain (Mercardante, 1996). Tricyclic antidepressants, for example amitriptyline, and anticonvulsants such as carbamazepine have proved effective in reducing these symptoms.

The use of antidepressants in children or teenagers for psychological reasons, rather than pain control, may be questioned, but they can be beneficial, in small doses, for an individual child. Reasons for the child remaining depressed once his or her general condition has improved should be investigated, and time should be spent in helping the child to communicate his or her anxieties. Relieving painful symptoms and improving quality of life will help the child to regain a feeling of well-being.

Sweating, which may or may not be associated with a raised temperature, can be a major problem for some children. It is more commonly seen when there is increased tumour load as the disease progresses, and it can be distressing. It may be helped by a low dose of corticosteroid (prednisolone or dexamethasone) or by naproxen.

Dyspnoea, which may be experienced by the child with lung metastases, is probably one of the most distressing sights for parents and carers to witness. The use of opiate drugs is invaluable as the child, although conscious, is unaware of his or her struggle for breath. There is no obvious respiratory depression when dyspnoea exists, and opiates can be used. Persistent coughs are often relieved by methadone. Antibiotics may be appropriate to treat chest infections if the child's general well-being will be improved, although if the child is unconscious, this may be questionable. Oxygen therapy may be indicated to help distressed breathing, and ensuring an adequate supply is essential. Helping the family cope with this situation demands empathy and understanding.

Table 16.1 Drugs currently used in syringe drivers that are compatible with diamorphine

	Examples
Antiemetics	Haloperidol (Haldol, Serenace)
	Metoclopramide (Maxolon)
	Cyclizine (Valoid)
Sedatives	Hyoscine (Scopolamine)
	Haloperidol
	Methotrimeprazine (Nozinan)
Bronchodilators	Salbutamol (Ventolin)
Antispasmodic agents	Hyoscine
	Midazolam
Agents to counteract excessive noisy secretions	Hyoscine

It is possible to administer co-analgesic drugs in conjunction with opiates via a syringe driver. Table 16.1 lists some examples of antiemetics, sedatives, bronchodilators and antispasmodic agents that can safely be mixed with diamorphine, thus relieving the child of further oral or intramuscular medication.

Fits, caused by cerebral metastases, are not uncommon and can be difficult to manage. They are also distressing for families to see and naturally cause great anxiety. They can usually easily be controlled at home with oral anticonvulsants or rectal diazepam, but they remain one of the most common reasons for a child's return to hospital for care or the control of symptoms.

Radiotherapy and chemotherapy both have a place in palliative care. A single fraction or a short course of radiotherapy can effectively treat bone pain caused by tumour infiltration and painful pressure symptoms caused by tumour bulk. Intrathecal drugs, for example methotrexate, hydrocortisone and cytosine, are used for children who have the symptoms of raised intracranial pressure, caused by leukaemic cell infiltration, and are experiencing severe headaches. Both forms of therapy necessitate a return to hospital for a brief period, which may be upsetting for the child – one must be sure that the benefits outweigh the disadvantages of the procedures necessary.

If nerve pain is localized and unresponsive to drug therapy, nerve blocks using local or phenol anaesthetic agents, and long-term epidural anaesthesia, all have a role. Experienced anaesthetists who have a special interest in pain control, usually found in symptom control clinics within hospitals, will advise and employ the most appropriate method of nerve blockade. The dosage of opiate drugs can often be reduced, and sometimes stopped, after this treatment. The experience of using nerve blocks in children is limited.

Transcutaneous electrical nerve stimulation (Seymour, 1995) is not widely used for the palliation of nerve symptoms in children. It may be useful as a non-invasive procedure, but as it involves personal control by the patient and its effect on pain is often brief, it is probably more suitable for an adolescent experiencing intermittent nerve pain, to whom its method and effect can more fully be explained.

The use of blood products may enhance quality of life and treat distressing symptoms in some children. Transfusions of packed cells may be given to a child who is generally well but in whom anaemia is resulting in tiredness and weakness. Platelets should be infused when thrombocytopenia is resulting in distressing or persistent bleeds or bruising. To see overt bleeding is upsetting and causes great anxiety for both parents and children so measures should be initiated to ensure that this is actively treated.

NUTRITIONAL NEEDS

There is a natural need for parents to provide food, warmth and comfort for their children so it can be difficult for them to accept their sick child's lack of interest or appetite for food. Progression of the disease, sore mouth or gums and an alteration in taste sensation caused by chemotherapy are some factors that will increase a child's reluctance to eat. Some children may 'pick' at small amounts of food but then decide they have had sufficient, whereas others will have 'fads' in which one food is constantly requested. Feeling that they are not providing sufficiently for their child can cause parents much anxiety. Food may be an issue on which they can focus their attention when they feel that they can do little else to help; it takes time and encouragement from carers to establish realistic expectations of their child's needs. The ambulant, active child may be encouraged with high-calorie drinks or ice-lollies, and a low dose of cortico-steroids may stimulate his or her appetite. The child who is less mobile, or sleeping for lengthy periods, will have different intake needs; this child's condition will determine when fluids alone may be sufficient.

Children and teenagers may themselves express their own desire to eat and may worry about their lack of appetite. Their nutritional intake may have been a focus of attention throughout their treatment. Special attention to their needs, and calorie supplementation of their food or drink, can alleviate some of their anxiety; a low dose of steroids may also be beneficial.

ORAL CARE

The pain and discomfort that are experienced when the child has a dry or sore mouth, ulcers, gingivitis or candidiasis will enhance his or her reluctance to eat. Particular attention should be paid to oral hygiene and any ulcers or infections treated. Soft toothbrushes will help if the gums have a tendency to bleed, and tranexamic acid mouthwashes may also be useful. Mouthwashes containing a locally acting analgesic, for example Difflam, may help the child to eat after a 'numbing' effect has been achieved.

Oral care packs, or soaked gauze wrapped around the fingers, should be used to cleanse the mouth when the child is unable to do this independently. When the child is drinking, fruit juices will encourage the mouth to feel fresh and will encourage salivation, fizzy drinks can reduce 'furring' of the tongue.

SKIN CARE

As children become progressively weaker and less mobile, care of their skin is important. Small children are easily lifted and their position changed, but this can be difficult for the parents of older children and teenagers or if the child is unconscious. Advice on techniques for moving or rolling the child will be appreciated. Children may also need help with bathing. If the child is thin and wasted, the use of a Spenco or other appropriate mattress is indicated.

It is much less common to see fungating lesions in a child than in adults, but if this is the case, appropriate cleansing agents and dressings should be used. Pressure sores may be a problem, and specific care must be given to the areas involved.

Parents are usually active in caring for their child's physical needs, and advice is often welcomed from nursing carers.

RESPONDING TO ONGOING NEEDS

The therapeutic effect of maintaining as normal a family lifestyle as possible should not be underestimated. Children enjoy playing with other children and having stories read to them in quieter moments. Their attention can be diverted as their symptoms become controlled. When they feel well, it may be appropriate for them to return to school for all or part of a day. If this is not possible, friends and teachers should be encouraged to visit and to include them in their daily life. As the child becomes weaker, his or her room may become a central place for family and friends. Where there is space, a downstairs room may be converted into the child's bedroom to prevent isolation from daily events. Being able to participate in games or conversation may help to distract the child and re-establish a sense of well-being.

EQUIPMENT

Parents have identified this as a particular area in which practical help is welcomed when caring for their child at home (Kohler and Radford, 1985). The provision of home nursing equipment has occasionally proved difficult, but community nurses are expert in mobilizing the resources available. The most commonly required items include mattresses, bedpans and urinals, commodes, back rests and bed cradles, wheelchairs or buggies and syringe drivers. Most oncology units have a small supply of equipment that is available for home use.

An item appreciated by many parents is a baby-listening device, which can be moved from room to room. This allows the parents to leave the child knowing that they will hear him or her, should they be needed. Also useful is an answerphone, which allows parents the space to screen calls and choose when they wish to answer.

EMPLOYMENT

Caring for a child who is dying is the most stressful experience for any parent. It imposes enormous physical and psychological strains on the individual and is a time when most of those in employment feel the need to be at home, to participate in care and to share the time left together as a family. Many employers are sympathetic, but a sick note needs to be obtained from an understanding general practitioner at this difficult time.

FINANCE

Caring for a sick child at home over what may be a prolonged period of time is expensive. Although this may seem of little importance, real financial hardship can be experienced if there are increased heating and telephone bills and loss of earnings when parents are at home.

It is possible to obtain an attendance allowance from the Department of Social Security under the Special Rules for terminal illness. Charitable organizations, the most well known being Sargent Cancer Care for Children, the Joseph Rowntree Family Fund and the Leukaemia Care Society, will often give direct financial assistance. There may also be local charities or ones associated with the oncology centre. It is important that the family is aware of all the allowances and grants available to them.

CONTACT, COMMUNICATION AND LIAISON

Throughout this chapter, the need for ongoing contact and communication between the carers has been stressed. If disciplinary boundaries and roles are minimized, and the channels of communication are established early and then maintained, optimal care can be provided for the child and family. The 'shared-care' management approach is most effective where there is continuing flexibility, good communication and close co-operation between oncology units and community teams (Figure 16.4).

DEATH

Caring for a child who is dying is both emotionally and physically exhausting. The 'anticipatory mourning' of parents from the time the child no longer receives active therapy encompasses the knowledge of their impending loss with hope that it will not happen, and despair that it is inevitable (Futterman and Hoffman, 1973). Families grieve at what is inevitable and may then reconcile themselves with thoughts of what their child has meant to them and given to others. Emotional detachment from the child as death becomes imminent is a recognition of the inevitability of death, that their child's life will end soon. The final stage, described by Futterman and Hoffman, is that of 'memorialization', in which the parents develop a mental picture of their dying child, one which may be idealized and not factual, but a picture that will remain with them.

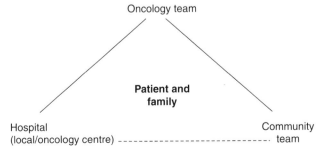

Figure 16.4 Flexibility, co-operation and communication

The duration of palliative care for children with cancer varies, usually lasting weeks or short months. When this time is prolonged, the time of waiting may for parents be fraught with other emotions. Parents have described how they mentally plan what will happen at the time of death, their plans for the funeral and what will happen afterwards, but when death does not happen immediately, they may feel guilty for 'wishing it would end', and empty of sadness or 'lost'. The waiting may seem endless. Others may feel a comfort in knowing that it will all end, that they can prepare for life again, with a different normality (Kübler-Ross, 1988).

The need for parents to know what will happen when their child dies is well described (Martinson, 1980; Kohler and Radford, 1985): 'How will it happen' and 'Will I know when the time comes?' are common questions. Parents fear that it will be traumatic, a struggle, or sudden with no time to prepare themselves and their family. The medical issues relating to the progression of disease and its effects should have already been addressed, but parents may want to know what happens when someone actually dies. It has been found helpful to have someone explain the physical changes, the changes in skin colour and breathing pattern (Martinson, 1980). These are the issues that many fear and for which most are unprepared.

Over the years, we have recognized and begun more fully to address parents' needs for information about what is happening to their child. It is now much less common for a nurse or doctor to be present at the time of death as parents recognize that death is occurring and are able to cope and share their feelings. It is also appropriate to describe the practical measures that need to be taken: the certification of death by a doctor, the registration of the death and the arrangements to be made with funeral directors for burial or cremation. Some units may have a prepared booklet or letter that describes the procedures to be undertaken.

The wishes and needs of parents at the time of death remain highly individual and must be respected. Some will want the formal procedures to begin immediately. Others may want to keep their children at home, wash and dress them, cuddle them or sleep holding them. They should be encouraged to do whatever they feel is right for them, to say their own goodbyes. For siblings, being able to be with their dead brother or sister and touch them or give them presents, and seeing that death is not frightening or a mystery, may help to allay their fears or fantasies and prevent their feeling excluded from the adults' grief.

BEREAVEMENT

The death of one's child has been described as the 'ultimate loss' (Lauer et al., 1989). It is a loss of part of oneself, of an individual and of hopes and dreams for the future. Many emotions may be experienced during the months and years after the death, but it may be more helpful to describe the tasks of mourning that must be accomplished before people can adjust to their personal bereavement.

TO ACCEPT THE REALITY OF THEIR LOSS

Families may initially experience feelings of relief and release from the stresses of their child's illness. This is often followed by numbness and shock as they begin the formalities of funeral arrangements and of informing relatives and friends. The practicalities serve to reinforce the issue of the child's death and allow for a time of saying goodbye and shared emotions.

TO EXPERIENCE THE PAIN OF GRIEF

The aching and longing for their child will be intense during this stage. Many parents describe their need to hold, hug and cuddle their child, but there is an emptiness that can be only partly filled by holding their other children. No one can replace the child who has died. The pain of grief can express itself in physical symptoms: anxiety, panic, breathlessness, lack of energy, insomnia and loss of appetite are just some of the symptoms described. Some will describe themselves as 'going mad'. They need the reassurance that their grief and feelings are being acknowledged and that these feelings are normal and will lessen with time. Parents also need to be encouraged to talk about themselves and their child.

TO ADJUST TO AN ENVIRONMENT IN WHICH THEIR CHILD IS MISSING

This task is one that cannot be completed early or easily as the daily reminders of their loss are constantly present. Favourite music or television programmes, the child's school friends growing up, an empty chair at a table, birthdays and anniversaries all enhance the grief that is never far away. If there are younger siblings, parents may have to go to all the places they used to visit with their other child – playgroups, school, swimming pools. One of the most difficult questions parents have to answer is 'How many children do you have?' Do they give a long explanation of why there are now two children rather than three, or do they just say, 'I have two children' and experience all the feelings of sadness and guilt at denying their dead child's existence. The process of adjusting to a new normality of family life takes years to accomplish.

TO WITHDRAW EMOTIONAL ENERGY AND REINVEST IT IN OTHER RELATIONSHIPS

The need to take up and enjoy life again may seem impossible. Parents may cling to the memory of their child, experience anguish when they feel unable to picture his or her face or remember his or her voice, and feel they can never truly enjoy life again. The differing needs of other family members can be hard to cope with when grief can be expressed in so many different ways. To smile or laugh may seem disloyal, and parents feel guilty when they realize that a period has passed when they have not thought about the child. Talking about the child, remembering happy times and being able to acknowledge and share emotions are part of the healing process. As time passes, they will be able to enjoy life again without displacing their memories.

It seems natural that one should try to protect children from the sadness around them, but we must recognize that they too have lost a family member and must also grieve. At a time when they most need the closeness of their family, it may be that other members are not able to fully respond, that their own grief is too intense. Research has shown that when children have been cared for in their own home, families cope better as a unit because they have shared the experience. There is less guilt, and they feel more able to share their sorrow with the rest of the family. This had led to a more positive and cohesive attitude for their future as a family.

Children will also express their sorrow in many ways. They too are individuals whose feelings must be acknowledged. They may be anxious or worried about being left alone, their security being threatened, or they may be concerned about their own health – are they too going to die? Insomnia, fear of the dark, nightmares and sleep-walking are not uncommon, nor is a regression to more childish behaviour, tantrums and bed-wetting. Parents have sometimes said that their other children never talk about their sibling: 'It's as if he never existed, she only wants his toys to play with.' They may recognize the need to keep something of the child who has died but not so easily recognize other behavioural problems as being related to the sibling's personal bereavement and grief.

Children must be encouraged to share their feelings, to know that it is all right to cry, to be angry or sad. When parents try to hide their own sadness, children feel that they too must deny it. They may feel responsible that the death has happened because of something they said or did, or believe that they are less important and unloved as attention has surrounded their dying sibling for so long. They need the reassurance and closeness of their family to know that they are loved for themselves and that their feelings are important too. Such feelings are encapsulated in the following poem.

STILL THERE, BUT GONE

To see him there,
When he's not,
Although he's there in my Mind,
I still Miss him a lot.

I can just imagine him there to say
"Go away,
leave me alone,
want to play"

When treatment time then came,
You could always hear his name,
It was Peter this,
Peter that,

Oh sigh!

It was like the talk of the World,
Envy and sometimes hate,
you'd think he had enough on his plate,

All the Attention.
But he is my brother,
And will be forever,
And I'll love him like never before.

Michael

Teachers and friends are a major part of a child's life. The death of a class-mate affects them all. Some children may be reluctant to return to school after their sibling has died. On their return, they may be easily distracted, disruptive and withdrawn or display what seem to be inappropriate emotions, all of which may be signs of inner distress and grief. A sympathetic teacher and close peer group can give the child support and security to talk about his or her feelings, or just be there when the child feels alone.

Bereavement following the death of a child lasts longer than after the death of an adult. One study reported that more than 20 per cent of families were experiencing their most intense grief 2 years after their child's death (Corr et al., 1985). A further 25 per cent said that their grief was most intense over the 12–18 months period. In many cases, the grief of siblings, especially adolescents, was experienced for longer than that of their parents.

It can be difficult for carers to know how best they can support families through this time. It is the practice of most oncology units for someone who has been closely involved with the family to attend the funeral: families appreciate the presence of someone who has helped them care for their child and who shows that the child also meant something to them. Maintaining contact by telephone calls and visits is essential. Strong bonds develop between the carers and the family as they share a unique experience. Families lose much of the regular contact and input from those around in the months after the death and need to share their feelings with those most closely involved. When contact is not maintained, families experience a 'double loss'; they need to feel that they and their child are still part of the staff's thoughts and that they do care.

More obvious times when contact should be made are birthdays and the anniversary of the death. These are very personal dates that belong only to their dead child and are usually seen as a great hurdle to be negotiated. Christmas is another difficult time, with its mixed emotions of the need to have a day that the other children will enjoy yet be able to grieve for the child who is not there. Other important occasions to be remembered by the family are personal ones such as the dates of diagnosis, scans, favourite holidays and events. Families will have many individual ways of spending these days, and acknowledgement by carers that these anniversaries are important may help them to feel less isolated.

Families are invited to come back to the oncology unit, usually a few weeks after the death, to talk to the physician who cared for their child. Most will welcome the opportunity to be able to talk about their child's illness, treatment and death. There may be many questions to be asked; some will come with prepared lists, as they did while their child was receiving treatment. The impact of actually returning to the hospital should not be underestimated, as it can be very traumatic to pass all the places they so often took their child. For some, this will be impossible, and an alternative office may need to be found to enable them to take the first steps of returning. They are encouraged to repeat the visit as often as they need and whenever they have questions to be asked. Many will visit 'socially' for coffee and a chat, thus maintaining their link.

Families will often direct their attention and energy into fund-raising for parents' groups and hospitals, finding a positivity in working for the benefit of other families. Some units may have groups for bereaved parents where they can meet others and share their experiences. Others may find locally run groups such as Compassionate Friends and Cruse helpful.

The reactions of other family members or friends can be difficult for parents to cope with. They may meet unhelpful comments, avoidance in the street and avoidance in mentioning the child's name, as well as coming into contact with people who are unaware of their loss. Parents' reactions to each situation will differ, depending on how they are feeling at any one time.

It is helpful for those visiting to show that they care and to allow parents to talk about the child as freely as they want. Parents need the reassurance that they did everything they could for their child.

CONCLUSION

To have a child die in one's community is a rare occurrence, especially when that child is dying from a malignant disease. The experience is a very personal one, one in which we may question our own feelings about death and its meaning. We may relate the child and parents to our own families and wonder how we would cope with such a situation. In sharing some of their anxieties and fears, we often feel inadequate and awkward, but it is in this sharing that carers have much to offer. It can be difficult when one feels one must be offering practical advice and performing tasks, but the most help we can give is by being with the family, establishing trust and being ready just to listen.

Resources are available from oncology units to help to manage specific problems that may be encountered, and we must seek to strengthen these links. In working as a team, our own feelings of isolation lessen. During palliative care and after the child's death, it is important that we too talk about our experience and our loss; it helps to share it both with those in our immediate unit and with others who have been involved in the care (McGoldrick, 1999). Despite the sadness of the situation, this can be a very positive and rewarding time.

REFERENCES

Arts, S.E., Abu-Saad, H.H., Champion, G.D. et al. 1994: Age-related response to lidocaine-prilocaine (E.M.L.A.) emulsion and effects of music on the pain of intravenous cannulation. *Paediatrics* **93**(5), 797–801.

Blum, R.W. 1989: The dying adolescent. In: Blum, R.W. (ed.) *Chronic illness and disabilities in childhood and adolescence*. New York: Grune and Stratton.

Bray, R.J., Woodhams, A.M., Vallis, C.J. et al. 1996: A double-blind comparison of morphine infusion and patient controlled analgesia in children. *Paediatric Anaesthesia* **6**, 121–7.

Burne, S.R., Francis, D. and Baum, J.D. 1984: Helen House – a hospice for children: analysis of the first year. *British Medical Journal* **289**, 1665–8.

Carrol, D. 1993: Managing cancer pain. *Nursing Times* **89**(38), 69–70.

Chambers, E.J., Oakhill, A., Cornish, J.M. and Curnick, S. 1989: Terminal care at home for children with cancer. *British Medical Journal* **298**, 937–40.

Clarke, J. and Cox, E. 1988: Heparinsation of Hickman catheters. *Nursing Times/Nursing Mirror* **84**, 51–3.

Corr, C.A., Martinson, I.M. and Dyer, K.L. 1985: Parental bereavement. In: Corr, C.A. and Corr, D.M. (eds) *Hospice approaches to paediatric care*. New York: Springer.

Crow, L. and Crow, A. 1965: *Adolescent development and adjustment*, 2nd edn. New York: McGraw-Hill.

Futterman, E.J. and Hoffman, I. 1973: Crisis and adaptation in families of fatally ill children. In: Anthony, E.J. and Koupernick, C. (eds) *The child in his family: the impact of disease and death*. New York: John Wiley.

Johansen, B.B. 1988: Care of the dying adolescent and the bereaved family. *Loss, Grief, Care* **2**(3/4), 59–67.

Kohler, J.A. and Radford, M. 1985: Terminal care for children dying of cancer – quantity and quality of life. *British Medical Journal* **291**, 115–16.

Koocher, G.P. and O'Malley J.E. 1981: *The Damocles syndrome*. New York: McGraw-Hill.

Kübler-Ross, E. 1988: *Living with death and dying*. London: Souvenir Press.

Lauer, M.E., Mulhern, R.K., Schell, M.J. and Camitta, B.M. 1989: Long-term follow up of parental adjustment following a child's death at home or hospital. *Cancer* (March 1), 988–93.

Lewandowski, W. and Jones, S.L. 1988: The family with cancer – nursing interventions throughout the course of living with cancer. *Cancer Nursing* **11**(6), 313–21.

Martinson, I.M. 1980: Dying children at home. *Nursing Times Occasional Paper* **76** (29), 129–32.

Martinson, I., Moldow, D.G., Armstrong, G.D., Henry, W.F., Nesbitt, B.E. and Kersey, J.H. 1986: Home care for children dying of cancer. *Research in Nursing and Health* **9**, 11–16.

Martinson, I., Nesbitt, M. and Kersey, Y. 1984: Home care for the child with cancer. In: Christ, A.E. and Flomenhaft, K. (eds) *Childhood cancer*. New York: Plenum.

McCallum, L. and Carr-Gregg, M. 1987: Adolescents with cancer. *Australian Nurses Journal* **16**(7), 39–43.

McGoldrick, L. 1999: Specialist palliative care nursing in the community. *Nursing Times* **95**(31), 5.

Mercandante, S. 1996: Ketamine in cancer pain – an update. *Palliative Medicine* **10**, 225–30.

Miser, A.W. and Miser, J.S. 1989: The treatment of cancer pain in children. *Paediatric Clinics of North America* **36**(4), 979–98.

Miser, A.W. and Narong, P.K. 1989: Transdermal fentanyl for pain control in patients with cancer. *Pain.* **37**, 15–21.

Northouse, L. 1984: The impact of cancer on the family – an overview. *International Journal of Psychiatry in Medicine* **14**, 215–43.

Norman, R. and Bennet, M. 1986: Care of the dying child at home; a unique co-operative relationship. *Australian Journal of Advanced Nursing* **3**, (4) 3–17.

Oakhill, A. 1988: *The supportive care of the child with cancer.* Bristol: John Wright.

O'Brian, M.E. 1983: An identification of needs of family members of terminally ill patients in a hospital setting. *Military Medicine* **148**, 712–16.

Papadatou, D. 1989: Caring for dying adolescents. *Nursing Times* **85**(8), 28–31.

Pfund, R. 1998: Palliative – implications for everyone's practice. *Paediatric Nursing* **10** (4), 12–15.

Reape, D. 1990: Children and pain (pain perceptions). *Nursing Standard* **4**(16), 33–6.

Sepion, B. 1990: Intravenous care for children. *Paediatric Nursing Journal* **2**(3), 14–16.

Seymour, J. 1995: Pain control – Tens machine. *Nursing Times* **91**(8), 51–2.

Spinetta, J.J., Rigler, D. and Karon, M. 1974: Personal space as a measure of a dying child's sense of isolation. *Journal of Consulting and Clinical Psychology* **42**, 751–7.

Spinetta, J. and Deasey-Spinetta, P. 1981: *Living with childhood cancer.* St Louis: C.V. Mosby.

Stein, A., Forrest, G.C., Woolley, H. and Baum, J.D. 1989: Life threatening illness and hospice care. *Archives of Disease in Childhood* **64**, 697–702.

Twycross, A. 1997: Nurses' perceptions of pain in children. *Paediatric Nursing Journal* **9**(1), 16–19.

Twycross, A. 1998: Children's cognitive level and their perception of pain. *Paediatric Nursing Journal* **10**(3), 24–7.

Tweddle, D.A., Windebank, K.P., Barrett, A.M., Leese, D. and Gowring, R. 1997: Central venous access use in UKCCSG oncology centres. *Archives of Disease in Childhood* **77**(1), 58–9.

Vickers, J.L. and Carlisle, C. 2000: Home care requirements for children and adolescents with cancer. *Journal of Paediatric Oncology Nursing* **17** (1), 45–9.

Wilson, D.C. 1985: Developing a hospice program for children. In: Corr, C.A. and Corr, D.M. (eds) *Hospice approaches to paediatric care.* New York: Springer.

Wilson, D.C. 1988: The ultimate loss: the dying child. *Loss, Grief, Care* **2**(3/4), 125–30.

Wong, D.L. and Baker, C.M. 1988: Pain in children: comparisons of assessment scales. *Paediatric Nursing* **14** (1), 9–17.

FURTHER READING

Adams, D.W. and Deveau, E.J. 1995: *Beyond the innocence of childhood*, Vols 1 and 2. Baywood.

Association for Children with Life-threatening or Terminal Conditions and their Families/Royal College of Paediatrics and Child Health. 1997: *A guide to the development of children's palliative care services.* Bristol: ACT.

Dent, A. *A child is dying – care of the family in illness and bereavement.* Penzance: Patten Press, Macmillan Education Centre.

Hill, L. (ed.) 1994: *Caring for dying children and their families.* London: Chapman & Hall.

Oakhill, A. 1988: *The supportive care of the child with cancer.* Bristol: John Wright.

Ward, B. and Associates. 1996: *Good Grief*, Vols 1 and 2, 2nd edn. London: Jessica Kingsley.

Part 4

PALLIATIVE CARE: VISIONS FOR THE FUTURE

chapter 17

THE PROPHETIC NATURE OF PALLIATIVE CARE

Sheila Cassidy

The most effective way to ensure the value of the future is to confront the present courageously and constructively.

Rollo May

American theologian Frederick Buechner defines 'prophet' as 'spokesman' rather than 'soothsayer', and I shall stick with his definition. When I describe the hospice, or rather the palliative care movement, as prophetic, I mean that it has become the spokesperson for a rag-tag group of people not unlike the early people of Israel: what the old Testament describes as the 'anawim'. The anawim are the little ones, the poor, the marginalized and disinherited, and God, it is said, has a special love for them, favouring them over the rich and powerful. The hospice movement does likewise.

Before I start irritating too many people, let me make it clear that I understand perfectly well the difference between the hospice movement and palliative care in general, and I would align myself with the latter, particularly as I lost my hospice job because it was considered that I spent too much time away from it lecturing on palliative care. There is, however, a certain divine madness, a passion for the dying, that one finds in hospices that is mostly absent from hospital or home palliative care. Hospital palliative care has expertise and efficacy, hospices have love and passion, and an *esprit de corps* that has made them unstoppable in their good work. Hospice work started life as a vocation, but it has matured into a profession. These are broad observations but I think they contain enough truth to provoke some thought.

A monk friend of mine who is something of a prophet in his own way described prophets as people who have felt called to leave the mainstream of society to live their lives on the margins. Thus, at one remove from family and friends, the prophet is able to see things more clearly, to reflect and then to comment on what is seen. The Old Testament prophets certainly fell into this category and, in commenting upon the manifold injustices they observed, became spokespeople for the oppressed. This description of the role of the prophet fits well the early hospice pioneers who ranted and raved at their colleagues about the inadequate treatment of the terminally ill.

They were heady days, back in the early 1980s when I first joined the 'movement'. Not that there has ever been a 'movement' as such for most of us were fiercely individual. Dame Cicely Saunders was the foundress, of course, and her biography by Shirley du Boulay is well worth reading. Cicely's passion was fuelled by committing the then unforgivable sin of 'getting involved' with her patients. As a young nurse, and later as a social worker, she spent many hours listening to her dying patients until her dream evolved: a 'home', in the true sense of the word, where terminally ill men and women could be skilfully and lovingly cared for until they died. One day, a Polish man, dying miserably in an open ward, gave her five hundred pounds towards the realization of her dream and told her 'I'll be a window in your home.'

To Cicely we owe the concept of 'total pain' – distress of body, mind and spirit – and the hospice philosophy that seeks to help people to live until they die. It is hard, 20 years on, to realize what this woman has accomplished, albeit with the help of many disciples over the years. Not only was pain control virtually non-existent, but also patients psychosocial needs were quite simply not considered – let alone thought important. Families were informed that their relative was dying, but patients themselves were deliberately lied to, ostensibly to spare them distress, but in reality because it was easier that way for the carers, personal and professional alike. Nurses were taught to make beds with 'hospital corners' rather than to sit on beds and put their arms around frightened or distressed patients. Psycho-oncology, my own speciality of the psychological care of cancer patients and their families, did not exist.

Then, like the tide slowly covering the sand, the hospice movement began: men and women, lay and professional, became concerned that their dying patients should be well cared for, and, as dreams became reality, hospices sprung up all over the UK. At the same time as this building boom, scientifically minded doctors such as Robert Twycross began to study the mechanism and pharmacology of morphine and diamorphine and to teach the basics of pain control to anyone who would listen.

I was among Twycross's early pupils at a week-long seminar in Oxford way back in 1982, preparing myself to be medical director of Plymouth's emergent hospice, St Luke's. It was there that I met Michael Kearney, who later moved from St Christopher's Hospice to be medical director at Our Lady's Hospice at Harrolds Cross in Dublin. Hospice was a small world in those early days, and we all knew each other. Macmillan Cancer Relief, who have done so much to establish palliative care in the UK, held a wonderful free residential conference for senior doctors and nurses each year, and we swapped experiences late into the night. I was in awe, in those days, of the elders of the movement: Derek Doyle from St Columba's in Edinburgh, Twycross from Oxford and Eric Wilkes of St Luke's in Sheffield. They were powerful, idiosyncratic men, as were most founders of hospices.

I would class myself as third-generation hospice, if Dame Cicely, Eric Wilkes and Ronnie Fisher were first generation, and Twycross, Doyle and Hillier second. Many of my generation of hospice 'founders' are still in post:

Andrew Hoy at the Princess Alice in Esher, Claud Regnard in Newcastle and Fiona Randall in Canterbury. Many of us have moved on, some retired and some been ousted by the newer generation who were impatient of their maverick forefathers. In hindsight, I think this is inevitable because the qualities needed to make a venture happen, in this case to establish a new hospice, are quite different from those needed for its maintenance.

The early founders of hospices and palliative care services needed a kind of evangelical zeal, which, although it got some people's backs up, set others on fire. More than anything, they needed a prodigious energy, working long hours at the bedside, teaching and fund-raising in their spare time. In my first year at St Luke's, I worked, or rather was on call, for around 90 hours a week while being paid for 18. Even then, I knew it was unjust, but I was carried along by the excitement of it all and my love for our small band of patients.

Those of us who worked in 'the old St Luke's', a converted house with seven, then 10, beds can remember those first patients as if it were yesterday. We knew them so well as patients and as people, and we learned from them how to practise hospice medicine. It was through listening to these patients, empathizing with their grief and their anger, that we fuelled ourselves to fight for the cause. It was the women in particular who moved me, partly through identification but also because the breast and gynaecological cancers wreaked such havoc on them. More than anything, there was the pain, especially the pain that we could not conquer – the neuropathic pain that was so poorly understood in the 1980s.

Worst of all were the young women with cancer of the cervix that had recurred following radiotherapy. They had what is called a 'frozen pelvis': advanced disease in the pelvis invading the sciatic nerve, vagina, bladder and rectum. This was before a new generation of gynaecologists trained in colposcopy and radical hysterectomy came to Plymouth, after which frozen pelvis seemed to become a rarity. Not only did these women suffer intractable pain, but they frequently also developed both faecal and urinary fistulae. Because none of these complications were in themselves life-threatening, these women were with us a long time, and we got to know them well. It was in conversation with them that we learned how bitterly they resented what they saw as the arrogance and lack of compassion of so many doctors. In those days, it never occurred to me that normal medical cool politeness could be perceived as lack of caring, but these women helped me to understand that when one is very frightened – and who with cancer is *not* very frightened? – one needs human warmth as well as courtesy. I believe that this has been one of the most important truths that hospice workers have fed back into mainstream medicine.

This is what I mean by the prophetic role of the hospice movement: we who were ordinary doctors and nurses, trained in the same medical schools as our fellows, have left mainstream medicine to work with the 'poor', the 'hopeless cases', and discovered that these 'cases' are men and women like ourselves with precisely the same needs and emotions as we have. My experience as a hospice doctor has completely changed the way I practise hospital medicine, has made me, quite unconsciously, adopt a much more informal, warmer style of relating to patients.

It is difficult, of course to separate the effect of ageing and experience. Now, in my sixties, perhaps I am much more at ease with people in general, but I believe that it is the hospice experience that has made me the kind of doctor that I am. There is something, too, about working with terminally ill people that forces one to draw upon one's own deepest psychological resources. I am reminded of the image of the wretched pelican pulling out its breast feathers until the blood flows to feed its young. On ward rounds, I had to be a chameleon, comforting one patient, teasing another and more or less doing handstands for another who was feeling down and needed cheering up. The changing style of one woman doctor is a small thing, but much more important is the change in style of whole institutions. During the past 7 years, I have seen a quiet revolution overtake our oncology department, a revolution that, I am convinced, had its seeds in our local hospice. Let me explain:

In 1980, I returned to the practice of medicine in the UK after a gap of some 9 years. Although over 40, I took a locum job as a senior house officer and spent most of my time talking to patients. Having neither husband nor lover, I spent many of my evenings sitting perched on the beds of my sickest patients, answering their questions and trying to alleviate their distress. What I learned almost at once from these people was that they wanted to know the truth about their illness and also about their prognosis. Being essentially a truthful sort of person, I told them and found that they neither became hysterical nor leaped out of the nearest window. Absurdly, it was usually I who was most frightened because it was my boss's policy to reassure his patients that all would be well. 'We'll give you some of my jungle juice', he would tell the women with advanced ovarian cancer whom we were treating with cis-platinum, and 'it'll kill any little cells that are left behind'. Because I spoke to both patients and their relatives, I learned at first hand just how damaging was the 'conspiracy of silence' in which doctors and family effectively ganged up on a patient, deciding it was not in his or her interest to know the truth.

Fearing to lose my job, I drew those patients to whom I had told the truth into another conspiracy, asking them not to tell my boss that they knew what was wrong with them. They became my loyal allies and we developed a kind of Morse code in which I would wink at them behind the boss's back or, engineering that I be the last person to leave the room, would administer a gentle squeeze to the big toe as a sign that we were co-conspirators. After 18 months as an elderly senior house officer, I was offered the job of medical director of the new hospice, seven beds in a converted suburban house. I initially had dreams of being an oncologist, but I fell asleep in all my tutorials and never really understood the physics anyway, so I decided that I should accept the invitation.

When St Luke's opened its doors to receive its first patient, a delightful farmer's wife called Cordelia, I was one of the few members of staff who had even been inside a hospice. I had spent 2 weeks as locum medical director at a hospice in Cornwall and done a sort of 'hospice crawl', visiting the great and the good in various famous centres. When we began, however, we had to make it up as we went along, responding to patient need as best we could. Nowadays, half a dozen patients would constitute a focus group and we would be praised for being patient centred. At the time, we just did what came naturally, asking people what they wanted and meeting their needs if we were able. Amazingly, it worked, and because we were working in a converted two-storey house, we achieved a sort of hybrid of home and hospital, expertise was coupled with friendship, an iron hand in a velvet glove.

Because the hospice was so small, the multi-disciplinary team had no option but to work together, and, with one or two exceptions, we became real friends. Most of the nurses were middle aged, lived locally and had returned to nursing after raising their children, so we all learned together. Having no medical colleagues and no junior doctor, I taught the senior nurses what I knew, and we unwittingly piloted an almost total breakdown of hierarchical barriers, quite different from our previous experience of playing doctors and nurses.

As I write this, I realize that relationships between doctors and nurses were changing anyway as a result of improvements in nursing education. When I say improvements, I really mean change, because sometimes I wonder whether the blurring of medical and nursing boundaries has really benefited either patients or nurses. This is not for one moment to deny the importance of recent advances in nursing or the intellectual work done by so many nurses; it is more a wistful retrospective look at the light-hearted nurses of my youth who threw themselves heart and soul into making patients comfortable without having to record it on a computer or write essays about it in their spare time. (It would also, I admit, be a nostalgic look back at the days when 'doctor's' word was not questioned and nurses made the coffee. We all have our shadow side.)

By the late 1980s, the hospice was bursting at the seams. The seven original beds had been increased to 10 during the first year, and the number of patients had steadily increased so that we were having to move people on to nursing homes rather than let them stay in the hospice until they died. The staff number had increased too because, as my workload increased, I had become more and more stressed, until a tearful outburst to the governors caused them to review medical staffing and spend precious money on more doctor hours. There was a social worker by then too, Carolyn, who later became lecturer in palliative care at the university. How we all fitted in, God only knows. I had a long narrow office in what had started life as a garage and then progressed to function as a mortuary until we realized that our friendly local undertakers provided such an efficient service that the space would be better used for the living.

In 1988, we moved home to a purpose-built, 20-bed unit overlooking Plymouth's harbour, and things were never the same again. Even now, after 18 years, the founder members whisper to each other, 'It's not like it was in the old hospice.' With 20 beds rather than 10, things had to change. The nursing staff doubled, as did the medical hours, and life inevitably became more hospital like. As our popularity grew, so did our turnover, until it became the norm for patients to stay only for 2 weeks before returning home or moving on to a nursing home.

Our educational endeavours were formalized too, with the building of a lecture room in the basement and the appointment of a full-time nurse teacher. It was here that we set out to reform the attitude to care of the dying in Plymouth, a feat that we, amazingly, accomplished. When I look back over the years, I marvel at how things have changed, and it is because of this that I dare to talk of the hospice's 'prophetic' role. In order to illustrate the impact of what we liked to think of as our philosophy upon medical and nursing care in the hospital and community, it is worth looking at four areas of treatment: pain and symptom control, communication, especially breaking bad news, emotional care and bereavement care.

Before I detail these changes, I should, however, stress that changes in these areas were taking place all over the UK. The soil was fertile and ready for the hospice 'word' to be sown. Patients, in particular, were demanding a different kind of care, as were new generations of nurses. We were merely the enthusiastic facilitators in a massive paradigm shift toward a more holistic approach to medicine, especially the treatment of cancer patients.

In the early 1980s, symptom control consisted mainly of doubling the dose of morphine and treating the resultant confusion with increasing doses of tranquilizers. I shudder to think how many patients died of constipation in the 'old days'. (One patient had certainly not moved his bowels for 6 weeks when I first met him.) The old myths were powerful and took a long time to debunk. 'You mustn't give morphine until the end', 'You mustn't tell him or he'll give up' and 'If you start her on morphine now, she'll get addicted and it won't work when she really needs it' were all 'truths' that everyone thought they knew, and it took a long time to convince the older doctors and nurses that things could and should be done differently.

Much of the success of the change in attitude resulted from the community specialist nurses, the Macmillan nurses, so called because the charity Macmillan Cancer Relief funded them for 3 years providing (and *only* providing) that the health authorities agreed to take over their funding. These nurses managed to convince the general practitioners, by a potent mixture of skill and guile, to try things the 'hospice way', until they too became believers. The real miracle, I have always thought, is that doctors learned to listen to nurses instead of expecting the reverse.

The second great change in care of the dying, which has now spread to all cancer patients, is the culture of openness, of truth-telling, unheard of in the late 1970s and early 1980s. This too was coming, a tradition of honesty having been firmly established in the USA for many years. British patients, however, were thought to be different, submitting passively to their medical carers without complaint. Many's the time I examined a patient with large abdominal scars who had no idea what, if anything, had been removed at surgery; some people's lack of understanding of their anatomy and physiology, particularly of their more intimate functions, is almost complete. The policy of outright lying slowly changed and then swung to the opposite pole so that people now complain that they have been told of their condition too brusquely and without compassion. In an attempt to rectify this, palliative care doctors and nurses have become specialists in 'breaking bad news'.

In Derriford Hospital, where I work, we have set up a 'rolling' programme for teaching senior doctors and nurses how to convey painful news. The courses are run by a team of nurses and doctors and are both well attended and appreciated; even so, a 4 hour workshop is not really long enough to do more than raise awareness and teach an outline of technique. It is, however, infinitely better than nothing. It is significant that this programme is funded by the hospital and taught by its own staff; the hospital has here learned from the hospice.

What I find exciting is the fact that this teaching, initially meant to improve the care of cancer patients, is impacting upon other disciplines. I have run a breaking bad news workshop for the whole of the X-ray department, and we have also had much interest from obstetricians and midwives, who of course have to tell patients about deformed and stillborn babies. It is in this way that skills learned on the periphery are being returned to the main medical body.

The third way in which I see palliative care as having influenced mainstream medicine lies in the area of psychological care. In some ways, I suspect, hospitals are forging head of their original teachers, and the time is coming when hospices will need to learn from them. I would like to illustrate this with the story of how psychosocial care has developed in Plymouth and how new techniques are being fed back to the hospice.

In 1994, David, the then business manager of the oncology department, mentioned to me that he would like to see a cancer support service as part of our department. As it happened, I was undercommitted and interested in doing a few more hours, so we hatched a plot that he would pay me for two more sessions and I would start a drop-in centre for our patients. We were lucky, very lucky, to have some extra space following a reduction in the number of beds, and we were able to set up our drop-in centre in a refurbished ward sitting room.

At first, of course, no one dropped in, and our nurses and volunteers sat about twiddling their thumbs. Gradually, however, the idea took on, and soon the Mustard Tree, as we christened it, was a going concern, around 10 patients a day dropping in. In 1998, the whole department moved to the main hospital site, and we were chosen by Macmillan to receive a grant to fund a purpose-built centre. Since then, the Mustard Tree Macmillan Centre, as it is rather clumsily called, has gone from strength to strength. We now have around 500 patients a month dropping in, a counselling service staffed by volunteers, massage, reflexology, healing and number of artistic workshops. I myself am engaged in a group programme for younger women with breast cancer and in another for children who have lost a parent.

Once again, it is the patients who have taught us what they want. The Mustard Tree set out to be a sort of friendly coffee shop with volunteer listeners and a few 'holistic therapies'. Listening, however, leads to an increased awareness of patient needs, and in responding to these the service has developed in ways that we never anticipated. The first development was the women's' group, Fighting Spirit, a psychoeducational group programme based upon the work of

American psychiatrists David Spiegel of Stanford and Fawzy Fawzy of Los Angeles. I should mention here that I have been, for some years, a member of the British Psycho-oncology Society and have, in attending their meetings and reading their journal, been exposed to a more rigorous view of psychosocial care than I had met in purely hospice circles.

It was not long after hearing Professor Fawzy lecture in London that I was approached by two young women with breast cancer who wanted to meet others in the same position. Luckily, I had spent lunchtime at the conference talking to Fawzy's wife Nancy, and she had sent me a workbook for the groups, so I told the women that if they could find a few more like-minded patients, I would run the group for them. We began a week later, my co-facilitator Kathy, and I embarking upon a journey that was to change our professional lives.

These were all young women, Fran, the youngest, being 29 and a single mum. The oldest was Rachel, a school teacher in her early forties, and the rest were in their early and mid-thirties. All had been diagnosed within the previous year, and all had children of school age or younger. Never had I met such passion, such determination to survive, and never before had I been so convinced that these women needed each other more than they needed us. In the past, I had vaguely suggested setting up a group, but my bosses had always been against it, saying that it was fine until someone died, and then they would all get terribly depressed. They could not have been more wrong. After 5 years, quite a number of the women have died, and although each death impacts upon other members, the morale of the survivors remains high.

This is not the place to give a detailed description of the work, but a brief account is relevant because I see these groups as being a direct offshoot of my hospice experience. It is not so much the groups that have their origin in hospice, but the way in which we run them, the way in which we relate to the women, that is shaped by our St Luke's days. Kathy Smeardon, my co-facilitator, was the nurse teacher at the hospice for many years, and we worked closely together, particularly in running the ENB 931 and 285 courses. Kathy has years of experience working with small groups of nurses and is more sensitive than I to issues of power and control. Together, we make a good team, moving easily from serious issues to light-hearted clowning. More than anything, we relate to the women as women rather than as doctor and nurse. I sometimes describe the groups as a cross between a seminar and a supper party, and they have that feel to them, the sharing of cake and coffee following the sharing of experience. When everyone has let off steam, we have about 40 minutes 'lesson' about cancer, treatment, psychological coping or whatever the women want – the educational component of the group.

It did not take us long to realize that the most important thing about the groups was the networking and friendship between the women. We meet with them for 6–8 consecutive weeks, providing a safe space and format for the sharing and ventilation of feelings. The teaching aims to equip them with enough information to demystify the illness and treatment, and, hopefully, to empower them to cope without too much unnecessary distress. When the group is finished, we set them loose to look after each other, like survivors in a lifeboat. They are told that they are welcome to contact either of us if they need help and that we will reconvene the group for a one-off meeting if they need it, but it is stressed that they will get the maximum benefit from the group if they stay in touch and care for each other.

After 5 years, we have run some 14 groups, and the evaluation by the women has been extremely positive. Around 10 out of the approximately 80 women have recurrent disease, and 5 have died. Some remain close friends, others prefer to leave the cancer experience behind them, but all who completed the group have found it a powerful experience and very supportive. Of the roughly 8 women convened for each group, 1 usually drops out because she finds the group is not for her, usually finding listening to other women's stories depressing rather than helpful. The format has remained the same though: the sharing of experience and feelings in the first hour, a coffee and cake break, and then 40 minutes of teaching – seems to work well.

As always, one thing leads to another, and our involvement with these women has led to a heightened awareness of not only their own difficulties, but also those of their families, especially their partners and children. We have, on a number of occasions, met with the women's partners, and although this has usually been a one-off event, some of the men have remained friends and have supported each other during a wife's terminal illness. Two older men, Andy and John, both now widowers, co-hosted a meeting of young men who had recently lost their wives. This last meeting, which I had thought might develop into a group programme, was not repeated because the men did not want it, but it has made us acutely aware of the difficulties of young, bereaved fathers.

This brings me, inevitably, as in all palliative care, to the issue of bereavement, the fourth area in which the hospice movement has influenced mainstream medicine. St Luke's Hospice Bereavement Service was established by Carolyn Brodribb, our social worker, who has become a national and international lecturer in the field. Carolyn selected and trained groups of volunteers as 'bereavement visitors' to accompany those experiencing normal loss and grief.

Feeling that the oncology department should have a similar programme, I helped to design a research study to select and train volunteers specifically to work with the families of our patients. The study was completed, but we had to widen it to include non-cancer bereavements because of the lack of participants. The 'package' devised during the research was developed into a service for people with complicated grief, which ran successfully until 2000, when funding was withdrawn on the pretext that general practitioner counsellors and psychiatric services were already being paid to provide such care. This decision has been challenged, and we await the results of this. Meanwhile, in the Mustard Tree, we do a limited amount of bereavement counselling, although we feel that we should provide a more formal service of assessment and treatment as needed.

Another development has been the establishment of a children's bereavement service, which we have named Jeremiah's Journey after one of my teddy bears, about whom I have written a story of grief and loss for teaching purposes. This is also a group programme, in which we meet with children and their parents in two separate groups. The children make memory boxes and undertake other tasks designed to help them think and talk about their feelings, with the unspoken message that it's OK to be sad and to talk about the person who has died, but it's also OK to have fun. The adults, usually six or seven and mainly women, talk about their loss and share their experience of difficulties that they encountered in coping with their children's grief. There are two facilitators for the adult group but many more for the children so that each child has some one-to-one time with a professional or a trained helper.

Each group lasts one-and-a-half hours and is held weekly for 6 weeks; we then have a day out together about a month later. We also hold an annual Christmas party for the children from Jeremiah's Journey and also for those of the Fighting Spirit participants. It is an occasion that is both joyous and poignant as we meet, sometimes for the first time, the children of the Fighting Spirit mothers and wonder whether they will one day be candidates for Jeremiah's Journey.

The children's progamme has been running around 5 years, and we usually see three groups of about 20–25 children each year. Both children and parents enjoy the groups, and there are few drop-outs. The teenagers are the least enthusiastic and tend to fall by the wayside if there is no one else of their own age. Not all the bereavements are caused by cancer: death by suicide is fairly common, and we have also worked with children whose fathers have been murdered.

A direct spin-off from the children's programme has been the establishment of a schools' liaison group and a schools' educational project. The liaison group consists of two school teachers, Jaqui Stedmon, the child psychologist who co-founded Jeremiah's Journey, an educational psychologist, the head of the city's educational welfare department, the lead worker in the Youth Enquiry Centre and myself. We have held one half-day seminar for secondary school teachers, which was well received, and one for primary school teachers as well as several 2-hour sessions.

There is no doubt that education has been one of palliative care's major contributions to British medical care, but what is less well known is the way in which the message has been spread abroad in both the developed and the developing world. Ann Merriman, a British doctor, has been active in setting up hospice care, initially in Singapore and more recently in Kenya. Gilly Burn, a nurse, has set up her own charity, Cancer Relief India, and has taught widely there. Robert Twycross has been particularly active in running courses for overseas graduates, and a group of doctors headed by Michael Minton goes each year to Poland to teach doctors and nurses from the Eastern European countries. Cicely Saunders' belief that men and women should be helped to 'live until they die' has formed ripples well beyond these shores.

In another 10 or 20 years time, many of the people I have mentioned will be forgotten, but their work will live on, built into the fabric of health care the world over. Before I end, however, I would like to highlight a way in which the original dream has failed to be incarnated, that is, in the provision of a safe harbour for the terminally ill to stay until they die. Symptom control has in fact become so skilled, so successful, that many people admitted to die can in fact be enabled to return home, often for many months. The demand for palliative care expertise has, however, grown so much that most hospices have a waiting list of patients needing admission for symptom control or general 'sorting out'. In order to meet this demand, it is now the norm in many hospices that patients stay no more than 2 weeks, those who cannot go home being moved on to nursing homes.

So what has happened to the original idea that once a dying person came to a hospice, he or she came to stay? Has the dream gone wrong? Has anyone done any research into the experience and feelings of those patients and their families who have been moved on from the hospice? The issue is complex, not least because hospices are free and nursing homes are not. Twenty years from now, will there be a revival of the original vision and the establishment of a new series of lower-demand, less-medicalized hospices? Who knows: we must await a new generation of prophets.

FURTHER READING

Buechner, F. 1994: *Wishful Thinking: A Seeker's ABC*. Continuum.

Boulay, S. der 1996: *Changing the Face of Death: The Story of Cicely Saunders*. Norwich: RMEP.

Cassidy, S. 1988: *Sharing the Darkness*. London: Darton, Longman & Todd.

Cassidy, S. 1995: *The Loneliest Journey*. London: Darton, Longman & Todd.

Kearney, M. and Saunders, C. 1996: *Mortally Wounded*. Dublin: Marino.

UNTANGLING THE WEB

John Sweeney

I think there's a world market for about five computers.
Thomas Watson, founder of IBM

The Internet, rooted as it is in the closeted worlds of the military and the academic, does not appear to have an immediate or obvious relevance to an area such as palliative care. Palliative care prides itself on human values, interactions, openness and honesty, and these seem at odds with those terms which spring readily to mind when we consider information technology and its uses: data collection, file transfer protocols, number-crunching, hypertext and encryption codes. However, as the Internet has moved from its beginnings as the work and plaything of a few individuals to become a tool used in the lives and work of many, it is clear that these two areas are moving closer together as we find ourselves placed ever more firmly in the information age.

If information and communication between individuals are an important part of palliative care, and they clearly are given the many thousands of words written about these topics, it would be unusual if current trends in society's approach to communication were not reflected within the discipline. Also, given the ever-closing link between the clinical world and that of research, it would again be unusual for this not to lead to some development and borrowing of methods of networking.

The Internet has been the major change over the last decade in how people communicate and seek for information on a variety of subjects. Pallen (1995) notes that it is more than simply a network of networks or 'a global information resource' (Hale, 1996), citing Rheingold's (1994) description of it as a 'vast community, larger than many nation states, that provides intellectual, psychological and social support for its inhabitants'. It offers a voice to many, from the single patient choosing to report their experiences online to sizeable collections of resources from sites such as Oncolink and the National Cancer Institute. Given the impact of the Internet on current society and the concerns its emergence has generated, it is worth glancing briefly at its historical development in order to gauge its relevance to communication within palliative nursing and to place some perspective on its growth.

In 1969, the Advanced Research Projects Agency, part of the US Department of Defence, established a network that connected computers at the University of California in Los Angeles and Santa Barbara, the Stanford Research Institute and the University of Utah. This network was known as Arpanet, other educational and research institutions soon becoming part of this development. Arpanet was designed to allow for continued communication in the event of a nuclear attack or natural catastrophe should one or more of these sites be destroyed. At this point, it was available to only a small number of scientists and engineers familiar with the language used to transmit information around the network.

Throughout the 1970s and 1980s, various different approaches were developed, leading to the birth of e-mail and newsgroups. What brought the Internet fully into the public domain was, however, the development of the World Wide Web (WWW) in 1991 by Tim Berners-Lee at CERN. The graphical interface used allowed many more people to experiment with the new medium, and its growth since then has been exponential, from the 130 websites available in 1993 to 3000 a year later and over 2 million by 1998 (Microsoft, 2000).

One of the most interesting and occasionally controversial features of the development of the Internet and the WWW has been its lack of regulation and an emphasis, at least in its early days, on information being shared freely between users. Although the growing commercialization of the WWW has in the past couple of years somewhat detracted from this it remains one of the least-regulated means of communication, and what standards there are exist to encourage developers to use common protocols, thus encouraging ease of use for the greatest number of people rather than limiting or attempting to control what is being said or exchanged.

Distinguishing between the WWW and the Internet is, although difficult, important as this reflects to some extent the difference between the display of information and its use. The WWW, with its ability to integrate different file formats such as text, images, sounds and video, and the options for interactivity that this affords, is very much now the public face of the Internet. Buried beneath this, however, is the structure of the Internet and other methods of communication, such as e-mail, newsgroups and discussion groups of every possible type. These methods offer a space in which the absolutely public information displayed on the WWW is put to use in ways that question definitions such as 'private' or 'public' by the ever-increasing number of us who have integrated this medium into our now 'wired' lives. For many users, these issues are as arcane as the workings of the motor car are to many motorists: there is no need to understand the workings of a machine or structure in order to use it, although there is no doubt a little knowledge can be useful when things go wrong.

Most users access information through the WWW, and the initial Internet experience essentially being one of 'visiting' a site and examining the information held there. The website sought is found through being aware of the location via a more traditional medium, via a link from another site, through an e-mail or more usually by having used a 'search engine' to find it. The use of these programs may sometimes be problematic as they do not in fact search the Internet but instead a database gathered from sites submitted by users and collected by the program's designers. Using a search engine may be ineffective if site developers have not been meticulous in submitting their sites to the many that now exist. The use of these search engines is fairly straightforward, although a common complaint is that the number of results returned is too large to be useful. This is, however, often not the great problem it appears to be since the most relevant results are listed first. Some methods of narrowing this process down are listed below using the words 'palliative', 'care' and 'cancer' as an example:

- palliative cancer: using these words will return documents containing either of these words;
- + palliative + cancer: will return documents containing both these words;
- + palliative − cancer: this will return documents that contain the word 'palliative' but not the word 'cancer';
- "palliative care": using the quotation marks turns any two words into a phrase and will return only documents that contain the words in that order.

A glance at the 'help' section of a search engine such as Alta Vista, from where the above information comes, is often helpful if difficulties arise. Many palliative care sites use a search engine provided by Growth House Inc. This can be a helpful starting place for the net-naïve as it is designed to look only for sites relevant to palliative care or related areas.

Once users have found what they are looking for, the information can be saved, downloaded, printed, cut and pasted, and many users, particularly those involved in research or teaching, tend to see the Internet as a document provider. Such limited approaches to Internet use may relate to issues of cost, which still vary widely depending on the nature of one's access, especially on whether it is personal or available through the workplace. To many, however, this defeats the purpose of the Internet as an information resource: after all, why *keep* the document if it is always there online? It may be that Internet use will bring about a shift in attitudes towards the ownership of information in ways that we cannot yet foresee, and it can be no coincidence that libraries, both public and academic, were among the early users of the Internet and have now largely integrated Internet access alongside their traditional book and journal stores. Just as Internet use has constantly increased since its inception, so too has the number of sites addressing health, in particular cancer and palliative care − recent searches of these terms produced a return of 1 456 287 documents.

Although the Internet, by definition, encourages networking and the development of connections between sites, many have a particular focus, and looking at what is available sees some clear groupings emerging. The main categories into which sites may be divided are:

- gateway sites
- clinical information
- education
- patients: experience and support
- promotion of palliative care
- networking.

GATEWAY SITES

Possibly the most useful for the Internet newcomer are those 'gateway' or portal sites in which an organization or individual has collected together a number of links to sites on a particular issue from around the WWW, the aforementioned Growth House Inc. being one such effort. Others include the Guide to Internet Resources for Cancer, which includes a remarkable number of links and thus saves users time and the need to familiarize themselves with a particular search engine. The Palliative Page takes this a little further by offering more by way of a description of sites for the user, thus again speeding up the process of finding the information sought.

Sites such as these have often begun as a WWW version of the developer's bookmarks or favourites list, and they hopefully allow users to take their first online steps, after which they can enjoy the process of 'surfing' from site to site. One of the major attractions of the Internet is that, by following a few links, information possibly more useful than that initially sought can be found. When time is limited, some discipline may of course have to be employed to avoid distraction.

CLINICAL INFORMATION

These sites include some very familiar names, and most journals are now available in an online form, the *British Medical Journal* providing what may be the best example of this type of publication. Its free, full-text articles are well referenced to other parts of the journal's archives, which allows an article to be easily followed up through related letters, editorials and replies.

Treatment guidelines are available in many countries, the Scottish Intercollegiate Guidelines Network, Australia's Multicultural Palliative Care Guidelines and the National Health Service National Institute of Clinical Excellence being good examples. Through a posting of draft guidelines on their websites, such organizations can encourage comments from a wider range of professionals and interested parties, thus allowing the finished product more fully to reflect the needs of those who will be using such approaches.

This open approach to information, and the ease with which it can be accessed, displayed and shared, is a major development, one not easily possible without internet use. Sites such as these indicate the cross-over between older media and the new, whereas specifically online sites such as Oncolink and the Edmonton Palliative Care Program, the development of which was detailed by Pereira et al. (1997), aim to use the new features of the WWW to encourage comments on their content. It may be the case that they will eventually offer options circumventing lengthy review and publication procedures while still holding to rigorous referencing criteria.

Oncolink in particular offers the full range of Internet technologies, from a vast repository of information on particular cancers, to advice on treatment protocols and areas within which patients and professionals can discuss their problems and situations, both by e-mail and through real-time chat rooms such as Oncochat. The Edmonton site remains a model of what a palliative care site can offer, both to its local service users and to the Internet community at large. Users can discover what is on offer, and staff can take advantage of the new media to publish advice on symptom matters for their peers.

EDUCATION

Plank (1998) describes the Internet as 'current, progressive, dynamic, accessible and time independent', all of which supports using online methods to address nursing education. It is important that we do not polarize this discussion in terms of 'online' versus 'traditional' but instead see the benefits that use of the Internet can offer and the problems it can often resolve. Indeed, the greatest support for Internet use in education comes from the current growth in distance learning and its wide acceptance in many fields, as exemplified by the work of the Open University in the UK. Plank points out that, with online testing and the generation of certification, the Internet offers ways of speeding up the process of students achieving their goals and suggests that if nursing does not adopt this technology, it will be left behind.

Importantly for employers, there are fewer difficulties with travel costs and with course times that rarely reflect the working hours nursing staff are used to. There is of course no doubt that employers may see this as an opportunity to opt out of any input into their staff's continuing development, but thoughtful employers may approach the issue of education differently, for example by providing Internet access in the workplace.

The key word here is flexibility, not all of the educational material online demanding this still formal approach. Many sites offer resources that can enhance traditional teaching methods and courses by offering a greater variety of materials that students can investigate in addition to more traditional references. A good example of this is the University of Washington's interactive site on ethical issues, which covers a number of areas of interest to palliative care nurses in a manner that brings the often hazy topic of ethical decision-making to life via case studies and interactive options offered to the user.

For the lecturer, notes and summaries of classes can be posted online, offering students accurate sources for revision and encouraging a more active use of time in class. Should some question the ongoing worth of this approach, it is worth noting the oversubscription to the online education program provided via the Edmonton site, which in addition hopes to explore just how useful these novel methods are. A growing number of educational units, including Macmillan's Education and Research Unit at the University of Dundee, now provide much of their material online, and accessing Macmillan's HELP package and other guidelines through, for example, hand-held PCs offers a chance to readily integrate educational material into the clinical world.

This also offers better scope for repeatedly updating material so that patients, doctors and nurses need not rely on sources that may have become outmoded or go through the lengthy process of checking this material against recent journals. Indeed, a growing number of textbooks are experimenting with CD-ROMs and related websites that allow research material to be updated, thus preventing the complete rewriting of a text when only specific developments need to be changed. In this way, the Internet is offering a glimpse of future ways of integrating media and of integrating education within our daily routines.

PATIENTS: EXPERIENCE AND SUPPORT

From those sites which detail the experience of illness and reflect on the care and management of their situation, to those which have been created to assist others in coping with their condition, patients too have taken to the Internet in a big way, and it is clear that they have much to teach us, even if their experiences are individual and subjective. Indeed, much valuable work has been carried out via qualitative approaches within palliative care research, and many efforts have been made to gauge the experience of illness and advanced disease on patients and their families (Bailey and Wilkinson, 1998; Ingleton, 1999).

These sites, and Internet use in general, have empowered patients to step forward and tell their story without its being relayed by a researcher so this type of site offers much to the novice nurse by way of insight into patients' the real day-to-day struggles. There is no doubt too that patients benefit from their online efforts; a good example of this can be found at Shadow in Tiger Country.

By these sites, patients often create a network that defies geography and allows them a further dimension in which to give and receive support. In the kind of research alluded to above, patients will often say that they had a need to tell their story from start to finish and be listened to, and it is clear that the Internet offers patients a direct way of doing just that.

In a more formal way many single-issue groups have also taken to the WWW to offer support in a number of ways, via e-mail networks of volunteers, chat rooms where real-time, text-based discussions can take place, and FAQ or 'frequently asked question' sites that address the often similar concerns that people may have about treatment or hospital procedures.

PROMOTION OF PALLIATIVE CARE

The promotion of better palliative care goes hand in hand with this type of specific information and is particularly evident on the National Council for Hospice and Specialist Palliative Care Services and Scottish Partnership Agency for Palliative and Cancer Care sites, both of which offer a variety of information on local and national approaches but which, through their online presence, offer models for other countries or areas to follow.

The efforts to place such information online are sometimes criticized as being a duplication of material already available through print, or as being available only for those with the money to afford an Internet connection. This view of the Internet as a device for the well informed and well off is, however, changing as patterns of use alter as a result of the rapid reduction in Internet cost that has recently been seen in the UK. Government plans to make Internet access more widely and freely available are also underway through school and community initiatives.

Such criticisms also miss the point that we do now live in a world in which the Internet is becoming a standard communication device and is no longer a plaything of computer geeks and boffins. The Internet is – in some form or other – here to stay, and to set up a service and not have at least some information available via this route seems now as short sighted as not having a telephone or a fax number. The growing commercialization of the Internet may also allow for such sites to be more easily accessed through media developments such as digital television, which will in a few years be the standard manner of broadcasting, thus allowing Internet access to be almost universal.

In addition, the major palliative care and cancer charities now all have some sort of online presence; these include the Prostate Cancer Charity and groups with strong links to service provision, such as Macmillan Cancer Relief.

NETWORKING

That these sites now offer web-based chat and opportunities for interactive support should remind us that the Internet is more than just the WWW and that much activity and many benefits can be found through e-mail activities and newsgroups or e-mail discussion groups.

Newsgroups such as alt.cancer and alt.nurse enable users to post messages and follow up replies, often being more informal than e-mail discussion groups or Listservs, one of the best known of which is palliative-medicine@mailbase.ac.uk. Listservs demand that users join a list by 'subscribing' to it, all subscribers receiving any messages posted, these messages often being moderated or screened to gauge their appropriateness for the list. This avoids the sometime random postings that clutter newsgroups even though newsgroup members often respond vigorously to inappropriate messages.

These groups reflect the real nature of the Internet as a community and its ethos of freedom of expression and empowerment. They are as opinionated, supportive and infuriating as any local community meeting might be, but they are a vital part of the Internet. An involvement in such groups does require some familiarity with online codes of conduct or 'netiquette', and many will use 'emoticons' or 'smileys' to assist in the full expression of their contribution (Shea, 2000).

Online counselling is now widely available, and although it may seem strange that a relationship can exist in a therapeutic way in sterile cyberspace, it is worth balancing this with the widespread and often government-funded acceptance of telephone helplines, telephone triage and the like.

The growth of discussion groups and online counselling and support in its many forms reminds us that the most common use of the Internet is not the bells and whistles of the WWW, but of e-mail and technologies based around this original 'killer app'. Hebda et al. (1998) note the pros and cons of e-mail use (Box 18.1).

We are at a point regarding the Internet at which it has yet to separate itself from the PC. Once this occurs more widely, for example through digital television and mobile phone networks, many more users will see it as less threatening and more relevant, and it will become, so to speak, invisible. Its function will then outweigh its novelty or the actual process of using it – how often do we consider the technology behind the telephone or the refrigerator? We will begin to forget about how it works and think more of how to use it.

As more of us see the spread of our skills into the developing countries of the world as the next step for palliative care, e-mail surely holds the key for the

---

BOX 18.1 E-MAIL: ADVANTAGES AND DISADVANTAGES

Advantages

- Eliminates telephone tag. Provides the ability to leave a written message
- Convenient. Can be sent or retrieved from multiple locations, including work, home, or while travelling. Can be used on a 24-hour basis
- Easy to prepare and send. Electronic mail requires less effort to prepare, address and send than the traditional means of dictation and mailing
- Saves time and money. Eliminates postage and paper expenses
- Delivery can be almost instantaneous. Eliminates the time-lag associated with traditional mail
- Messages are time and date stamped. Provides documentation of the actual time of the mail transaction. Can also provide a log of when the message was received, read and answered

Disadvantages

- Interpretation of messages without the voice inflection. Unlike telephone conversations, e-mail eliminates the additional information that may be communicated through verbal cues
- High volume of messages sent and received. E-mail's popularity and ease of use have resulted in the generation of large numbers of messages including copies, forwarded messages and junk mail
- Viral contamination with e-mail attachments. Attached files that contain a virus may contaminate the recipient's computer
- Security concerns related to maintaining confidentiality
- E-mail is easily intercepted and forwarded and may be read by unintended parties. Employers have the right to read e-mail transmitted using company resources. In addition deleted messages may be retrieved during system backups

From Hebda et al. (1998)

dissemination of specific information between those experienced in palliative care and those less familiar with the discipline. Groups such as the International Association for Hospice and Palliative Care and the Australasian Palliative Link Index, along with nursing groups such as the International Palliative Nursing Network and the International Society of Nurses in Cancer Care, address this through their sites and facilitate much online networking.

To many, the above usage demands some standardization and control, although patients themselves are rarely in the forefront of such complaints, and it often appears that many groups feel threatened by the freedom of access that the Internet affords (Chambers, 1997). It must, however, be accepted that patients now use the Internet and will continue do so in ever-increasing numbers.

One frequent concern of professionals is the informed patient (don't we as nurses always say we make the most difficult patients!), and the Internet has been criticized for providing patients with mountains of information that may or may not be relevant to their own situation, wreaking emotional havoc and providing false hopes of treatment options or recovery. This view of the Internet as threat is really no different from the threat offered by the patient whose wife or brother is an oncologist or whose sister is a Macmillan nurse, or by someone who has read in the papers about some nascent research project that will lead to a cure for cancer.

The desire for information that some patients show, with their sheaves of downloaded web pages, should thus not be dismissed as a problem but instead be seen as a need for information that we are all too aware is not readily met. It is surely in both our own and our patients' interests to adapt positively to this and see it as a starting point for discussion and an opportunity for clarification. This certainly has implications for time and a need for full and considered ways of disclosing information. It may well be the case, however, that patients will expect doctors and nurses to be familiar with the ways of the WWW and to assist in their search for information or support rather dismiss it as not being relevant to their care or country.

Guidelines do exist though, and it is worth having some kind of structure for assessing sites should one accept the challenge of working with the best of the Internet and assisting patients in its use. Pereira et al. (*1997*) cite the University of Alberta's evaluation criteria (1997), which concentrate on the scope and content of a site, its authorship, design and currency along with the ease of its use. Another widely used set of principles are propounded by the Health on the Net Foundation (Box 18.2).

Patients' use of the Internet and the embrace of the WWW by all sections of society – news media, government, education and individuals – are the reasons why nurses should grasp the flexible and exciting opportunity afforded by this new and exciting technology. Indeed, the Internet has shown such potential over the past few years that if our point of criticism is that it cannot achieve what we wish it to, we should begin thinking of how we can use it to achieve exactly that goal. By so doing, we will be able to produce areas of the Internet with which we can feel more comfortable and with which we can develop methods of use

BOX 18.2 PRINCIPLES FOR INTERNET USE

1. **Authority**   Any medical or health advice provided and hosted on this site will only be given by medically trained and qualified professionals unless a clear statement is made that a piece of advice offered is from a non-medically qualified individual or organisation.

2. **Complementarity**   The information provided on this site is designed to support, not replace, the relationship that exists between a patient/site visitor and his/her existing physician.

3. **Confidentiality**   Confidentiality of data relating to individual patients and visitors to a medical/health Web site, including their identity, is respected by this Web site. The Web site owners undertake to honour or exceed the legal requirements of medical/health information privacy that apply in the country and state where the Web site and mirror sites are located.

4. **Attribution**   Where appropriate, information contained on this site will be supported by clear references to source data and, where possible, have specific HTML links to that data. The date when a clinical page was last modified will be clearly displayed (e.g. at the bottom of the page).

5. **Justifiability**   Any claims relating to the benefits/performance of a specific treatment, commercial product or service will be supported by appropriate, balanced evidence in the manner outlined above in Principle 4.

6. **Transparency of authorship**   The designers of this Web site will seek to provide information in the clearest possible manner and provide contact addresses for visitors that seek further information or support. The Webmaster will display his/her E-mail address clearly throughout the Web site.

7. **Transparency of sponsorship**   Support for this Web site will be clearly identified, including the identities of commercial and non-commercial organisations that have contributed funding, services or material for the site.

8. **Honesty in advertising and editorial policy**   If advertising is a source of funding it will be clearly stated. A brief description of the advertising policy adopted by the Web site owners will be displayed on the site. Advertising and other promotional material will be presented to viewers in a manner and context that facilitates differentiation between it and the original material created by the institution operating the site.

Version 1.6, April 1997, Health on the Net Foundation

that offer our patients more choice, more involvement and an opportunity for better care.

FURTHER SURFING

Breast Cancer Care   www.breastcancercare.org.uk
Edmonton Palliative Care Program   www.palliative.org
International Association for
  Hospice and Palliative Care   www.hospicecare.com
Macmillan Cancer Relief   www.macmillan.org.uk

Macmillan Education and Research Unit	www.dundee.ac.uk/meded/MERU/welcome.htm
Multicultural Palliative Care Guidelines	www.pallcare.asn.au/mc/index.html
National Cancer Institute	www.nci.nih.gov
Oncochat	www.oncochat.org
Oncolink	www.oncolink.com
Prostate Cancer Charity	www.prostate-cancer.org.uk
Scottish Intercollegiate Guidelines Network	www.sign.ac.uk
Scottish Partnership Agency for Palliative and Cancer Care	www.palliativecarescotland.org.uk/
Shadow in Tiger Country	www.shadowdiary.com
The Palliative Page	http://homepage.dtn.ntl.com/johnsweeney

REFERENCES

Bailey, K. and Wilkinson, S. 1998: Patients' views on nurses' communication skills. *International Journal of Palliative Nursing* 4(6), 300–8.

Chambers, P. 1997: The web can be a trap. *Bacup News*, 28, 1–2.

Hale, C. (ed.) 1996: *Wired Style: Principles of English Usage in the Digital Age*. San Francisco: Hardwired.

Hebda, T., Czar P. and Mascara C. 1998: *Handbook of Informatics for Nurses and Health Care Professionals*. California: Addison Wesley Longman.

Ingleton, C. 1999: The views of patients and carers on one palliative care service. *International Journal of Palliative Nursing* 5(4), 187–96.

Microsoft 2000: A Brief History of the Internet. http://channels.microsoft.com/insider/internet/articles/history.htm

Pallen, M. 1995: Guide to the Internet: introducing the Internet. *British Medical Journal*, 311, 1422–4.

Pereira, J., Macmillan, A. and Bruera, A. 1997: Launching a palliative care homepage: the Edmonton experience. *Palliative Medicine* 11, 435–43.

Plank, R.K. 1998: Nursing online for continuing education credit. *Journal of Continuing Education in Nursing* 24(4), 165–72.

Rheingold, G. 1994: The virtual community. In: Pallen, M. 1995: Guide to the Internet: introducing the Internet. *British Medical Journal* 311, 1422–4.

Shea, V. 2000: http://www.albion.com/netiquette/index.html

University of Alberta 1997: Critical evaluation of resources on the Internet. In: Pereira, J., Macmillan, A. and Bluera, A. 1997: Launching a palliative care homepage: the Edmonton experience. *Palliative Medicine* 11, 435–43.

chapter 19

ETHICAL ISSUES

Alan Winchester

> Dear Lord,
>   I expect to pass through this world but once;
>   and any good thing, therefore, that I can do
>   or any kindness that I can show to any fellow creature,
>   let me do it now;
>   let me not defer or neglect it,
>   for I shall not pass this way again.
>
> Stephen Grellet (1773–1855)

This chapter will outline the essential background theories that form the basis of ethical reasoning. Examples of clinical situations facing practitioners in palliative care will wherever possible, be interwoven with the theoretical principles so that the reader will be able to connect the theory with his or her everyday practice with patients, families and colleagues.

It is emphasized that the study of ethics in palliative care, or indeed elsewhere within the practice of medicine or nursing, is not intended to furnish the reader with a formulary of set prescriptive answers to practice-related moral issues. Instead, one may think of studying ethics rather like one studies anatomy and physiology: these subjects, although fascinating in themselves, serve the practitioner as background maps to the human body so that diagnosis and treatment may be carried out in an informed way.

In a similar way, a working knowledge of ethics is desirable in order for a team of health-care professionals to reach the best contextual decision in situations in which perhaps competing factors or differing views on what is right or wrong may cloud the central moral issues affecting a patient's care.

A practical definition of ethics has been suggested by David Stone (1998), writing in the Christian Medical Fellowship files:

> Ethics and morality concern the decisions we make about whether something is right or wrong: first about how we make such decisions and secondly about how we carry them out in practice.

This definition would appear to fit with the practice of the palliative care professional. It clarifies how ethics is firmly placed within practice, at the hospital or hospice bedside, in the consulting room or in the intimacy of the patient's home, including of course the support provided for the bereaved person after the patient has died.

CENTRAL MORAL THEORIES

There are two great categories of moral theory. The first claims that people act in an ethically acceptable manner when they carry out actions because of the obligations and duties that apply to them. This theory is termed *deontology* (from the Greek *deon*, meaning duty). The aim is therefore to determine which duties the palliative care professional has towards the person concerned in any given situation, whether a patient, colleague, relative, student or other party with whom a relationship exists.

The professional regulatory bodies, the General Medical Council (GMC) for doctors and the United Kingdom Central Council for Nursing, Midwifery and Health Visiting (UKCC) for nurses, set out guidelines designed to protect the public and clarify the duties and responsibilities of their practitioners. Other professions have similar sources of regulation and guidance.

In addition to the professional aspects of duty, there exists a more fundamental set of duties related to being a member of a societal group, functioning as a citizen, a parent or someone's son or daughter, brother, sister, partner, husband or wife. There may also be obligations on someone who is a member of a particular religious belief system or who participates in some form of public office, such as a magistrate. The same duties clearly do not apply to all these situations: people engaged in a particular activity are ethically required to identify the *relevant* duties that need to be observed with regard to what they are engaged in.

The philosopher Immanuel Kant (1724–1804) had a towering influence over deontological thinking in the Enlightenment period of history. He was famous for his prolific writings on such diverse subjects as mathematics, geography and cosmology, as well as for his contributions to moral philosophy. Kant's legacy to ethics may be described in terms of some of what he wrote in his celebrated work *The Categorical Imperative*. Stated plainly, but hopefully not simplistically, three main themes emerge (Strathern, 1996):

1 We should always behave in such a way as we wish all other people to behave.
2 We ought never to treat other people *exclusively* as a means to an end.
3 People everywhere ought to be regarded as ends in themselves.

These ethical proposals, especially the second and third themes – that patients should always be regarded as persons of inherent worth – resonate well with the practice of palliative care. We are reminded of Dame Cicely Saunders' famous statement 'You are worthy because you are you', and in our dealings with patients, especially in relation to treatments or changes needing an element of consent, it is necessary to ensure that their consent is valid.

The second central category that warrants description is the theory arguing that the moral rightness of an action is determined by the overall balance of the good and bad consequences that result from it. This theory is commonly known as *consequentialism*. As the title suggests, it is results that count. With regard to its application to palliative care, it is easily recognized that consequentialist ethics are used whenever symptom control is applied to the care of a patient or when 'a good death' is hoped for. This may involve the proper use of medication and the practice of interpersonal skills, both of which are targeted towards maximizing comfort or creating the conditions for death to be peaceful. The chief proponents of consequentialist theory were John Stuart Mill (1806–1873) and Jeremy Bentham (1748–1832), both of whom were philosophers from the Enlightenment period.

Consequentialism attempts to perform a calculation in order to decide what action to undertake. The good consequences of each action are set against the sum total of the bad ones, and a decision is made based on which action yields the greatest good for the greatest number or, as a microcosm of this, the greatest good for one person.

A recent example of consequentialism in medicolegal and ethical argument was the tragic case of the conjoined twins Jodie and Mary. There was an initial disagreement between the parents and the clinical team over which course of action to take. The first option was to provide only pain relief and supportive care, the projected result being the death of both twins. The clinical team did not consider this to be a viable ethical or clinical option, for two reasons. First, Mary did not have a functioning cardiorespiratory system although Jodie did. Second, Mary suffered from an underdeveloped nervous system, one judged to be, by expert opinion, incapable of improvement, whereas Jodie demonstrated normal reflexes and had a chance of, with help, a good quality of life. The second option was surgical separation, which would inevitably result in Mary not surviving but would enable Jodie to have a good chance of a full life. The parent's wish was that supportive care only be provided, and the case was brought to court for a legal adjudication because of the disagreement. This case illustrates that in cases where there is never going to be a 'good' outcome, the decision should focus on the least bad outcome, in this case surgical separation, with of course the death of Mary.

The remainder of this chapter draws heavily on Stone (1998), Gillon (1992) and Strathern (1996), and the reader is also directed to the further reading list at the end of the chapter.

THE CLUSTER OF FOUR PRINCIPLES

In the introductory part of this chapter, the foundations of ethical theory were explored in order to align these with the work of the health professional. The American ethicists Tom Beauchamp and James Childress (1994) have devised a model of ethical principles that is apposite to palliative care but also applicable across most speciality boundaries. Their four principles are outlined below.

BENEFICENCE

Most if not all health professionals aim to do good in dealing with their patients, the minimum of pain being inflicted when carrying out procedures. In the practice of communication, empathy and sensitivity co-exist with telling bad news or discussing a patient's concerns. It should be noted that beneficence is not kindness: it is doing good for the benefit of another, involving acts that do not have to be accompanied by any particular emotion.

Health professionals and management claim to put the patient first, but is that always true? Readers may be able to recall situations in which the reverse has actually occurred; can it sometimes be that one's ego and professional position get in the way of someone receiving effective pain control? The challenge is to recognize any inconsistency and do something about it.

Is clinical governance sufficiently developed to ensure support for the nurse with a concern on his or her mind? These and many other issues impinge on the concept of actually putting the patient first.

NON-MALEFICENCE

This is probably the oldest injunction placed upon health professionals: '*primum non nocere*' – first do no harm. Originally Hippocratic, this was adopted and quoted many generations later by Nightingale, in relation to conditions in military hospitals in the Crimea.

In contemporary practice, it is, with the rapidly increasing potential of modern therapeutics to interfere with or alter, if not cure, disease processes, easy to do harm. Everyday we are faced with the question: we can but should we? This question is posed on the basis of the benefit/burden equation. How much meaningful good is possible and at what cost to the patient's quality of life? It may be possible to give another course of chemotherapy, but what is going to be the realistic effect on the disease process and perhaps on improving some symptoms, balanced against the toxicity of the drug and its effect on the individual's total good?

RESPECT THE AUTONOMY OF OTHERS

This principle ranks highly in contemporary health care. We live in an age of liberal individualism within which the rights of the individual sometimes assume the highest priority; certainly, the claim 'I can do what I choose' (sometimes at the expense of the freedom of another) can be heard stridently in our society.

Autonomy means self-governing (from the Greek *autos*, meaning self, and *nomos*, meaning law). The possession of autonomy rests largely on the state of the patient's mental capacity and competence. One may be autonomous in terms of thought, will or action.

During illness, it is unlikely that many of us would be able to claim the complete ability to be self-governing; indeed, that is probably true of life outside health care as well. In cancer, many factors may be present which threaten a person's autonomy – pain and other symptoms, fear of treatment and of the future, concerns about family, job and money, being in awe of staff, previous bad experiences with doctors or nurses. In palliative care, when the illness is not curable, psychospiritual concerns and anticipatory grief, which of course apply to both patient and family, come into focus.

Autonomy, and its respect may be considered within health care to be primarily concerned with:

- the revealing of clinical information;
- consent to treatment;
- negotiating the nature and direction of care.

In palliative care, we often claim to be particularly sensitive to the patient's need to control his or her life as far as possible. In claiming to respect autonomy, particular attention needs to be paid to the supply of understandable information, bearing in mind that so-called autonomous decisions are not autonomous if the decisions are made in ignorance or are based on misunderstandings. It is appropriate to emphasize that respect for autonomy is not synonomous with obedience. As mentioned in connection with consent, those who are autonomous do not always have to make sensible decisions about themselves, but the health professional has a clear obligation to place before the patient, with kindness and empathy, enough information to enable the patient to consider what action is right for him or her.

JUSTICE AND FAIRNESS

These aspects may be considered under the following headings:

- *Distributive justice* is concerned with the allocation of fair, equitable and appropriate distribution in society, determined by justified norms that structure the terms of social co-operation. Examples are the right to vote and freedom of speech. This category also includes the appropriate and proportionate amount of time that the palliative care practitioner allocates to individual patients as opposed to other commitments.
- *Criminal justice* refers to the just infliction of punishment on those who have transgressed the accepted norms of behaviour of the particular society, this usually being administered by the approved criminal legal system.
- *Rectificatory justice* refers to compensation claims related to cases of transactional or contractual breaches of, usually civil, law, including malpractice cases.

When considering justice within the field of palliative care, it may be worth considering the topical issue of the referral of non-malignant conditions. This produces a serious challenge for most palliative care services in terms of how they propose to modify their referral protocols and caseloads to accomodate this cohort together with their continuing commitment to cancer care.

RELATIONSHIP-BASED ETHICS

Although traditional biomedical ethical theory is concerned with the application of such concepts as laws, rules, rights, obligations and prima facie principles, relationship-based ethics attempts to approach the subject from the perspective of human relationships, recognizing that the concept of caring for each other is central to good moral activity within helping relationships. This concept of caring may be present both within society and as part of the professional therapeutic relationship existing within health-care settings.

The central concept, that of *responsibility,* is described by Harbison (1992) as being pivotal to understanding Professor Carol Gilligan's theory of relationship-based ethics. The conventional understanding of responsibility means making a commitment and standing by it. Gilligan suggests that this could be extended by an awareness of others and their feelings, and further asserts that a moral agent is characterized as one who 'responds to need and demonstrates a consideration of care and responsibility in relationships' (Harbison, 1992).

An example in palliative care practice is that of the patient who has just had bad news of a recurrence revealed by the oncologist. The patient cannot get to sleep that night, the nurse on night duty in such a situation has two options: to block the patient in expressing his concerns and anxieties by a 'Let me get you a hot chocolate, then you will feel better' response, or to engage empathically and encourage the vocalization of feelings and concerns individual to that person.

Chapter 12 in this book draws attention to counselling skills, it is recommended that the reader consult this for further guidance on the subject.

PRACTICE-BASED ETHICAL ISSUES

DECISION-MAKING

Figure 19.1 (Kaye, 1999) outlines a guide designed to assist the health professional in making contextual ethical decisions.

THE DISCLOSURE OF INFORMATION ON DIAGNOSIS AND PROGNOSIS

Telling the news of a diagnosis or discussing the results of hearing such news commonly falls within the remit of a hospital clinical team, palliative care team, community palliative care team, hospice ward or day centre team, or a general practitioner and district nurse. Whatever the setting, the ethical issues concerned with this situation centre around who owns the information, who possesses information that may be relevant and, last but not least, how such information may best be disclosed to the patient. Winchester (1999) suggests that, whatever the clinical circumstances, a five-step model of sharing bad news may be helpful and applicable across clinical boundaries:

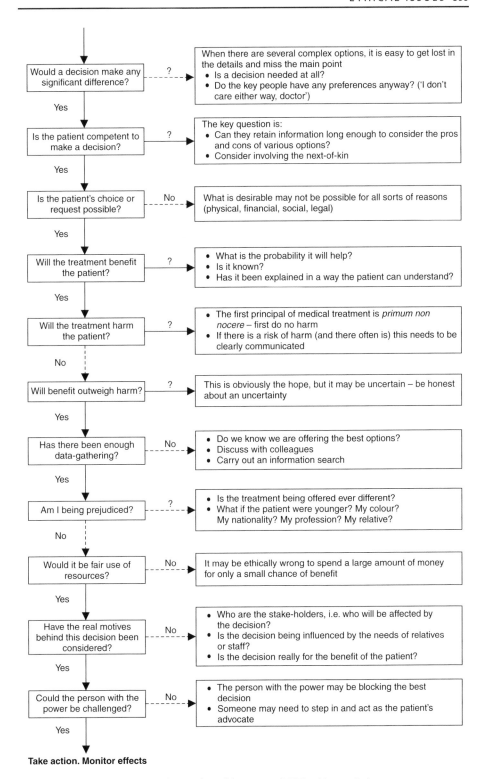

Figure 19.1 Ethical decision-making. Adapted from Kaye (1999) with permission

1 *Pay attention to the setting or environment* in which the interview is to take place. Issues such as privacy, quietness, having the notes available, and telephones and bleeps being removed, all contribute to the patient feeling valued and respected.

2 *Assess the level of the patient's knowledge.* Start a dialogue, encouraging the patient to say what he or she not only thinks, but also feels. Start communicating empathically.

3 *Develop a connection with the patient.* This means deepening the level of empathy in order to try to create conditions in which the patient feels understood. A 'warning shot' needs to be fired, for example, 'The results are more serious than we had hoped.' Continue listening and responding empathically.

4 *Offer information,* the key word here being 'offer'. This is a vital part of the consultation. There is a chronic tendency for health-care staff to oversupply factual information (Faulkner, 1998), giving no time for the patient to 'catch up' with this. Medical facts need to be given in manageable chunks and the importance of patients having an opportunity to express their feelings and emotion related to the news recognized.

5 *Balance bad news with the assurance of support.* Although the prognosis may be poor, the disclosure of bad news should not leave the patient without hope of supportive and helpful services. There is no justification ever to say or imply 'Nothing more can be done.'

Ethically, the relevant duties of the health professional are related to preventing psychoemotional harm by telling the news in such a way as to be in congruence with the patient's speed of acceptance and to assure him/her of continuing support in the future. It is also relevant to consider the consequentialist aspects of telling bad news. Enabling patients, to know what is causing their symptoms, giving permission for them to express their feelings about this and providing an avenue for continued support make it possible for the patient to catch up emotionally with the reality of the clinical facts and adapt to a changing lifestyle. Goldie (1982) argues that the moral issue concerns *how* the patient is told his particular truth.

COLLUSION (OR THE CONSPIRACY OF SILENCE)

This usually applies to a situation in which a patient's relative requests or demands that a health professional either withholds or alters the nature of medical information, with the objective of preventing the patient knowing the true nature of that information. In other words, the nurse or doctor is being requested by a relative to *deceive* the patient.

From a duty-based perspective, lying to a patient is not permissible. If he or she is mentally competent, the ownership of information is undisputed – it belongs to the patient – and, rather like disclosing bad news (which it may well also be), the central issue concerns how it is done.

The reader is referred here to Chapters 7 and 12 because the motivation underlying this is almost always based on a love for and protection of the sick person. The relative demanding a collusive situation may be crying out for understanding, and negotiation rather than deserving merely a description of our GMC or UKCC rules about not lying.

ETHICS IN RELATION TO SYMPTOM MANAGEMENT

Managing distressing symptoms is the cornerstone of palliative care. When the meaning of the term 'palliative' is discussed, words such as 'alleviate' and 'relieve' are frequently mentioned. The reader is referred to the introductory chapters of this book for a discussion on the origins and philosophy of palliative care, but suffice it to say that a considerable number of doctors, nurses and other health professionals have entered, and indeed are still entering, the palliative care field with a vocational desire to improve the lot of patients with distressing symptoms.

In general terms, symptom management is aimed at maximum relief coupled with the minimum of undesirable side-effects (of the particular treatment or drug regime), this being accepted as good medical or nursing practice. The reader is referred to specific chapters of this book for information related to areas of symptom management in detailed terms. It is sufficient, however, to say that in the last years, months or indeed hours of a person's life, the main consideration ought to be the maximization of total good for the patient.

THE RULE OF DOUBLE EFFECT

This ethical rule (or doctrine as it was originally called) is a concept of Roman Catholic moral theory. It was intended to clarify the moral dilemma encountered when a bad effect (i.e. death) resulted unintentionally following the performance of an act or acts that were intended to produce a good effect as their primary aim. A contemporary example in palliative care is that of the patient who has a brain tumour causing convulsions, the intent of the doctor in prescribing parenteral benzodiazepine medication being to produce a situation of comfort for the patient and calm for the family. If the dosage has to be increased in order to control the convulsions, it is possible that the respiratory depth and rate may be compromised, which *may* lead to an earlier death if a chest infection then occurs in this seriously and terminally ill person.

The rule of double effect asserts that such action in prescribing relevant medication to alleviate suffering is morally permissible provided that the intention of the prescriber was, in the first place, to alleviate suffering. Four conditions apply to this rule (Gillon, 1992)

1 The intention must be good in itself.
2 The bad effect may be foreseen but not intended.
3 The good effect must not be achieved through the bad effect.
4 Proportionality must exist; in other words, there must be sufficient reason to risk, as a possibility, the occurrence of the bad effect.

CONSENT

The issue of consent is an example of a subject in which the law and ethics have a common application. Consent may be expressed or implied (Sheldon, 1996). There is a general principle here involving the mentally competent adult described thus by Lord Donaldson:

> An adult patient who suffers from no mental incapacity has an absolute right to choose whether to consent to medical treatment, to refuse it or to choose one rather than another of the treatments being offered....This right of choice is not limited to decisions which others might regard as sensible. It exists notwithstanding that the reasons for making the choice are rational or irrational, unknown or even non-existent.

> Lord Donaldson MR in Re T (1992)

A transgression of this general principle may give rise to two possible civil law actions: battery and negligence (Sheldon, 1996).

It is clear that mental competence is a key issue in consenting to treatment, and that understanding the relevant information, rather than the mere existence of a signature, is pivotal to consent being valid. In situations in which competence is clearly absent, that is during unconsciousness, and where no valid advance directive exists, the law empowers the treating doctor to take decisions in what is considered to be the patient's best interests. Relatives or other interested parties, albeit involved in the situation, do not have the legal right to make decisions about the patient's welfare that may conflict with the doctor's clinical judgement. This general legal position also applies to the care of dying patients when they become unable to order their own affairs because of the natural advancement of the dying process.

This is not to say that families ought to be excluded from decision-making – just the reverse in fact – and, within palliative care, emphasis is placed on their support. With this in mind the reader is directed to Chapters 7 and 12, which address the relevant communication issues.

LIVING WILLS

So-called 'living wills' may be divided into advance statements and advance directives. From an ethical standpoint, the concept of making provision in terms of stating one's wishes for future medical treatment rests largely on the principle of respect for autonomy.

Advance statements

These are essentially expressions of preferences held by the patient and documented when during autonomy, the intention being for those preferences to apply to future clinical situations when incapacity makes it impossible for the patient to make such decisions. It is emphasized that advance statements clarify certain wishes or values held by the patient, the usefulness of such statements lying in clarifying to the clinical team what the patient would have wished in certain circumstances. Advance statements are *not*, however, binding on health professionals.

Advance directives

These consist of specific *refusals* of certain medical treatments in certain clinical circumstances that may occur in the future, and are, provided the directive is correctly drawn up and is valid, binding on health professionals. Advance directives are as legally binding as contemporaneous refusals made by a competent adult. In cases in which there is a combination of statements of preferences and refusals in one document, the refusals may have legal force (British Medical Association, 1995).

There is no doubt that some people view advance statements and directives as a significant way of retaining some control over how they may be treated when they are unable to order their own lives. In order to ensure as far as possible that living wills reflect the actual current wishes of the person, it is recommended that advance directives and statements are drawn up with both legal and medical guidance, including provision for updating on a regular basis.

For general advice on drafting such documents, the reader is referred to British Medical Association (1995).

EUTHANASIA

The literal translation of euthanasia is 'good death' (from the Greek *eu* and *thanatos*). In contemporary times, euthanasia may be defined as the deliberate bringing about of someone's death in situations in which it is preferable to be dead than to continue living. Euthanasia may be classified in the following way (Wilkinson, 1993):

- voluntary euthanasia: requested or agreed to by the subject;
- Imposed euthanasia: not requested or agreed to by the subject;
  - Imposed involuntary: agreement can be obtained but is not;
  - Imposed non-voluntary: agreement cannot be obtained because of the subject's physical or mental state.

The act of euthanasia is illegal in every country in the Western world with the exception of Holland, whose parliament fully legalized the practice of voluntary euthanasia in 2001. From an ethical standpoint, euthanasia may be seen as the ultimate respect of someone's autonomy: authorizing and indeed assisting in controlling the circumstances and timing of one's own death is a powerful concept indeed.

There is some confusion in pro-euthanasia circles surrounding issues related to suffering, pain and the nature of what palliative care can offer. It is easy to form the impression that the opinions of some supporters of euthanasia are in fact based on an incorrect set of assumptions, leading of course to the question of how autonomous a decision can be, if it is based on an inadequate or incorrect raft of information. From the perspective of a balanced discussion on this subject within a textbook on palliative care, it is perhaps helpful to raise the following questions for the reader's reflection, as well as to encourage further reading, debate in small groups and a general opening-up of a topic that is crying out for debate between interested parties. The pertinent questions would seem to be:

- Why the need for euthanasia in the first place?
- What duties does society owe to those who suffer?
- What might be the results for society if euthanasia were to be permitted?
- Are there circumstances in which euthanasia might be permitted?
- Is the doctrine of the sanctity of life at all relevant, or are we the undisputed masters of our existence?
- What may be the consequences for the bereaved if, after the trauma of a being alongside a loved one throughout a distressing illness, they collude in the active taking of life (albeit to stop suffering)?
- Finally, are we directing palliative care in the *broadest* sense towards those who need our claimed skills in physical and psychospiritual support?

CONCLUSION

In conclusion, this chapter has explored the pivotal concepts that form a base for ethical reasoning, namely duties and consequences. It has then attempted to place these concepts within two working models – principle-based ethics and relationship-based ethics – which may be used in an analytical way to tackle clinically-based moral questions. Ethics in health-care practice is essentially that, it is *within* practice, so it follows that all health professionals need a working knowledge and the ability to construct a reasoned argument in support of actions that they believe to be right.

It is not enough simply to have an instinctive feel for what is right or wrong. Reasoned argument is the main implement in the toolkit of the ethicist, and if this chapter has whetted the reader's appetite, academic training may be the way forward for some. Another plan gaining popularity in forward-looking National Health Service trusts is the establishment of clinical ethics committees, forums or groups, small groups of doctors, nurses, chaplains and others who make themselves available to consult with the treating doctor and team with the specific remit to assist in helping with difficult medicomoral decisions. If there is one thing, in addition to knowledge, that is crucial to good moral decision-making, it is communication and open consultation with colleagues and of course the patient.

REFERENCES

Beauchamp, T.L. and Childress, J.F. 1994: *Principles of Biomedical Ethics*, 4th edn. Oxford: Oxford University Press.
British Medical Association 1995: *Advance Statements about Medical Treatment*. London: BMJ Publishing Group.

Faulkner, A. 1998: *When the News is Bad: A Guide for Health Professionals*. Cheltenham: Stanley Thornes.

Gillon, R.A. 1992: *Philosophical Medical Ethics*. Chichester: John Wiley.

Goldie, L. 1982: The ethics of telling the patient. *Journal of Medical Ethics* 8, 128–33.

Harbison, J. 1992: Gilligan, a voice for nursing? *Journal of Medical Ethics* 18, 202–5.

Kaye, P. 1999: *Decision Making in Palliative Care*. Northampton: EPL.

Sheldon, S. 1996: Law Tutorials. Unpublished document, Department of Law, University of Keele.

Stone, D. 1998: *Introduction to Ethics*. Christian Medical Fellowship Files. London: CMF.

Strathern, P. 1996: *Kant*. London: Constable.

Wilkinson, J. 1993: Ethical issues in palliative care. In Doyle, D., Hanks, G. and MacDonald, N. (eds) *The Oxford Textbook of Palliative Medicine*. Oxford: Oxford University Press.

Winchester, A. 1999: Sharing bad news. *Nursing Standard* 13(26), 48–52.

INDEX

Note: Page numbers in *italics* refer to tables, page numbers in **bold** refer to figures.